Prostitution, Trafficking, and Traumatic Stress

Prostitution, Trafficking, and Traumatic Stress has been co-published simultaneously as *Journal of Trauma Practice,* Volume 2, Numbers 3/4 2003.

Prostitution, Trafficking, and Traumatic Stress

Melissa Farley, PhD
Editor

Prostitution, Trafficking, and Traumatic Stress has been co-published simultaneously as *Journal of Trauma Practice*, Volume 2, Numbers 3/4 2003.

HMTP

The Haworth Maltreatment & Trauma Press®
An Imprint of The Haworth Press, Inc.

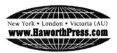

New York • London • Victoria (AU)
www.HaworthPress.com

Published by

The Haworth Maltreatment & Trauma Press, 10 Alice Street, Binghamton, NY 13904-1580 USA

The Haworth Maltreatment & Trauma Press is an imprint of The Haworth Press, Inc., 10 Alice Street, Binghamton, NY 13904-1580 USA.

Prostitution, Trafficking, and Traumatic Stress has been co-published simultaneously as *Journal of Trauma Practice,* Volume 2, Numbers 3/4 2003.

Cover design by Jennifer Gaska.

Cover photograph by Melissa Farley. ©Melissa Farley 2000. All Rights Reserved. For photo permission contact Melissa Farley, Box 16254, San Francisco, CA 94116-0254 or email: mfarley@prostitutionresearch.com

Library of Congress Cataloging-in-Publication Data

Prostitution, trafficking, and traumatic stress/ Melissa Farley, editor.
    p.; cm.
    "Simultaneously published as Journal of trauma practice, volume 2, numbers 3/4 2003."
    Includes bibliographical references and index.
    ISBN 0-7890-2378-4 (hardcover : alk. paper)–ISBN 0-7890-2379-2 (softcover: alk. paper)
    1. Post-traumatic stress disorder. 2. Prostitution.
    [DNLM: 1. Prostitution. 2. Stress Disorders, Post-Traumatic. 3. Domestic Violence. WM 170 P966 2003] I. Farley, Melissa.
RC552.P67 P745 2003
616.85′21–dc22   2003018824

Dedicated to Aileen Carol Wuornos

A prostituted woman who was executed
by the state of Florida, October 9, 2002

Melissa Farley's statement about the cover photograph

I originally interviewed these three women in Mexico City as part of research on the effects of prostitution (that data is found in "Prostitution and Trafficking in Nine Countries" in this volume). They told me about a ceremony honoring women who had died in prostitution that took place during the Mexican holiday, Day of the Dead.* Seeking nonexploitive images of prostitution that would illustrate its harm, I returned to Mexico City to photograph the Day of the Dead festivities.

The three women assisted me in taking a number of photographs. Two of them were homeless, living in a small Mexico City park. After a number of hours of working together, one of the women chose the cover photograph's location in front of a horror mask shop.

Although we seemed to have a friendly, easy rapport, like other survivors of human-inflicted trauma, they never really trusted me during the hours we spent together. Although I was a woman, I was also forever apart from them because I was protected by the privileges of class, race, and education. People encountered in their world, especially those with more power than they, could never be assumed to be safe. Until the end, the women assumed that I was eventually going to ask them to take their clothes off. They were sure that we'd proceed to the last photograph and I'd change into the familiar john/pornographer with: "OK girls, keep the masks on and take your clothes off."

Having been prostituted for many years, the three women assumed the constant inevitability of sexual exploitation. This left me with a sadness in my heart.

*The Mexican Day of the Dead is a traditional fall holiday that bears only a slight resemblance to Halloween. Rather, it is a deeply spiritual community event that honors the dead. Its spohisticated perspective on death is playful, humorous, and especially ironic.

Prostitution, Trafficking, and Traumatic Stress

CONTENTS

Preface: Prostitution, Trafficking, and Traumatic Stress   xi
Melissa Farley

Introduction: Hidden in Plain Sight:
Clinical Observations on Prostitution   1
Judith Lewis Herman

UNDERSTANDING PROSTITUTION AND TRAFFICKING
AS ORGANIZED INTERPERSONAL VIOLENCE

Sister Oppressions:
A Comparison of Wife Battering and Prostitution   17
Christine Stark
Carol Hodgson

Prostitution and Trafficking in Nine Countries:
An Update on Violence and Posttraumatic Stress Disorder   33
Melissa Farley
Ann Cotton
Jacqueline Lynne
Sybille Zumbeck
Frida Spiwak
Maria E. Reyes
Dinorah Alvarez
Ufuk Sezgin

Prostitution and Trauma in U.S. Rape Law   75
Michelle J. Anderson

Gay Male Pornography's "Actors":
  When "Fantasy" Isn't   93
    Christopher N. Kendall
    Rus Ervin Funk

Prostitution Online   115
    Donna M. Hughes

From Duty to Despair:
  Brothel Prostitution in Cambodia   133
    Wendy Freed

Prostitution and Trafficking of Women and Children
  from Mexico to the United States   147
    Marisa B. Ugarte
    Laura Zarate
    Melissa Farley

Prostitution and Trafficking in Women:
  An Intimate Relationship   167
    Dorchen A. Leidholdt

HEALING FROM PROSTITUTION AND TRAFFICKING

Emotional Experiences of Performing Prostitution   187
    Lisa A. Kramer

Dissociation Among Women in Prostitution   199
    Colin A. Ross
    Melissa Farley
    Harvey L. Schwartz

Providing Services to African American Prostituted Women   213
    Vednita Carter

The Importance of Supportive Relationships
  Among Women Leaving Prostitution   223
    Ulla-Carin Hedin
    Sven Axel Månsson

PEERS:
  The Prostitutes' Empowerment, Education
  and Resource Society   239
    Jannit Rabinovitch

Been There Done That:
  SAGE, a Peer Leadership Model
  Among Prostitution Survivors   255
    Norma Hotaling
    Autumn Burris
    B. Julie Johnson
    Yoshi M. Bird
    Kirsten A. Melbye

Living in Longing:
  Prostitution, Trauma Recovery, and Public Assistance   267
    Margaret A. Baldwin

Ten Reasons for *Not* Legalizing Prostitution
  and a Legal Response to the Demand for Prostitution   315
    Janice G. Raymond

Author Index   333

Subject Index   341

Preface:
Prostitution, Trafficking, and Traumatic Stress

Melissa Farley

Former victim of prostitution Claude Jaget described her experience of being picked out of a brothel lineup:

> I'd freeze up inside . . . It was horrible, they'd look you up and down. That moment, when you felt them looking at you, sizing you up, judging you . . . and those men, those fat pigs who weren't worth half as much as the worst of us, they'd joke, make comments. . . . They made you turn and face in all directions, because of course a front view wasn't enough for them. It used to make me furious, but at the same time I was panic-stricken, I didn't dare speak. I wasn't physically frightened, but it shook my confidence. I felt really [demeaned]. . . . I was the thing he came and literally bought. He had judged me like he'd judge cattle at a fairground, and that's revolting, it's sickening, it's terrible for the women. You can't imagine it if you've never been through it yourself. (Jaget, 1980)

The internal ravages of prostitution have not been well understood or analyzed in psychology. Even in the field of traumatic stress, there is a dearth of literature that addresses the experience of prostitution for the prostitute. For exam-

Melissa Farley, PhD, is at Prostitution Research & Education, Box 16254, San Francisco CA 94116-0254 USA (Email: mfarley@prostitutionresearch.com).
Printed with permission.

[Haworth co-indexing entry note]: "Preface: Prostitution, Trafficking, and Traumatic Stress." Farley, Melissa. Co-published simultaneously in *Journal of Trauma Practice* (The Haworth Maltreatment & Trauma Press, an imprint of The Haworth Press, Inc.) Vol. 2, No. 3/4, 2003, pp. xvii-xxviii; and: *Prostitution, Trafficking, and Traumatic Stress* (ed: Melissa Farley) The Haworth Maltreatment & Trauma Press, an imprint of The Haworth Press, Inc., 2003, pp. xi-xxii. Single or multiple copies of this article are available for a fee from The Haworth Document Delivery Service [1-800-HAWORTH, 9:00 a.m. - 5:00 p.m. (EST). E-mail address: docdelivery@haworthpress.com].

ple, there is a failure to comprehend or even to see what Jaget describes: the traumatic revulsion at being repeatedly lined up for selection, with johns making their choices much like butchers select cows.

In 1995 I spoke with Sara, a woman prostituting in what was called a high-class brothel in Johannesburg, South Africa. She asked me why I was there. I told her the truth: I thought that prostitution caused tremendous harm to women, but since there were few studies that asked about the experience of prostitution across different cultures, I wanted to know about her (and others') experiences of rape, physical assault, psychological distress, and childhood trauma. We talked about posttraumatic stress disorder and we talked about her lack of trust in people, including psychologists. Looking over the research questionnaires, she said that there were things inside her that she'd never tell anyone. Sara told me how difficult it was to get out of prostitution. As I talked with her, I felt as if I had jumped into a bunker in the middle of a war, asking questions about stress reactions to combat. I spoke to her about my concern that I would be asking about her life at a moment in time when it would cause her additional distress. She said that if her responses helped others, it would be worth it to her.

We had a conversation about our children. She had a son who was seven years old at the time; he was the reason she wanted to stay alive. She was very proud that she could afford to send him to the best school in town. She was adamant that she never, ever wanted her son to know that she was working as a prostitute. With eyes that were empty with pain, she told me about one of the most anguished moments in her life. One evening after her childcare worker arrived to spend the night at her home caring for her son, she changed into her prostitute clothes and makeup. Assuming that her son was asleep, she quietly opened the front door to leave the house. Unexpectedly, her son woke up and ran to her. Seeing her, he stopped in his tracks crying, "Mommy, I'm scared of your eyes. Where are you?" Sara was devastated. She had switched into someone who was not herself in order to prostitute and her young son saw that. As has been well documented in psychological investigations of other forms of torture, overwhelming human cruelty results in fragmentation of the mind into different parts of the self that observe, and react, as well as those that do not know about the harm. Sara's dissociation was an escape strategy to handle overwhelming fear and pain by splitting that off from the rest of her self (see Ross, Farley & Schwartz, this volume).

This harm is made particularly difficult to see because of the invisibility of prostitution's harm to women in the mainstream media. A woman in prostitution told me that the one line in the movie *Pretty Woman* that was *not* a lie was when the john (Richard Gere) asked the prostitute (Julia Roberts) what her name was, and she responded "Anything you want it to be." In prostitution, she is depersonalized; her name and identity disappear. She shuts down her feelings to protect her self. She becomes "something for him to empty himself into, acting as a kind of human toilet" (Hoigard & Finstad, 1986). Whether she is coerced at gunpoint, or whether she "acts the part" in order to survive for so long that the mask takes over–either way, she doesn't stay a whole person. She constructs a self that conforms to the masturbatory fantasies of johns, a self that smilingly accommodates verbal abuse, sexual harassment, rape and torture. Over time, the prostituted self takes over more and more of the rest of her. She is disappeared. The harm she experiences in prostitution is made invisible, described not as sexual harassment, not as rape, not as intimate partner violence, but as "sex." The cruelty of prostitution intensifies when it is presented as "something else, when the context has been radically altered, and [its] cruelty is exhibited as something humorous or sexy" (Millett, 1994, p. 158).

One motivation for this denial of the harm of prostitution is clearly economic. Approximately 14% of the gross domestic product of Thailand (US $27 billion per year) was supplied by sex businesses (Lim, 1998). In 2000, an organization for prostituted adolescents reported that one girl was worth Canadian $250,000.00 a year to her pimp.

The articles in this collection describe what being prostituted or trafficked is like for the women, men and children in it. Some describe the physical and emotional sequelae of prostitution and trafficking. Others analyze these experiences from a feminist perspective, building on the existing literature on incest, rape, battering, and other forms of male violence. Several contributions describe programs to support women in escaping and healing from prostitution.

In this volume we attempt to answer some of the many questions that have arisen about prostitution and trafficking. What life experiences precede entry into prostitution? Are there gender or race/ethnic or socioeconomic demographics that increase vulnerability to entry into prostitution? What social structures and events channel women into prostitution or to being trafficked? What are the similarities and differences in the prostitution transaction and other encounters between men and women? Does violence occur in prostitution, and if so, what kinds of violence? What conceptual models are useful in understanding the institution of prostitution? Does the literature on incest, rape and intimate partner violence apply to prostitution? What is the emotional experience of prostitution for the woman performing sex acts for pay? Once out of prostitution, what are the psychological and physical consequences of prostitution? What are the needs of those in prostitution, and how can we meet those needs? What are the former prostitute's needs with respect to stable housing, physical healthcare, treatment for addictions, psychotherapy, vocational training, and social supports?

As the work in this volume shows, the acts perpetrated on women in prostitution cause not only physical harm, they also psychologically define her as object, as degraded, as "cunt," as "filthy whore." Her self, her individuality, her humanness is systematically attacked and destroyed in prostitution. She is reduced to vagina, anus, breasts and mouth. She acts the part of the thing men want her to be (Dworkin, 1997). Despite the clarity of many analysts on this topic, there is a lack of knowledge among clinicians regarding the systematic methods of brainwashing, indoctrination (called "seasoning" by pimps), and physical control that are used against women in prostitution. These techniques are specifically aimed at eliminating any corner of mental space for her to exist in. The strategies of political torturers: debilitation, dread, and dependency, read like a pimp's manual. The unpredictable and extreme violence in prostitution, like that in torture, is not only used for economic and sadistic reasons. It ultimately physically impresses upon the woman that she is utterly worthless and that she is socially nonexistent except as a prostitute. As her civilian identity fades, these techniques ensure that she loses her resistance and that she will comply with customers' and pimps' demands. Terror gets the job done; it makes her controllable.

Normalized in most cultures, prostitution is nonetheless what might well be described as a "harmful traditional cultural practice," a term applied internationally to female genital mutilation that refers to customs that are "based on the idea of the inferiority or the superiority of either of the sexes or on stereotyped roles for men and women" (MacKinnon, 2001; Wynter, Thompson & Jeffreys, 2002).[1] As of 2003 prostitution is sponsored by the state in the Netherlands, Germany, Australia, and New Zealand, among others. Where it is not state-sponsored, it is culturally promoted even in states where laws against prostitution are in place, such as the United States and Mexico.

A number of writers have analyzed prostitution as violence against women and children and also as a gross violation of human rights.[2] In their book about the sex industry in Thailand, Ryan Bishop advises coauthor Lillian Robinson on her first visit to Bangkok that she has to visit the sex shows in Patpong: "You have to do it," he tells her, "you have to go there the way you have to visit Dachau" (Bishop & Robinson, 1998, p. 6).

Elisabeth, from Norway, described her experience of the human rights violations of prostitution in graphic detail:

> They see you as a whore, never as someone they'd want to know . . . I'm nothing and no one they feel connected to. I'm only the genitals that they use. They could just as well have bought themselves one of those blown-up dolls. I'm nothing. I'm just a piece of shit. . . . I'm no one there's any reason to know. . . . I use tampons all the time. Even when I'm

not having my period. It's because I'm afraid of stinking. I never sit too close to people. I wash my ears ten times a day because I'm afraid guck is running out of them. (Hoigard & Finstad, 1992, p. 112-113)

The similarity between the experiences of women in prostitution in San Francisco to those of women in the conflict in Bosnia-Herzegovina are striking (Farley, Munczek & Weine, 1995). The dailiness of the rapes of San Francisco women in prostitution appeared chillingly similar to the rapes of women during that genocide. Gutman (1993) documented the existence of rape/death camps (survivors' term) in which Muslim and Croat women were kidnapped, humiliated, raped, tortured, deliberately impregnated by Serbs, and sometimes killed. Stiglmayer (1994) and Vranic (1996) interviewed survivors of brothel-like camps in Bosnia where women described being treated with a contempt, objectification, and violence that was very much like that in San Francisco massage parlors and street prostitution.

The struggle to understand prostitution is being waged, among others, on international legal fronts. Is prostitution a form of sex in need of freedom, or is it sexually exploitive and discriminatory, in need of abolition? (MacKinnon, 2001, p. 1396). The enactment of a 1999 Swedish law is cause for optimism.[3] Viewing prostitution as a social phenomenon that should be abolished, the Swedish government criminalized *the buying of sex but not the selling of sex.* Understanding that without the demand for purchased sexual access to women and children, prostitution and trafficking would not flourish, the 1999 Swedish law criminalized the customer himself as well as pimps, procurers, and traffickers, but *not the prostituted person.* The Swedish law recognized that "in the majority of cases . . . [the woman in prostitution] is a weaker partner who is exploited" and allocated funding for social services to "motivate prostitutes to seek help to leave their way of life".[3]

The effects of the law thus far seem beneficial. Two years after the law's passage, a Stockholm taskforce reported that there was a 50% decrease in women prostituting and a 75% decrease in men buying sex. Since the law was implemented, trafficking of women into Sweden has decreased as well, with pimps and traffickers apparently transporting women to nearby states that tolerate or legalize prostitution, such as the Netherlands, Germany, and Estonia (Ekberg, 2001).

Directly challenging the expansion of the global prostitution industry, and squarely recognizing the inextricability of trafficking from prostitution, Swedish Minister for Gender Equality Margareta Winberg asked:

Shall we accept the fact that certain women and children, primarily girls, often those who are most economically and ethnically marginalized, are

treated as a lower class, whose purpose is to serve men sexually? . . .
[E]fforts to combat prostitution and trafficking in women can only succeed if we refuse to be the stooges of the international proprostitution industry. . . . [W]e must take a stand against a society in which women and
children are regarded as commodities for trade, against the purchase of
women and children by men, and for a future in which all women and
children are given equal opportunities and in which their human rights
are respected. (Winberg, 2002)

Prostitution is to the community what incest is to the family. Incest and
prostitution are the bedrock of male domination of women, with incest functioning as "bootcamp" for prostitution (Dworkin, 1997). And just as there are
political movements to keep incest invisible (such as organizations that accuse
people of making up "false memories" about incest), there are also organizations that obscure the harm of prostitution by presenting it as a form of labor, as
if it were just another job.

Our thinking about prostitution and trafficking has been deeply affected by
the perspective of johns, pornographers, and their collaborators. Information
and disinformation about pornography and prostitution is still generated by
sexologists and libertarians–those who have historically tended to maintain the
status quo regarding women's sexuality. Pornography is a specific form of
prostitution, in which prostitution occurs and is documented. For its consumers, including the mainstream media, pornography is often their original experience of prostitution. Through pornography, misinformation about women,
including women in prostitution, and misinformation about women's sexuality, is widely promoted and ultimately incorporated into male sexuality via the
prostitution/pornography industry. A significant literature on the effects of
consumption of pornography suggests that pornography is frequently the basis
not only of how prostitutes are seen but how all women are seen and often
treated.

Prostitution today is a toxic cultural product, which is to say that all women
are socialized to objectify themselves in order to be desirable, to act like prostitutes, to act out the sexuality of prostitution. In western popular culture, the ex-
perts on women's sexuality are in fact prostitutes. For example, a 2002 issue of a
young women's magazine (*Marie Claire*) contained an article about women's
sexuality co-authored by a prostitute in a Nevada brothel and by a woman who
had prostituted in more than 50 videos. In another example of the effects of
cultural promotion of prostitution, a 3-year old girl at a San Francisco daycare
center bragged, "I'm a pimp." Children and adolescents learn to view pimps as
powerful, cold, in-charge rebels. When asked what pimp meant the child responded, "he has a lot of hoes." And that was a good thing: someone who has a
lot of hoes.

Sex trafficking occurs either within or across international borders, thus women may be domestically or internationally trafficked. In reality, girls are trafficked–meaning taken and sold for sexual use–from the countryside to the city, from one part of town to another, and across states' borders to wherever there are customers. For many centuries, women have been transported and sold in prostitution, in actual slavery or slavery-like practices (Barry, 1979).

Despite the illogical attempt of some to distinguish prostitution and trafficking, trafficking is simply the global form of prostitution. The economic dependence of countries on multinational corporations promotes and exacerbates prostitution and trafficking by creating conditions for women to sell their own sexual exploitation at far better rates of pay than other forms of labor (Hernandez, 2001). In any country with a high rate of unemployment, women (but not men) are channeled into prostitution. Despite some descriptions of prostitution as a reasonable job for poor women, the actualities better describe multiple violations of human rights (MacKinnon, 1993; Leidholdt, 1993).

Women and adolescents who have been trafficked across international borders are often in an unfamiliar culture, without social support and without friends who speak their language. They may have had their passports stolen, and are often kept in conditions of debt bondage. But there is no logic to the argument that if she is hurt *somewhat less or in different ways* in strip club prostitution than when she is trafficked from another country into a brothel, then strip club prostitution is not harmful. There is equally little sense to the notion that if she is coerced in a different way into prostitution in one location than when she is trafficked half way around the world, then that means that street prostitution is freely chosen. The fact that some injuries and forms of force are more severe than others does not mean that the marginally less severe forms are not harmful and should not be recognized as such. Physical assault is legally actionable harm, even though it is not murder.

Prostitution is made invisible when it is called *entertainment, work, hostessing* or when it is antiseptically described as the *sex sector* of a country's economy. It is made invisible by being glibly described as the *world's oldest profession*, or when prostitution is dismissed with *boys will be boys* or *it's a dick thing*. There is a virtual dictionary of lies that conceal the harm of prostitution: *voluntary prostitution*, words that imply that she consented when in fact, almost always, she had no other survival options than prostitution. The redundancy of the term *forced trafficking* insinuates its opposite–that somewhere there are women who volunteer to be trafficked into prostitution.

The following words lead to confusion regarding the nature and reality of prostitution. The increasingly common US/UK/Dutch expression *sex work*, suggests that prostitution is a normal job, rather than violence against women. The term *migrant sex worker* blends prostitution and trafficking and implies that both are harmless. Women in prostitution are called *escorts, strippers,* and *dancers.* The Chinese words, *beautiful merchandise* conceal in flowery language the objectification and commodification of women in prostitution. The expression *socially disadvantaged women* (allegedly used to destigmatize prostitutes) removes any hint of the sexual violence intrinsic to prostitution. The physical and verbal sexual abuse in strip club prostitution have been reformulated as *sexual expression* or *freedom* to *express one's sensuality* by dancing. Brothels are referred to as *short-time hotels, massage parlors, saunas,* and *health clubs.* Older men who buy teenagers for sex acts in Seoul call prostitution *compensated dating.* In Tokyo prostitution is articulated as *assisted intercourse.*

Prostitution has been described as a *business venture.* Men who buy women in prostitution are called *interested parties* or *third parties,* rather than johns or tricks, which is what women call customers. Pimps have been called *boyfriends* or *managers.* One pimp recently referred to the *brief shelf life* of a girl in prostitution, meaning that he knew the extent of the damage in prostitution and realized that she will not be saleable (if alive) after a few years. In the United States, the usage of the word *'ho* interchangeably with *women* reflects the view that all women are whores.

Counteracting disinformation about prostitution, the organization WHISPER distributed a tongue-in-cheek job description that brilliantly demystified prostitution.[4] "Advertising" a career working with people, with no experience needed, the WHISPER ad "warned" that benefits would only be provided at management discretion, and that there was no redress for nonpayment of services or for STDs. Accusations of rape were to be treated as an employee breach of contract.

I began research on prostitution in 1994 after San Francisco formed a Task Force on Prostitution. A former victim of prostitution was being kicked off the Task Force, and a friend of hers called me and asked me to write a letter of protest. I did, but I was confused. Why would a task force on prostitution not want to hear from someone who had been in it and gotten out?

I discovered that the goal of the San Francisco Task Force was to promote prostitution by eliminating legal barriers to its expansion. Members of the Task Force did not want to hear testimony about how brutally prostitution hurt women. The Task Force was carefully composed of those who promoted prostitution or who pimped other women, including a vocal minority who said prostitution was a fun and sexy job. When I offered to contribute papers from WHISPER and the Council for Prostitution Alternatives, two agencies that offered services for women escaping prostitution as well as an analysis of prostitution as violence, I was politely told that there was no room for that type of material in the Task Force library.

Two years later, the Task Force produced a report that advocated decriminalization of prostitution (Leigh, 1999). Decriminalization of prostitution would remove all laws against buying women and children for sex, sending a legal welcome to pimps, johns and especially traffickers. Not surprisingly, politicians on all sides ignored the San Francisco Task Force recommendations.

It is no accident that neither WHISPER nor Council for Prostitution Alternatives is in existence today. Groups that work for the human rights of formerly prostituted women are desperately underfunded, and the stress of the work sometimes causes bitter political infighting.

Since that political awakening I have learned some things about prostitution. Those who promote prostitution–and by extension, trafficking–are politically connected and well financed. Misinformation about prostitution is widespread–in the media, in academia, in social service agencies, and embedded in the healthcare system. This can only happen because real voices of former victims of prostitution are systematically silenced. It also happens because knowing the truth about prostitution might interfere with men's comfort and pleasure in using women in prostitution. It is also because prostitution itself is horrible: People don't want to hear details about it, just as they don't like to hear about torture. People tend to feel uncomfortable, powerless, guilty, and sometimes retraumatized by hearing about prostitution.

US slavery at its height was normalized as unpleasant but inevitable, yet it is now considered to be an institution that violated human rights. Perhaps we will at some point in the future look back on prostitution/trafficking with a similar historical perspective. It is my hope that the contributions in this volume will assist the reader in understanding prostitution and trafficking and in how to help women and children escape it.

NOTES

1. A United Nations General Assembly resolution (A/RES/54/133, 7 Feb. 2000) addressed the harm of female genital mutilation using language from the The Committee on the Elimination of Discrimination Against Women (CEDAW). The resolution requires states' parties to take all appropriate measures "to modify the social and cultural patterns of conduct of men and women, with a view to achieving the elimination of prejudices and customary and all other practices which are based on the idea of the inferiority or the superiority of either of the sexes or on stereotyped roles for men and women." For further information on these concepts see C.A. MacKinnon (2001) *Sex Equality*, page 1590-1591.

2. For a summary of some of those who have described prostitution as violence against women and as human rights violation see M. Farley and V. Kelly (2000) Prosti-

tution: A Critical Review of the Medical and Social Sciences Literature. *Women & Criminal Justice*, 11 (4): 29-64.

3. For information about Swedish laws regarding prostitution and trafficking, see http://naring.regeringen.se/pressinfo/faktablad/PDF/n2001_038e.pdf or http://www. prostitutionresearch.com/swedish.html

4. The following material is Copyright© WHISPER (Women Hurt in Systems of Prostitution Engaged in Revolt) & Evelina Giobbe. All Rights Reserved.

HELP WANTED: WOMEN AND GIRLS DO <u>YOU</u> WANT THIS JOB?

Prostitution has been euphemized as an occupational alternative for women, as an answer to low-paying, low skilled, boring dead-end jobs, as a solution to the high unemployment rate of poor women, as a form of sexual liberation, and a career women freely choose.

Are you tired of mindless, low skilled, low-paying jobs? Would you like a career with flexible hours? Working with people? Offering a professional service?
- No experience required. No high school diploma needed.
- No minimum age requirement. On-the-job training provided.
- Special opportunities for poor women–single mothers–women of color.

Women and girls applying for this position will provide the following services:
- Being penetrated orally, anally, and vaginally with penises, fingers, fists, and objects, including but not limited to, bottles, brushes, dildoes, guns and/or animals;
- Being bound and gagged, tied with ropes and/or chains, burned with cigarettes, or hung from beams or trees;
- Being photographed or filmed performing these acts.

Workplace: Job-related activities will be performed in the following locations: in an apartment, a hotel, a "massage parlor," car, doorway, hallway, street, executive suite, fraternity house, convention, bar, public toilet, public park, alleyway, military base, on a stage, in a glass booth.
- Wages will be negotiated at each and every transaction. Payment will be delivered when client determines when and if services have been rendered to his satisfaction.
- Corporate management fees range from 40-60% of wages; private manager reserves the right to impound all monies earned.

Benefits: Benefits will be provided at the discretion of management.

No Responsibility or Legal Redress for the Following on-the-Job Hazards:
- Nonpayment for services rendered;
- Sexually transmitted diseases or pregnancy;
- Injuries sustained through performance of services including but not limited to cuts, bruises, lacerations, internal hemorrhaging, broken bones, suffocation, mutilation, disfigurement, dismemberment, and death.

Note: Accusations of rape will be treated as a breach of contract by employee.
Name of applicant: _____
Signature of manager on behalf of applicant:_____

Printed with permission.

REFERENCES

Bishop, R. and Robinson, L.S. (1998). *Night Market: Sexual Cultures and the Thai Economic Miracle* Routledge, New York and London.

Barry, K., Bunch, C., Castley, S. (editors) (1984). *International Feminism: Networking Against Female Sexual Slavery.* Report of the Global Feminist Workshop to Organize against Traffic in Women Rotterdam, the Netherlands April 6-15 1983) International Women's Tribune Centre, In, UN Plaza, NY, NY.

Barry, K. (1979). *Female Sexual Slavery.* New York: New York University Press.

Dworkin, A. (1997). Prostitution and Male Supremacy in *Life and Death* p. 139-151. New York: Free Press.

Ekberg, G.S. (2001). Prostitution and Trafficking: The Legal Situation in Sweden. Paper presented at Journées de formation sur la mondialisation de la prostitution et du trafic sexuel, Association québécoise des organismes de coopération internationale, Montréal, Québec, Canada. March 15, 2001.

M. Farley and V. Kelly (2000). Prostitution: A Critical Review of the Medical and Social Sciences Literature. *Women & Criminal Justice*, 11 (4): 29-64.

Farley, M., Munczek, D. & Weine, S. (1995). Research as resistance to genocide and its psychological sequelae. Presentation at 11th Annual Meeting of the International Society for the Study of Traumatic Stress Studies. Boston, MA. November 4, 1995.

Gutman, R.A. (1993). *Witness to Genocide.* New York: MacMillan.

Hernandez, T.K. (2001). Sexual Harassment and Racial Disparity: The Mutual Construction of Gender and Race, *U. Iowa Journal of Gender, Race & Justice* Volume 4: 183-224.

Hoigard, C. & Finstad, L. (1986). *Backstreets: Prostitution, Money, and Love.* Pennsylvania State University Press, University Park, PA.

Jaget, C. (1980). *Prostitutes–Our Life* Bristol UK: Falling Wall Press.

Leidholt, D. (1993). Prostitution: A violation of women's human rights. *Cardozo Women's Law Journal* 1 (1): 133-147.

Leigh, C. (1999). A First Hand Look at the San Francisco Task Force Report on Prostitution. *Hastings Women's Law Journal* 10: 59-90.

Lim, L.L. (ed) (1998). *The Sex Sector: The economic and social bases of prostitution in Southeast Asia.* International Labor Organization, Geneva.

MacKinnon, C.A. (1993). Prostitution and Civil Rights. *Michigan Journal of Gender and Law* 1: 13-31.

MacKinnon, C.A. (2001). *Sex Equality.* New York: Foundation Press.

Millett, Kate (1994). *The Politics of Cruelty an essay on the literature on political imprisonment.* WW Norton, New York.

Stiglmayer, A. (ed) (1994). *Mass Rape: The War against Women in Bosnia-Herzegovina,* University of Nebraska Press, Lincoln.

Vranic, S. (1996). *Breaking the Wall of Silence: The Voices of Raped Bosnia.* Zagreb: antibarbarus.

WHO (1996). Female Genital Mutilation: Report of a WHO Technical Working Group. Geneva: WHO, 1996 WHO/FRH/WHD/96.10.

Winberg, M. (2002). Speech. Seminar on the Effects of Legalisation of Prostitution Activities–A Critical Analysis. Artikelnr N3006. Regeringskansliet. Stockholm: Naringsdepartementet.

Wynter, B., Thompson, D. & Jeffreys, S. (2002). The UN Approach to Harmful Traditional Practices. *International Feminist Journal of Politics* 4: 72-94.

Introduction: Hidden in Plain Sight: Clinical Observations on Prostitution

Judith Lewis Herman

Prostitution is everywhere. Everyone knows this; we just don't particularly want to know (MacKinnon, 2001). Who can bear to think for too long about a worldwide enterprise that condemns millions of women and children to social death (Patterson, 1982), and often to literal death, for the sexual pleasure and profit of men? The choice to avoid knowing operates at the edges of our consciousness; this is how dissociation is practiced as a social norm.

Thirty years ago, rape, domestic violence, and incest were similarly invisible, despite their high prevalence. A mass movement was required to bring these abuses into public awareness. In the social analysis developed by feminists, these crimes were understood as intrinsic features of a system of male dominance. It was recognized that the purpose of these crimes is to impose power, and that the methods used in furtherance of this goal are essentially the same as the methods of torture practiced in political prisons worldwide (Amnesty International, 1973; Russell, 1984).

One question that this analysis left unanswered was how individual batterers and sex offenders came to learn these often quite sophisticated methods of domination. In state-sponsored political violence, the practice of torture is or-

---

Judith Lewis Herman, MD, is affiliated with Harvard Medical School. She is at Victims of Violence Program, Department of Psychiatry, Cambridge Hospital, 26 Central Street, Somerville, MA 02143.
Printed with permission.

[Haworth co-indexing entry note]: "Introduction: Hidden in Plain Sight: Clinical Observations on Prostitution." Herman, Judith Lewis. Co-published simultaneously in *Journal of Trauma Practice* (The Haworth Maltreatment & Trauma Press, an imprint of The Haworth Press, Inc.) Vol. 2, No. 3/4, 2003, pp. 1-13; and: *Prostitution, Trafficking, and Traumatic Stress* (ed: Melissa Farley) The Haworth Maltreatment & Trauma Press, an imprint of The Haworth Press, Inc., 2003, pp. 1-13. Single or multiple copies of this article are available for a fee from The Haworth Document Delivery Service [1-800-HAWORTH, 9:00 a.m. - 5:00 p.m. (EST). E-mail address: docdelivery@haworthpress.com].

http://www.haworthpress.com/store/product.asp?sku=J189
10.1300/J189v02n03_01

1

ganized within secret police forces and "irregular" military units, who presumably teach these methods to carefully selected new recruits. Knowledge of these methods may be shared among clandestine military units of different countries; indeed, according to declassified documents, such methods have been taught in the US at the notorious School of the Americas (Haugaard, 1997; Nelson-Pallmeyer, 1997). But this mode of transmission can not account for the widespread practice of methods of coercive control in sexual and domestic life. Powerful as they may be, secret military and police units are relatively small in number even within dictatorships, whereas batterers and sex offenders are legion, not only in authoritarian political systems, but also in democratic societies.

It is theoretically possible, of course, that each abuser might spontaneously re-invent the basic methods of coercive control for himself, but this seems quite unlikely, given the constancy and uniformity of these practices across class and culture. It is more likely that this knowledge is transmitted within all-male groups that promote an ideology of male dominance and contempt for women, what Brownmiller (1975) calls the "men's house culture." It is already known that sexual assault is common among young men who belong to groups such as sports teams and fraternities (Koss, 1987). In such groups, the exchange of women or a shared visit to a brothel is often the means by which male bonding and solidarity is affirmed. The ritual display of the power to command sex from women is also a common custom in many business and political enterprises and, of course, in armies worldwide (Johnson, 2000; Goldstein, 2001). It is conceivable, then, that the prostitution industry, which operates in virtually every society, might be a primary vector for socialization in the practices of coercive control, and the pimp might be among the world's most common instructors in the arts of torture.

For helping professionals, it is difficult enough to face the reality of sexual and domestic violence as it operates in a single family, and to engage in a therapeutic relationship with a battered woman or abused child. How much more difficult, then, to face the reality of sexual violence as exercised by an organized criminal enterprise that operates freely in every community, hidden in plain sight, and to engage with victims who have been systematically reduced to the condition of slavery. Even those of us who are seasoned clinicians may find ourselves overcome with feelings of disgust, fascination, or pervasive dread, reactions which interfere with the formation of a successful therapeutic alliance. Like bystanders everywhere, we may choose not to see, hear, or speak about what in fact we already know.

Recently, when preparing a lecture for a conference on trauma, I proposed to address the subject of prostitution. The conference organizer was not pleased with my suggestion. Most of the program was devoted to the response to terrorist attacks and the formation of a national center for traumatic stress in children. Here was plenty of "clean" trauma, with many innocent victims whose plight aroused general sympathy. Prostitution, by contrast, was embarrassing, shameful, in a word, dirty. Did it even make sense to speak of victims? Wasn't prostitution, after all, a "victimless crime?"

I noted that our staff at the Victims of Violence Program (Department of Psychiatry, The Cambridge Hospital, Cambridge, MA) were seeing a remarkable number of patients who had been used in prostitution, and that these were among the most cruelly abused people we had ever treated. My colleague acknowledged that he, too, had seen such cases, but surely they were unusual. I suggested as an empirical test that we poll the audience at the conference. If few of the participants had seen such cases, I promised not to pursue the subject any further.

At the start of my lecture, with about 600 people in attendance, I asked how many had treated or were currently treating patients who had been used in prostitution. By my rough visual estimate, 450 people (75%) raised their hands. It was a moment of surprise, not only for my colleague, the conference organizer, but for those in the audience as well. Here was a common experience that by common, unspoken consent was simply not discussed in public, not even by a group of mental health professionals who had already amply proved their willingness to bear witness to terrible stories. It was also a moment of illumination and relief, as members of the audience looked around and realized they had lots of company. With the acknowledgement and support of colleagues, perhaps we clinicians could overcome our own resistance to engagement with victims who are generally viewed as neither "clean" nor "innocent."

We have a great deal to learn from these patients. The complex traumatic syndromes from which they suffer are among the most difficult to understand and the most challenging to treat. They define for us the far edges of the spectrum of traumatic disorders, and the frontiers of our current knowledge.

Secrecy is the first and most serious obstacle to forming a therapeutic alliance. People engaged in prostitution, if they seek treatment at all, are likely to conceal or minimize their involvement in prostitution. The shame and stigma attached to prostitution are so severe that most people will go to great lengths to hide this aspect of their experience, even in a confidential therapy relationship that depends for its success on frank and full disclosure (Baldwin, this volume). Given the widespread prevalence of prostitution, it would seem advisable for clinicians to learn to incorporate questions regarding this experience into routine history-taking (for examples see Stark & Hodgson, this volume). Clinicians working with trauma populations should be especially alert to this possibility, given the vulnerability of childhood abuse survivors to revictimization in general (Coid et al., 2001), and to recruitment for pornography and prostitution in particular (Russell, 1986).

People in prostitution also commonly suffer from serious neurobiological and personality disorders that hinder the formation of a cooperative working relationship. Moreover, the realities of their daily lives are often so precarious and dangerous that without sustained and well-organized social intervention, ordinary therapeutic measures are unlikely to have any meaningful effect. Some of the problems encountered in treating this group of patients are illustrated by the following case vignettes, drawn from the records of the Victims of Violence Program. Details that might permit identification of individuals have been omitted or disguised.

NEUROBIOLOGICAL PROBLEMS

These include very complex and confusing ego states (Ross, Farley, & Schwartz, this volume), and severe forms of emotional and bodily dysregulation. While somatic and affective dysregulation are commonly seen in complex PTSD (van der Kolk et al., 1996), the conditions of prostitution exacerbate this problem. Control of bodily functions is an established method of coercion well known to clandestine police forces and criminal organizations worldwide. It is systematically practiced by pimps and traffickers in the sex industry, not only to intimidate victims and break their resistance, but also to train them for sexual performance.

The ultimate goal in this, as in all systems of domination, is to destroy the autonomy of the victim and induce as far as possible a state of willing submission. This may require the intentional induction of altered states of consciousness and the development of dissociated ego states in which the enslaved person is given a new name and a new identity as a whore (Stark & Hodgson, this volume). An example can be found in the autobiographical account of Linda Marciano, who describes being first raped and beaten into submission, and then trained with the aid of hypnosis to suppress her gag reflex, in order to perform her role as "Linda Lovelace" in the famous pornographic film *Deep Throat* (Lovelace & McGrady, 1980). Here the colonization of the body extends to the suppression of the most basic autonomic functions.

Under conditions of prostitution, autonomous self-regulation of any sort is a form of insubordination; it is expressly forbidden and actively suppressed. In the absence of normal self-soothing, substance abuse provides the most accessible route to bodily calm and emotional comfort. Addiction further complicates an already complicated clinical picture. When chemical means of self-regulation fail, self-harming behavior, and suicide attempts are often the last resort.

CASE EXAMPLE ONE

Jenny, a 35-year-old-single woman, entered outpatient treatment complaining of depression and post-traumatic stress symptoms. She was living alone in a condominium owned by her father and working part time in the office of one of her father's business associates. She complained of feeling controlled and bullied by her father, who had sexually abused her when she was a child, but depended on him for financial support.

The initial treatment plan focused on stabilization of symptoms and development of a workable safety plan. Ostensibly, Jenny agreed with this plan and seemed highly motivated to carry it out. However, despite her best efforts and those of her treatment team, apparently well-crafted safety plans were repeatedly and inexplicably breached. Her sense of desperation and helplessness deepened, and she became actively suicidal. Her treatment team was puzzled by her deteriorating condition. Clearly, some major piece of information was missing.

Finally, two years into her treatment, it was recognized that "Jenny" was the host personality in a patient with Dissociative Identity Disorder. Our experienced clinicians had previously failed to make the diagnosis, despite their general familiarity with dissociative disorders and a high index of suspicion in this particular case. It became clear that the patient had intentionally concealed her dissociative symptoms. Some of her numerous alters disclosed that they had been actively collaborating with the father, who operated a private sex ring. The patient reported that her father had been pimping her since the age of 14, rewarding her with money and cocaine. He was fully aware of her dissociative disorder and routinely summoned specific alters, who identified themselves as willing prostitutes, to perform the desired sexual activities.

In his original study of 100 cases of Dissociative Identity Disorder, Putnam (1986) noted that the average length of time between entry into the mental health system and correct diagnosis was six years. The two year delay in diagnosing this case, while it might represent an improvement over the norms of 20 years ago, certainly leaves much to be desired. It seems clear in retrospect that the key to the diagnosis in this complex case was recognition of the patient's ongoing involvement in prostitution. Specific questioning regarding prostitution might have uncovered this essential fact earlier.

CHARACTEROLOGICAL PROBLEMS

Victimization does not generally improve a person's character. Personality disorders are a common feature of the complex traumatic syndrome that results from prolonged and repeated trauma in relationships of coercive control (Herman, 1992). Many survivors develop a stigmatized, negative identity and have difficulty establishing stable, cooperative and mutually rewarding relationships. Identity and relational problems reflect the degree of moral degradation to which the person has been subjected, and the resultant shame, resentment, and mistrust which she brings to any new relationship. It is common for survivors to engage in a pattern of intense, unstable, and highly conflictual relationships.

Even when the prostitution secret has been revealed, other forms of dissembling and dishonesty may continue. People who have been used in prostitution are keenly aware of the hypocrisy of the supposedly respectable people who seek out their services. They are further exposed to the ideology of the criminal class that exploits them, in which every sort of immoral behavior is rationalized and even glorified, on the grounds that the whole society is exploitative and corrupt, and the only way to preserve one's dignity is to "beat the system." Relationships, including the therapeutic relationship, are often approached with the assumption that people are generally selfish or perverse, and that only a limited number of roles are possible: One can be a perpetrator, an accomplice, a well-meaning but useless bystander, a victim, or, perhaps, a rescuer. The concept of a freely chosen, honest and fair relationship, in which both parties work hard to fulfill their responsibilities and both parties benefit, may be completely foreign to the patient's world-view or experience.

To counter this cynical and despairing view of human relationships, the rules of engagement in psychotherapy must be clearly explained, and the therapist must make it clear that both parties are accountable for honoring them. Honesty, fairness, and respect are mutual obligations. The patient should be encouraged to voice any complaints she may have about her treatment, especially any behavior that she views as unjust, dishonest or disrespectful. Similarly, the therapist should deal openly with dishonest or disrespectful behavior on the part of the patient, both in and outside of the office. Treating patients with dignity includes the expectation that they take reasonable responsibility for their actions.

In general, clinicians aspire to create a therapeutic climate that is accepting, warm and non-judgmental. Confronting a patient's unacceptable behavior, while maintaining an attitude of caring and respect, is one of the therapist's most difficult and challenging tasks. When working with people in prostitution, clinicians may bend over backward to avoid seeming prudish or judgmental. In the effort to overcome their own prejudices, clinicians may be tempted to overlook or excuse antisocial behavior. This stance, while well-intentioned, ultimately undermines the therapy relationship. Patients do not appreciate being patronized. On the contrary, patients often express their appreciation for therapists who recognize them as moral beings, using expressions such as "she never let me get over on her," or "he believed in me."

CASE EXAMPLE TWO

Katarina is a 24-year-old mother of a two-year-old son. In the course of her treatment, she had successfully ended a relationship with a pimp and was living in a small apartment with a new boyfriend, who, like herself, was a recovering addict. She supported herself by providing home daycare for several children. Daily contact with the children reminded her of how profoundly neglected she had been as a child and how deeply she longed for both attention and material possessions. She acknowledged that she missed the extravagant spending that was part of her life in prostitution, even though she recognized that her pimp controlled all the money and that she herself had always been desperately poor.

Just before Christmas, Katarina reported that while in a store with her son she had impulsively stolen a bracelet. Her initial feeling of entitlement and triumph had quickly given way to shame and regret as she realized how seriously she had put herself and her child at risk. She was very relieved that she had not been caught, but getting away with shoplifting didn't feel right either; now she couldn't even stand to wear the bracelet.

The therapist was glad Katarina had confided in her, and told her so, but also made it clear that she did not approve of stealing. She asked whether Katarina had considered returning the bracelet. This idea came as a complete surprise to the patient, who had never entertained the possibility that she could make things right. Her eventual choice to return the bracelet gave her a new sense of agency and self-respect.

In this case, the therapist was able to maintain the distinction between moral and therapeutic neutrality. To clarify the distinction: Moral neutrality means declining to take a stand on the abstract question whether stealing is right or wrong. Therapeutic neutrality means declining to take a stand regarding the patient's inner conflicts about stealing. Here, the therapist was able to convey a clear moral position against shoplifting, while maintaining a confidential and accepting stance toward the patient. This allowed the patient to explore her conflicted feelings about what she had done and come to her own resolution of her dilemma. The therapeutic alliance was enhanced, to the mutual satisfaction of patient and therapist, and the therapy progressed well.

In other cases, however, where crimes against persons rather than property crimes are at issue, neutrality of any sort may be impossible to maintain. If the patient's behavior is putting others at risk, the therapist may be morally or even legally obligated to take a stand, even at the cost of violating confidentiality or jeopardizing the therapy relationship.

CASE EXAMPLE THREE

Nicole, a 22-year-old single mother, came to the clinic seeking medication to help her panic attacks and counseling to help her cope with the behavior of her five-year-old daughter. She had recently moved into the home of a wealthy, divorced older man whom she had met at the nightclub where she worked as a stripper. She saw this move as a great improvement in her life. She was estranged both from her abusive parents and from the father of her child, who had beaten her and had never provided any financial support. Her new boyfriend treated her "like a queen." The only problem was her daughter, who had turned into a "brat." The child had become alternately clingy and defiant, had started wetting the bed, and was refusing to accept her new "daddy." Over time Nicole disclosed that this man had a prior conviction for rape and was currently under permanent court order to have no contact with his two teenage daughters, who had accused him of incest. Nicole believed his assurances that in both cases he had been falsely accused by conniving women who were after his money. She frequently left her daughter alone in his care, despite the child's protests.

The therapist expressed his concern about the situation. He attempted to engage Nicole's protective feelings for her daughter and to raise her awareness regarding the possibility of abuse, but Nicole adamantly refused to entertain the idea that her child could be in any danger. The therapist shared his dilemma with the patient. He explained that he did not want to take action without her consent, but he could not remain a passive bystander when he suspected that the child might be at risk. He reminded Nicole how much she had longed for someone to intervene when she herself was being abused as a child. In this case, he explained, there were clear warning signals, and he would be negligent if he failed to pay attention. Furthermore, as a mandated reporter he was required by law to bring his concern about the child's safety to the attention of protective services. Enraged, Nicole called the therapist a "fucking pig" and stormed out of the office. An investigation by the state Department of Social Services confirmed sexual abuse, and the child was placed in foster care.

In this case, despite the therapist's best efforts, it was not possible to engage the patient in the project of establishing safety. The treatment alliance failed, and the therapist was obliged to act unilaterally. Though the intervention was necessary, the outcome was tragic for both the patient and her daughter. It was also painful for therapist, who was placed in an untenable position, forced to choose between passive complicity in the ongoing abuse of a child and drastic action that invoked the intervention of the state. In general, because violence and exploitation are an intrinsic part of the daily lives of people in prostitution, therapists who work with them may often be placed in the uncomfortable position of a bystander and faced with similar moral dilemmas regarding intervention.

SOCIAL PROBLEMS

The numerous social problems encountered by people in prostitution are reviewed by several authors in this volume (Carter; Hedin & Manson; Hotaling et al.; Rabinovitch). Of particular concern are the dangers and practical difficulties of leaving prostitution. Like battered women, prostituted women can expect an escalation of violence should they attempt to escape from their abusers, and may need a great deal of assistance to obtain shelter and rudimentary physical safety. Several attempts may be necessary before safety is achieved. Caregivers who assist women attempting to leave prostitution may feel frustrated and overwhelmed by the complexity of the task; they may also occasionally feel threatened and endangered along with their patients.

CASE EXAMPLE FOUR

Yvette, a 28-year-old woman with a 15 year history of prostitution and drug addiction, finally made a decision to leave her pimp. Support for this decision required intensive involvement and sustained cooperation among numerous agencies. She was hospitalized on several occasions, first for detoxification and then for severe depression. She was eventually granted disability on the basis of psychiatric impairment and was assigned a case manager. Supervised housing was arranged through the state Department of Mental Health. A victim advocate assisted her in seeking a court order to prevent the pimp from pursuing her in her new location.

For several months after the court order was granted, Yvette had no contact with her pimp and was consistently abstinent from drugs and alcohol for the first time since early adolescence. Safety was maintained until she was discharged (against her therapist's advice) from the halfway house where she had been living and moved to an unsupervised apartment in an unfamiliar community. Within two weeks she relapsed and called one of the pimp's associates, looking for drugs. Shortly thereafter she was found by the police wandering on the street at night, dazed and bleeding, and brought to the local emergency room. She initially stated that her pimp had tracked her down and beaten her, but soon retracted her story and refused to cooperate further with law enforcement.

When she recovered from her injuries, Yvette was discharged from the hospital to a secure residential placement. She is currently sober and to the best of our knowledge has had no further contact with her pimp. In therapy she acknowledges that was indeed the pimp who attacked her, but she is afraid that he might kill her if she ever dared to press criminal charges against him. Her therapist considers this to be a reasonable fear.

Consultation was sought with the victim witness advocacy service in the district attorney's office, regarding potential danger to the therapist as well as the patient. In the advocate's judgment, the pimp appeared to be a rational criminal entrepreneur who was unlikely to risk attacking a person with professional status and a strong social support network. Nevertheless, the therapist has taken additional security precautions to protect herself and her family.

The investment of service resources in this case was extraordinary. The financial and emotional costs of this one case were very high, and while significant progress has been made, the patient's recovery is still quite fragile. Premature attempts to move the patient to a less intensive (and less costly) care environment resulted in relapse and placed her in serious danger. Though this case may represent an extreme, some comparable degree of resource mobilization may be necessary for many people in prostitution. Effective recovery programs are likely to require coordination of many types of service, including health, mental health and addiction services, disability or other forms of public assistance (Baldwin, this volume), housing support, and victim advocacy. Any social policy approach to this problem must include a realistic appraisal of the cost and cost-effectiveness of rehabilitation services.

This case also raises philosophical and legal questions regarding responsibility, and choice. Should a criminal case be brought against the pimp, despite the patient's refusal to cooperate, based on her initial "excited utterance" in the emergency room and her documented injuries? Would such an "evidence-based" prosecution be in her best interest, or would it further disempower or endanger her? Given the extreme degree of coercive control exercised by pimps, and the general reluctance of their victims to testify against them, is such paternalistic intervention ever warranted (Buzawa & Buzawa, 2003; Epstein, 1999; Mills, 1998)?

Finally, most people who attempt to leave prostitution are also very poor and lack basic education or the rudimentary job skills that might enable them to support themselves independently. They also frequently lack the social skills required for participation in ordinary, non-exploitative relationships. The code of "getting over," although it might conceivably be adaptive within highly stigmatized social groups, is completely maladaptive for a person attempting to enter into the "straight" world. A structured peer support group may offer the most meaningful opportunity for the survivor to develop a new identity as a valued and responsible member of a community (see, for example, Carter, this volume; Rabinovitch, this volume; Hotaling et al., this volume).

CASE EXAMPLE FIVE

Kevin, a 21-year-old man, had escaped from his abusive family at the age of 17 by running away to live with an older man whom he met in an Internet chat room. At first, the relationship seemed very romantic, and Kevin was "happier than I had ever been in my life." Gradually, however, he became disillusioned, as his partner began to pressure him into prostitution, threatening to throw him out of the house if he refused. Kevin became increasingly frightened as the men his partner brought home insisted on increasingly risky and painful sexual practices. Finally, feeling lost and betrayed, he fled to a homeless shelter and sought psychiatric treatment.

In the course of his recovery, Kevin moved into a rooming house, got a job at a fast-food restaurant, and entered a program to get his high school diploma. Though he had succeeded in getting safe, he complained that he was lonely and bored and acknowledged that he was strongly tempted to return to "tricking." He reported a dream in which he escaped from a swamp filled with dangerous creatures, only to find himself all alone in a cold, antiseptic swimming pool. It became apparent that Kevin had no idea how to make friends with people his own age, let alone how to form an intimate relationship. He felt that he didn't belong anywhere.

With his therapist's encouragement, Kevin joined a group for male survivors of sexual abuse. In this group he experienced a sense of belonging and felt understood by his peers, and he was able to explore complicated issues such as confusion about his sexual orientation. He also gained self-respect from the experience of being supportive to others. After some time in the group, he began volunteering at an animal shelter, where he found that he could bond with others who shared his concern for abandoned and mistreated animals.

These case vignettes suggest that the basic principles of trauma treatment–establishing safety, working through the trauma, reconnecting with a community–are potentially useful and effective for survivors of prostitution. Many of the issues illustrated in these case examples are already familiar to clinicians working with trauma survivors. Themes of secrecy, social alienation and stigma are common to victims of many types of oppression, particularly those forms that are socially condoned. Even seasoned clinicians, however, may be shocked to discover the extent of prostitution in their own communities and horrified by the extreme violence and degradation to which people in prostitution are subjected. The contagion of trauma produces a range of predictable countertransference reactions that mirror the symptoms of the posttraumatic disorders. Hyperarousal reactions may include heightened anxiety, embarrassment, fascination, or even sexual excitement. Numbing reactions may include denial, disgust, aversion, and avoidance. These intense countertransference reactions have slowed recognition of the problem of prostitution within the trauma field. Furthermore, clinicians are not immune to the prejudices of the larger community. The dishonor attached to prostitution is so profound that it affects all social interactions, including the therapy relationship.

This collection of papers is designed to raise awareness of prostitution among clinicians and to foster public conversation on a subject that has hitherto largely been avoided. For the three out of four clinicians who have already worked with survivors of prostitution, but have done their work in isolation, this volume is designed to build support and community. For the one out of four who has not yet (knowingly) treated a patient with a history of prostitution, this volume is designed as preparation for an encounter that is very likely to happen sooner or later. Clinicians who work with traumatized people have borne witness to many kinds of atrocity; we are capable of facing this one, too, as long as we do not have to face it alone.

REFERENCES

Amnesty International (1973). *Report on Torture*. New York: Farrar, Straus, & Giroux.

Baldwin, M.A. (2003). Living in longing: Prostitution, trauma recovery, and public assistance. In M. Farley (ed.) *Prostitution, Trafficking, and Traumatic Stress*. Binghamton: The Haworth Press, Inc.

Brownmiller, S. (1975). Against Our Will: Men, Women, and Rape. New York: Simon & Schuster.

Buzawa, E.S. & Buzawa, C.G. (2003). Domestic Violence: The Criminal Justice Response (Third Edition). Thousand Oaks, CA: Sage.

Carter, V. (2003). Providing services to African-American prostituted women. In M. Farley (ed.) *Prostitution, Trafficking, and Traumatic Stress*. Binghamton: The Haworth Press, Inc.

Coid, J., Petruckevitch, A., Feder G., Chung, W-S., Richardson, J., & Moorey S. (2001). Relation between childhood sexual and physical abuse and risk of revictimization in women: A cross-sectional survey. *The Lancet*: 358; 450-454.

Epstein, D. (1999). Effective intervention in domestic violence cases: Rethinking the role of prosecutors, judges, and the court system. *Yale Journal of Law and Feminism:* 11; 3-50.

Goldstein, J. (2001). *War and Gender: How Gender Shapes the War System and Vice Versa.* New York: Cambridge University Press.

Haugaard, L. (1997). *Declassified Army and CIA Manuals Used in Latin America: An Analysis of Their Content.* Washington, D.C.: Latin America Working Group.

Hedin, U.-C., & Mansson, S.A., (2003). The importance of supportive relationships among women leaving prostitution. In M. Farley (ed.) *Prostitution, Trafficking, and Traumatic Stress.* Binghamton: The Haworth Press, Inc: 223-237.

Herman, J.L. (1992). *Trauma and Recovery.* New York: Basic Books.

Hotaling, N, Burris, A, Johnson, BJ, Bird YM, Melbye, KA, (2003). Been There Done That: A peer leadership model among prostitution survivors. In M. Farley (ed.) *Prostitution, Trafficking, and Traumatic Stress.* Binghamton: The Haworth Press, Inc: 255-265.

Johnson, C. (2000). *Blowback: The Costs and Consequences of American Empire.* New York: Metropolitan Books.

Koss, M. (1987). Hidden rape: Sexual aggression and victimization in a national sample of students of higher education. In AW Burgess (Ed.): *Rape and Sexual Assault*, Vol. 2. New York: Garland: 3-26.

Lovelace L. & McGrady, M. (1980). *Ordeal.* Secaucus, NJ: Citadel.

MacKinnon, C.A. (2001). *Sex Equality.* NY: Foundation Press. Chapter 10 Trading Women, pp. 1381-1661.

Mills, L. (1998). *The Heart of Intimate Abuse: New Interventions in Child Welfare, Criminal Justice, and Health Settings.* New York: Springer.

Nelson-Pallmeyer, J. (1997). *School of Assassins: The Case for Closing the School of the Americas and for Fundamentally Changing U.S. Foreign Policy.* Maryknoll, NY: Orbis Books.

Patterson, O. (1982). *Slavery and Social Death: A Comparative Study.* Cambridge, MA: Harvard University Press.

Putnam, F.W., Guroff, J.J., Silberman, E.K. et al. (1986). The clinical phenomenology of multiple personality disorder: Review of 100 recent cases. *Journal of Clinical Psychiatry* 47: 285-293.

Rabinovitch, J. (2003). PEERS: The prostitutes empowerment, education and resource society. In M. Farley (ed.) *Prostitution, Trafficking, and Traumatic Stress.* Binghamton: The Haworth Press, Inc: 239-253.

Ross, C.A., Farley, M., & Schwartz, H.L. (2003). Dissociation among women in prostitution. In M. Farley (ed.) *Prostitution, Trafficking, and Traumatic Stress.* Binghamton: The Haworth Press, Inc: 199-212.

Russell, D.E.H. (1984). *Sexual Exploitation.* Beverly Hills, CA: Sage.

Russell, D.E.H. (1986). *The Secret Trauma: Incest in the Lives of Girls and Women.* New York: Basic Books.

Stark, C. & Hodgson, C. (2003). Sister oppressions: A comparison of wife-battering and prostitution. In M. Farley (ed.) *Prostitution, Trafficking, and Traumatic Stress.* Binghamton: The Haworth Press, Inc: 217-232.

van der Kolk, B.A., Pelcovitz, D., Roth, S., Mandel, F., McFarlane, A., & Herman, J.L. (1996). Dissociation, affect dysregulation and somatization: The complexity of adaptation to trauma. *American Journal of Psychiatry: 153 (Festschrift Supplement): 83-93.*

*UNDERSTANDING
PROSTITUTION AND TRAFFICKING
AS ORGANIZED INTERPERSONAL VIOLENCE*

Sister Oppressions:
A Comparison of Wife Battering and Prostitution

Christine Stark
Carol Hodgson

SUMMARY. Little has been written about the similarities between domestic violence and prostitution. It is important for those who come in contact with prostituted women and girls, especially people working in battered women's shelters, homeless shelters, rape crisis centers, and health care professions, to understand prostitution as the battery of women and girls. The similarities between domestic violence and prostitution are discussed here, including the techniques of control used by batterers and pimps, homelessness, physical injuries from battering, healthcare barriers, and substance abuse. Finally, solutions to assist prostituted women and girls are outlined.

INTRODUCTION

A father rapes and beats his daughter throughout her childhood. As an adult she gets into a relationship with a man who beats her, rapes her, and

Christine Stark is at P.O. Box 11925, Minneapolis, MN 55411 (E-mail: christine.stark-1@mnsu.edu).

Carol Hodgson is affiliated with Recollections–Capturing Memories, British Columbia, Canada (Email: Recollections@uniserve.com).

This is dedicated to our mothers: Linda Grussendorf and Bernadine J. Upton. Printed with permission.

[Haworth co-indexing entry note]: "Sister Oppressions: A Comparison of Wife Battering and Prostitution." Stark, Christine, and Carol Hodgson. Co-published simultaneously in *Journal of Trauma Practice* (The Haworth Maltreatment & Trauma Press, an imprint of The Haworth Press, Inc.) Vol. 2, No. 3/4, 2003, pp. 17-32; and: *Prostitution, Trafficking, and Traumatic Stress* (ed: Melissa Farley) The Haworth Maltreatment & Trauma Press, an imprint of The Haworth Press, Inc., 2003, pp. 17-32. Single or multiple copies of this article are available for a fee from The Haworth Document Delivery Service [1-800-HAWORTH, 9:00 a.m. - 5:00 p.m. (EST). E-mail address: docdelivery@haworthpress.com].

http://www.haworthpress.com/store/product.asp?sku=J189
10.1300/J189v02n03_02

threatens to kill her. He does this in order to control her and to keep her in line. He says she deserves it because she did not do the dishes the way he wants or because she painted her fingernails like a whore or because she went bowling with her friends and did not check in with him. His friends monitor her activities when he is not around. The money is his even though she earns it. He calls her names like whore and slut to intimidate her and he threatens to hurt their children. He tells her he owns her and that no one else would want her by now, and she believes him. This woman feels helpless and exhausted all the time. Friends and family say she chose to be in the relationship or they say it could not be that bad because if it was that bad she would just leave. Some days, she thinks this must be true. Beside herself with terror and desperation, she dials the number of an advocacy center and asks for help.

If you have identified this woman as a battered woman, you are correct. But have you also identified her as a prostituted woman? Most of the time prostituted women and girls tell advocates and health care workers only part of what is going on in their lives, because to reveal involvement in prostitution can be dangerous, even to those who understand other issues of sexual exploitation.[1] It is important to consider what you would say to a woman if she told you her husband also sells her to other men for sex or makes pornography of her. Would you help her, or would you turn away? If you decided to help her, what services in your community are available to her? Although prostituted women and girls are victims of sexual violence, battered women's shelters, rape crisis centers, therapists, homeless shelters, and healthcare workers have not understood prostitution as battery, thus they have not consistently been able to assist prostituted women and girls. We will discuss the similarities between battering and prostitution, including the victims, the perpetrators, and solutions that advocates can implement to assist prostituted women and girls.

DOMESTIC VIOLENCE

Domestic violence is a pattern of behavior whose purpose is to control women (Walker, 2000). Men are the abusive partners in 95% of domestic violence cases (Island & Letellier, 1991). U.S. men batter four million intimate partners each year (City Club of Portland Report, 1997). Abusive men shove, slap, kick, rape, hit, or bite their partners. They also beat women up and they use weapons to maintain control. Women sometimes die at the hands of their partners, particularly when they try to leave after years of brutal abuse. Our U.S. culture creates a viciously woman-hating environment that supports the rights and privileges of men who abuse women. This violence is a means of controlling women.

> Rape and assault on the street keep women controlled and imprisoned by fear. The war waged against women every minute of every day to maintain male domination permeates society so completely that it is invisible to most people as water is to the fish who swim in it, or air is to those of us who breathe it. Batterers are the home guards of this war. (Garrity, 2002)

Like the battering of women in the home, prostitution is embedded in this culture.

PROSTITUTION

Prostitution is a global industry in which sex is traded for money, clothing, food, drugs, shelter, or favors. Prostitution is an industry of exploitation that includes strip clubs, massage parlors, saunas, pornography, street walking, live sex shows, phone sex, prostitution rings, international and domestic trafficking, internet pornography, escort services, peep shows, ritual abuse, and mail order bride services. Pimps are men who batter, rape, and sell women for sex; they control the systems of prostitution. In the U.S., it has been estimated that over 90% of prostitutes are controlled by pimps (Giobbe, 1993). Tricks are men who buy women and girls for sex; they also batter, rape, and murder prostituted women and girls. Few studies have been done about pimps and tricks, but prostituted women and girls know that they are average, everyday, all-American men.

THE CONNECTION BETWEEN DOMESTIC VIOLENCE, PORNOGRAPHY, AND PROSTITUTION

While some has been written about the connections between rape and prostitution (Russell, 1993, Farley, Baral, Kiremire, & Sezgin, 1998), racism and prostitution (Nelson, 1993), incest and prostitution (Silbert & Pines, 1981, Dworkin, 1988, Hotaling, 1999), little has been written about the connections between domestic violence and prostitution. Women and girls in prostitution can trace their involvement in prostitution to sexual violence that began in the home as physical, verbal, and sexual violence directed at wives, girlfriends, sisters, daughters, and granddaughters. In the U.S. only 10% to 20% of prostitution is street-based

(O'Leary & Howard, 2001). These studies belie the myth that most prostitution occurs on urban street corners. Prostitution that occurs in escort services, strip clubs, and massage parlors is generally assumed to be safe for prostituted women. However, violence is prevalent in all systems of prostitution. One woman, who was used for over thirty years in various systems of prostitution, described being repeatedly beaten and gang raped in the back rooms of strip clubs, in hotel rooms while on out call, and in massage parlors. In more than thirty years, she never prostituted on the streets. In fact, prostitution occurs behind closed doors in homes and businesses, and in suburban and rural areas more frequently than it does on inner city streets.

In addition to domestic violence, most prostituted women also have histories of neglect and abuse from families, social isolation, sexual, psychological and physical abuse, drug and alcohol abuse, and limited alternatives for escaping the abuse (Council for Prostitution Alternatives, 1991). Some people view women as the property of one man in marriage, whereas in prostitution women are the property of many men. Husbands and boyfriends commonly use wives and girlfriends in systems of prostitution, especially pornography. Sometimes prostituted women and battered women are one and the same. For instance, a woman who was battered by her husband for many years was also forced by her husband into prostitution. She testified, "He would read from the pornography like a textbook, like a journal. And most of the scenes where I had to dress up or go through different fantasies were the exact scenes that he had read in the magazine" (Dworkin & MacKinnon, 1998, pp. 113-114).

Pornography's role in domestic violence and prostitution tends to be overlooked. In photographs, articles, and cartoons, pornography depicts many different kinds of violence as erotic, including wife beating, the exploitation of women and girls in prostitution, incest, ethno-rape (abuse committed against a woman or girl based on her skin color or ethnicity), and workplace sexual harassment. Pornography trivializes wife beating by treating physical assault as a joke. For instance, *Hustler* published a photograph of a man pulling a woman covered in batter out of a deep fryer with tongs. The caption read: "Battered Wives. Now he's going to have to beat her just to smooth out all those lumps" (Russell, 1993, p. 43). *Playboy* published a Romanian article titled "How to Beat Your Wife . . . Without Leaving Prints," which gave men instructions as to how they could beat their wives without getting caught (Playboy Romania, 2000). The trivialization of wife battering in pornography contributes to social attitudes that condone wife battering, articulate wife battering as humor instead of a crime, and generally teach men to view their wives as whores.

Pornography is itself pictures of acts of prostitution, including the beatings and rapes of prostituted women. Men masturbate to pictures of prostituted women being beaten and raped, and some of them act out what they see in the pornography on their wives and girlfriends. Men also produce pornography of their wives and girlfriends in their homes. These pictures and videos of women being sexually tortured in the home are sold, and according to definition, these women are prostituted women. The rise of the Internet and the availability of related technology have made it easy for men to turn their wives, girlfriends, daughters, and granddaughters into pornography. There is a large market for these amateur videos and pictures. Amateur pornography websites are prevalent on the Internet with titles like Turning Wife Into A Whore, Forced White Wife: Watch as this Housewife is Raped and Humiliated, and Wives That Whore From Home (forcedwhitewife.com, 2002). These sites encourage men to view their wives as whores, and to treat them like whores are treated.

Pornography is central to the battering of prostituted women. Pimps use pornography to season women and girls to acts of prostitution. Thirty percent of the women in one research project reported that their pimps compelled them to imitate scenes from pornography to teach them how to be prostitutes (Giobbe, 1990). One woman, prostituted as a teen and as an adult, said, "The man who prostituted me showed me pictures of what he was going to do to me and he would 'practice' on me what was happening in the picture. That's how I learned what to do for the trick. The hard thing is, I know the pornography he made of me is being used to hurt others" (Stark & Leighton, 2002). In effect, pornography is a training manual that pimps use to show women and girls how to become prostitutes. Pornography is also a record of the sexual torture of prostituted women and girls.

SIMILAR TECHNIQUES OF CONTROL USED BY BATTERERS AND PIMPS

The techniques of control used by batterers to ensure the compliance of their wives and girlfriends parallel the tactics pimps use to recruit and keep women trapped in prostitution. These maneuvers, commonly referred to in shelters as tactics of power and control, include isolation of the woman; minimization and denial of her abuse; the exercising of male privilege; threats and intimidation; and emotional, sexual, and physical violence (Giobbe, 1993). Men who batter women in their homes and pimps who batter women in prostitution use torture techniques consistent with those described in an international summary of torture, in which torturers deprive their victims of social support, eliminate stimuli other than those controlled by the captor, and block noncompliant behaviors (Jones, 1994). Batterers and pimps socially isolate women, thereby diminishing their ability to resist. Many who work with prostituted women have noted the captors' use of extreme violence to demonstrate the futility of resistance (Giobbe, Harrigan, Ryan, & Gamache, 1990; Minnesota Coalition Against Prostitution, 1997; Holsopple, 1999). Like other batterers, pimps attempt to maintain complete control over "their" women and ensure that the women are too terrified and too psychologically and physically broken down to contemplate escape.

Like pimps, men who batter in the home also exploit their wives and girlfriends economically to maintain control over them. They do this by preventing women from getting or keeping jobs, making them beg for money, giving allowances, taking all their money away, or preventing the women from having access to the family's income (Pense & Paymor, 1993). Some batterers even go to the women's workplaces on payday to collect paychecks; and batterers often do not allow women to have money for essentials like shampoo, tampons, or baby food. Batterers may also destroy the women's possessions, and threaten to hurt or murder them, their pets, or their children if the women try to leave. Often battered women flee their homes, leaving behind their belongings and pets. Women frequently come into shelters with only their purses and the clothes they are wearing.[2]

Pimps break women down emotionally, psychologically, and physically before they turn women out into prostitution.[3] This involves battering her, including hitting, punching, kicking, starving, raping, verbally abusing her, telling her she chose to be in prostitution, and telling her she is good for nothing but sex. Pimps socially isolate prostituted women, threaten to blackmail them with pornography made of them, and keep them from getting jobs outside of prostitution.

Many prostituted women lack job experience and have very little education because they entered prostitution at a young age. This makes it easier for pimps to keep prostituted women in prostitution and out of the work force. Pimps economically exploit prostituted women by keeping all or most of the money the women get in prostitution, and by making the women beg for money. Often pimps do not let prostituted women out of their sight, watching them from across the street or even following them to the emergency room and sitting with women after beating them. As one formerly prostituted woman said, "That's his gravy train. He's not going to let her out of his sight."

Pimps control her sense of self, often to the extent of completely controlling her identity. It is not uncommon for pimps to change the names and appearances of the women once they begin to prostitute. This reinforces the idea that they not only own the women, but have actually created a new woman specifically for the purpose of prostitution. Pimps promote the idea that prostituted women's exclusive function is to be used sexually by men. Pimps often tell prostituted women, "once a whore, always a whore" in order to establish a sense of futility and separation from other people and society.

A pimp will typically establish a relationship with the woman or girl he wants to turn out in prostitution. He may tell the woman or girl that he is her "man," or her boyfriend, or promise marriage. Establishing a connection and ownership through traditional husband and boyfriend relationships allows pimps to gain women and girls' trust and begin the process of coercion. Like other battered women, prostituted women become dependent upon and controlled by the abusers, and escape becomes difficult and dangerous. If the women try to leave, pimps beat, rape, threaten to murder, murder, and steal or destroy prostituted women's belongings. Most women who escape prostitution leave with few, if any, belongings. One woman, describing her exodus from twenty years of legalized prostitution in Nevada, escaped with no money or possessions (Stark & Hanson, 1998).

Not only are prostituted women battered by pimps, they are also battered and sexually assaulted by the men who buy them for sex. A prostituted woman may be battered and raped by thousands of men every year. It must be recognized that being repeatedly battered by tricks or pimps is similar to being battered by husbands or boyfriends, except that prostituted women have multiple batterers where non-prostituted women have one batterer.

> Unless human behavior under conditions of captivity is understood, the emotional bond between those prostituted and pimps is difficult to comprehend. The terror created in the prostituted woman by the pimps causes a sense of helplessness and dependence. This emotional bonding to an abuser under conditions of captivity has been described as the Stockholm Syndrome. Attitudes and behaviors which are part of this syndrome include: (1) intense gratefulness for small favors when the captor holds life and death power over the captor; (2) denial of the extent of violence and harm which the captor has inflicted or is obviously capable of inflicting; (3) hypervigilance with respect to the pimp's needs and identification with the pimp's perspective on the world (an example of this was Patty Hearst's identification with her captor's ideology); (4) perception of those trying to assist in escape as enemies and perception of captors as friends; (5) extreme difficulty leaving one's captor/pimp, even after physical release has occurred. Paradoxically, women in prostitution may feel that they owe their lives to pimps. (Farley, 1998, citing Graham, Rawlings, & Rigsby, 1994)

HOMELESSNESS AND BATTERING

Battered women and prostituted women have another experience in common. Both groups of women have high rates of homelessness, and there is much crossover between battered women, homeless women, and prostituted women. When women battered in their homes leave abusers, they may end up on the streets, at homeless shelters, or with relatives and friends. Lack of affordable housing and long waiting lists for assisted housing mean that many women and their children are forced to choose between abuse at home or on the streets (National Coalition for the Homeless Fact Sheet, 2002). Homelessness leaves battered women and their children vulnerable to economic instability as well as further physical and sexual abuse since many homeless women are sexually assaulted. In one study, 89% of homeless mothers previously experienced some kind of abuse in their lives, including childhood physical and sexual abuse, adult physical and sexual abuse including being beaten up by a partner, and sexual assault, including rape (Goodman, 1991). Another study found that half of all homeless women were beaten by their partners or husbands. This figure is more than twice that of housed women (Goodman, 1991). Many homeless women end up in prostitution, and many prostituted women become homeless, making homelessness both a cause and a result of prostitution. In another study, 90% of prostituted women were homeless for an average of 6.3 years (Council for Prostitution Alternatives, 1991). Violence in the home, specifically wife battering, is for many women the beginning stage of entry into prostitution.

PHYSICAL INJURIES FROM BATTERING IN GENERAL AND FROM BATTERING IN PROSTITUTION

Battered women and prostituted women suffer similar injuries and often have similar experiences with healthcare services when they seek care for injuries inflicted by husbands, boyfriends, tricks, and pimps. Physical injuries among non-prostituted battered women vary widely, and include hematomas, lacerations, contusions, fractures, head injuries, dislocations, burns, and miscarriages (Loring & Smith, 1999). Battered women frequently go to emergency rooms with injuries inflicted by boyfriends and husbands. It is estimated that 40% of all injured women in emergency rooms are injured by an abusive partner (Loring & Smith, 1999).

Prostituted women also have serious physical injuries resulting from rapes and beatings by pimps, tricks, and partners. Like battered women, prostituted women seek emergency care for broken bones, burns, fractured skulls, and other physical injuries (Raymond, Hughes, & Gomez, 2001). In a midwest study, half of the women were physically assaulted by a john, and a third of these experienced assaults at least several times a year. Twenty-three percent of those assaulted by a john were beaten severely enough to have suffered a broken bone and two women reported assaults so vicious that they spent time in a coma (Parriott, 1994). Another study of 475 prostituted people in five countries found that 73% reported physical assault in prostitution (Farley et al., 1998).

HEALTHCARE BARRIERS FACED BY BATTERED WOMEN AND PROSTITUTED WOMEN

Battered women face many barriers to accessing services, particularly healthcare. Isolation, finances, naive interview questions, blaming the battered woman herself, trauma symptoms, denial, and negative attitudes of emergency room personnel–all prevent intervention on behalf of battered women and contribute to the high recidivism rate (Loring & Smith, 1999). If they are asked, battered women are willing to talk with health care providers about violence in their lives. However, they are often not asked about battery or threat of violence. A 1999 survey found that only 29% of health maintenance organizations in the United States had policies or protocols for domestic violence (Family Violence Prevention Fund Survey, 1999). Ninety-two percent of women who were physically abused by their partners did not discuss these incidents with their physicians; 57% did not discuss the incidents with anyone (Commonwealth Fund Survey, 1993). Yet, in several different studies of survivors of abuse, 70 to 80% of the patients studied reported that they would like their healthcare providers to ask them privately about intimate partner violence (Caralis & Musialowski, 1998; McCauley, Yurk, Jenckes, & Ford, 1998).

It is not known what percentage of women seeking help for injuries are prostituted women, but many of those working with prostituted women believe that a significant percentage of women presenting at psychiatric units and other health care facilities have been in prostitution. Many prostituted women are disabled as a result of years of physical, emotional, and psychological abuse (see Baldwin, 2003, this volume). According to one estimate, a third of prostituted women are disabled from emotional traumas and physical injuries, including brain injury, suffered in prostitution (Parker, 1998). Prostituted women are typically apprehensive about disclosing to health care workers that they are or have been in prostitution. They fear loss of custody of their children, loss of "straight" jobs, judgmental attitudes, and revictimization at the hands of health care providers. According to Parriott (1994), only 35% of the women who had access to primary health care had told their provider about their experience in prostitution.

SUBSTANCE ABUSE

Many battered women report that they began to use drugs and alcohol as a way to cope with terror (Flitcraft & Stark, 1988). Using substances functions as an analgesic for physical pain from battering and rape. Battered women who are also addicted, reported that every aspect of their behavior comes under scrutiny while the batterer's behavior, his addiction, and his contribution to her addiction tend to be ignored. Women interviewed in shelters have told the authors that batterers encouraged substance abuse while simultaneously using her drug use as a reason to verbally or physically abuse her. As a means of control, batterers sometimes curtail their partners' attempts to seek treatment for substance abuse. Batterers may prevent the women from attending meetings or keeping appointments, or they may escalate violence in order to control the women. The addicted battered woman is then likely to leave treatment in response to the increased danger (Haver, 1987). Battered women may lack access to shelters, because of their substance abuse, since some shelter policies exclude addicted women (Bennett & Lawson, 1994). Women are usually prevented from returning to the shelter while intoxicated, and simply referred to substance abuse programs.

Drug or alcohol addictions function both as a way to survive the violence and as a barrier to escaping prostitution. Most women must be high in order to endure prostitution (see Kramer, 2003, this volume). Being high permits them to detach from the experience of sexual exploitation and to distance themselves from the constant fear of overt violence. Pimps deliberately create addictions by paying women for their prostitution with crack cocaine or other drugs (Maher, 1997; Miller, 1986). Seventy-six percent of the women in one study were paid with crack for prostitution (Parriott, 1994). Some pimps addict women to crack cocaine, hold them captive in drug houses, and force them to submit to other men in exchange for an hourly crack hit. These women may be forced to "sexually service" up to twenty men a day, which is equivalent to being raped twenty times a day. Some men have recruited women into prostitution by addicting wives or girlfriends to drugs and then coercing them into prostitution and other rape scenarios in exchange for drugs. In this instance, there is an intimate relationship between marital battering, prostitution, and drug addiction.

Prostituted women who are addicted may encounter barriers when they seek treatment for alcoholism and other drug addictions. At 12 Step meetings men often exploit prostituted women when the women disclose involvement in prostitution. Prostituted women urgently need their own 12 Step meetings to address addictions. They need to have the freedom to talk about the emotional, physical, and sexual abuse (Stark & Mitchell, 2002).

SOLUTIONS

Currently, the harm of prostitution is culturally, socially, and politically invisible. Solutions to prostitution must be rooted in the understanding that prostitution is violence against women and girls. This knowledge must be brought into public awareness, made into public policy, and structurally implemented in mental health services, homeless shelters, rape crisis centers, battered women's shelters, and public health care.

Understanding prostitution and pornography as battering requires a shift in our way of thinking. Currently, we speak of "domestic violence" or "violence against women in intimate relationships" to describe the battering of a woman by her male partner. These phrases, which reflect an awareness of violence, generally exclude prostituted women in spite of the fact that prostituted women are battered by multiple perpetrators. We recommend the use of more inclusive terms such as "violence against women" or "battering of women" to describe the battery and rape suffered by prostituted and nonprostituted women alike.

Ignorance about prostitution and deliberate misinformation disseminated by pimps, tricks, and their apologists create obstacles for battered women and prostituted women, who are blamed for remaining in violent relationships. There is still little understanding of the brutal terror inflicted by abusers. Battered women's lives are in constant danger from their male partners and prostituted women are in danger from pimps and tricks. No one asks why prisoners of war stay with their captors, yet the question "Why doesn't she just leave?" is regularly asked of women. Attempting to leave a batterer is dangerous and the consequences of doing so may include torture and execution. The argument that women choose to be in prostitution is not an acceptable way to dismiss the harm of prostitution. We do not dismiss rape and battery by saying that women choose to walk down the street alone at night. Or, if a woman chose to get married, we do not dismiss the battery that occurs within the marriage by saying she chose to be with him.

An understanding of sexual abuse, as applied to battered and raped women, can and must be applied to prostituted women. The differences between women battered in their homes and prostituted women are only in the more extreme violence and multiplicity of perpetrators against prostituted women. All abused women and girls, not only those battered outside of prostitution, should receive assistance.

An understanding of prostitution as violence must be structurally implemented in organizations so that the organization itself addresses the issues, for example in its mission statement, rather than its being addressed haphazardly by individuals who may not be long term employees. Posters stating that prostitution is violence should be visible. Screening questions should ask whether she has ever been involved in prostitution, had sexually explicit pictures taken of her, and whether pornography played a role in the assault(s).[4] Women and girls who are in or have been in prostitution will rarely be forthcoming with that information because of social ostracism, and also because they may not recognize what happened to them as prostitution. It is helpful to actually list different types of prostitution, including pornography, strip clubs, massage parlors, saunas, escort services, live sex shows, peep shows, trafficking, phone sex, ritual abuse, mail order bride services, prostitution tourism, and street prostitution.

Anti-rape organizations, homeless shelters, and health care facilities need to reach out to prostituted women, letting them know that the agency understands prostitution as harm, and that help is offered for that harm. The burden cannot be on individual women and girls to risk their emotional or physical safety by disclosing involvement in prostitution. Organizations can reach out to prostituted women and girls on the streets, in schools, in strip clubs, at truck stops, and other areas frequented by prostituted people. Articles, pamphlets, and books with information about prostitution can be placed in libraries and schools.

Programs specifically for prostituted women and girls must be developed in conjunction with battered women's shelters and homeless shelters.[5] These programs must comprehensively address the multiple needs of prostituted women, which include housing, psychotherapy, physical healthcare, job training and placement, help with disabilities, clothing, food, and treatment for alcohol and drug dependence. The programs need to be culturally sensitive to language, race, class, ethnicity, sexual orientation, and nationality. A national toll free line should offer information regarding services available for prostituted women and girls.

Laws should criminalize pimping and buying women, but it should not be a crime to prostitute or be prostituted. Court outreach advocates must learn to sensitively assess prostitution among women and girls, who are frequently arrested on drug charges rather than prostitution charges.

In summary, social justice organizations and health care services must publicly state that prostitution and pornography are forms of violence against women and girls and their services must be extended to the prostituted. Those prostituted must be humanized, because after all, it is difficult to advocate on behalf of a group of women that is feared, stigmatized, and "other." It is a matter of social justice that all abused women and girls receive the help they need and deserve, not only those battered outside of prostitution.

NOTES

1. Prostituted women and girls are in constant danger from pimps and tricks. Pimps threaten to hurt prostituted women and girls if they tell anyone about their situation. Pimps and tricks often hurt the women and girls by beating, raping, slapping, punching, stalking, and killing them. A Canadian study found that prostituted women and girls have a mortality rate 40 times higher than non-prostituted women and girls (cited in Baldwin, 1992).

2. While shelter staff can provide clothing and personal items, it is often a long, difficult process to obtain police accompaniment so that the women can return for their belongings.

3. Being prostituted is one of the ways that men debilitate women psychologically, emotionally, and physically. A man could verbally berate a woman, pressure her into prostitution, and then use the prostitution itself as a method to break her down further.

4. The way in which these questions are phrased is important. Girls and women use many different phrases to describe their involvement in prostitution and it is important to know what terms are used locally to talk about prostitution. The phrases used to talk about prostitution can vary even within a city; these variations can be attributed mainly to race and cultural differences. It is also common for women in stripping and "escort services" to not identify what they are doing as prostitution and so it is important to meet them on their terms rather than demanding that they have to identify as a prostitute.

When talking with girls and women about prostitution it is important to let her describe her involvement in prostitution in her own words and on her own terms. If she says, "I wouldn't call it that," then say, "How do you describe it?" Statements such as "A lot of people have been approached by people asking them to be in prostitution, or asking if people if they know anyone who might do prostitution. Do you know anybody who has done this? Have you done that?" will help the girl or woman feel less threatened.

The girls and women will want to know the reason why they are being asked about involvement in prostitution. Is the person asking the questions asking because she wants to call the girl or woman a prostitute, or because the person cares about the girl or woman's well being? As one girl said: "It's like breathing air, everybody does it and you're trying to put me into a box and call me a prostitute." It may take some time and trial and error to figure out the best way to approach prostituted women and girls. Often a neutral question such as "Have you ever traded sex for money, gifts, drugs, or survival needs?" is a good beginning (Stark & O'Leary, 2002).

5. A battered women's shelter in Massachusetts recently obtained funding to extend their services to prostituted women. They are using existing organizations that specifically help prostituted women as models to develop their own program. In this way, the shelter is acknowledging prostituted women as battered women and it is creating appropriate services to insure that the needs of prostituted women will be met in the shelter.

Health care facilities can make their services available to prostituted women by including questions on their intake forms, making sure that they interview the women and girls alone in a room without their pimps present, and taking steps to insure that their staff is trained on issues of prostitution to eliminate judgmental attitudes and increase awareness of the physical and emotional harm endured in prostitution.

REFERENCES

Baldwin, Margaret A. (1992). Split at the Root: Prostitution and Feminist Discourses of Law Reform. *Yale Journal of Law and Feminism* 5: 47-120 citing: Special Committee on Pornography and Prostitution 1985: *Pornography and Prostitution in Canada*, 350.

Baldwin, M.A. (2003). Living in Longing: Prostitution, Trauma Recovery, and Public Assistance in M. Farley (ed.) *Prostitution, Trafficking, & Traumatic Stress*. Binghamton, NY: The Haworth Press, Inc.

Bennett, L., & Lawson, M. (1994). Barriers to Cooperation Between Domestic Violence and Substance Abuse Programs. Families in Society. *The Journal of Contemporary Human Services* 75(5): 277-286.

Caralis, P., & Musialowski, R. (1997). Women's Experiences with Domestic Violence and Their Attitudes and Expectations Regarding Medical Care of Abuse Victims. *Southern Medical Journal*: 90: 1075-1080.

City Club of Portland Report (1997). *Domestic Violence: Everybody's Business*, 2nd Edition, August. Portland, City Club of Portland.

Commonwealth Fund Survey of Women's Health (1993). New York: Commonwealth Fund.

Council for Prostitution Alternatives (1991). Characteristics of 800 CPA Participants. In R. Weitzer (ed.), *Sex for Sale: Prostitution, Pornography, and the Sex Industry*, (pp. 139-155). New York: Routledge.

Dworkin, A. (1988). *Intercourse*. New York, Free Press.

Dworkin, A., & MacKinnon, C. (1998). *In Harm's Way: The Pornography Civil Rights Hearings*. Boston: Harvard University Press.

Family Violence Prevention Fund, (1999). *National Survey of Managed Care Organizations*. National Health Resource Center on Domestic Violence: San Francisco, CA.

Farley, M. (2003). Prostitution and the Invisibility of Harm. In M. Banks & R. Ackerman (eds.) Special Issue on Women and Invisible Disabilities, *Women & Therapy* 26 (1-4).

Farley, M., Baral, I., Kiremire, M., & Sezgin, U. (1998). Prostitution in Five Countries: Violence and Post-Traumatic Stress Disorder. *Feminism & Psychology* 8(4): 405-426.

Flitcraft, A., & Stark, E. (1998). Violence Among Intimates: An Epidemiological Review. In V.D. Van Hasselt, R.L. Morrison, A.S. Bellack, & M. Hersen (eds). *Handbook of Family Violence* (pp. 159-99). New York: Plenum Press.

Forced White Wife <www.forcedwhitewife.com>. Accessed online 1-12-02.

Garrity, R. (2002). Movement Activism Versus Professionalism. Domestic Violence Offender Programs as Tools of Oppression: How Cooptation Works To Silence Truth and Excuse Men's Violence Against Women, Unpublished Paper, Binghamton, New York.

Giobbe, E. (1993). An Analysis of Individual, Institutional, and Cultural Pimping. *Michigan Journal of Gender and Law*, 1: 33-57.

Giobbe, E. (1990). Confronting Liberal Lies About Prostitution, In D. Leidholdt & J. Raymond (eds), *The Sexual Liberals and the Attack on Feminism* (pp. 67-80). New York: Elsevier Science Ltd.

Giobbe, E., Harrigan, M., Ryan, J., & Gamache, D. (1990). *Prostitution: A Matter of Violence Against Women.* Minneapolis, WHISPER.

Goodman, L.A. (1991). The Prevalence of Abuse Among Homeless and Housed Poor Mothers: A Comparison Study. *American Journal of Orthopsychiatry* 61: 489-500.

Graham, D.L.R., Rawlings, E., & Rigsby, R. (1994). *Loving to Survive: Sexual terror, men's violence and women's lives.* New York: New York University Press.

Haver, B. (1987). Female Alcoholics: IV. The Relationship Between Family Violence and Outcome 3-10 Years After Treatment. *Acta Psychiatric Scandinavia* 57, 449-56.

Holsopple, K. (1999). Pimps, Tricks and Feminists *Women's Studies Quarterly* 27 (1-2): 47-52.

Hotaling, N. (1999). Making the Harm Visible. In Hughes, D. & Roche, C. (eds.) *Making the Harm Visible: Global Sexual Exploitation of Women and Girls* (pp. 227-232). Rhode Island: Coalition Against Trafficking in Women.

Island, D., & Letellier, P. (1991). *Men Who Beat the Men Who Love Them.* New York: Harrington Park Press.

Jones, A. (1994). Next Time, She'll Be Dead. Boston: Beacon Press Books.

Kramer, L. A. (2003). Emotional Experiences of Performing Prostitution in M. Farley (ed.) *Prostitution, Trafficking, and Traumatic Stress.* Binghamton, NY: The Haworth Press, Inc.

Loring, M. T., & Smith, R. W. (1999). Health Care Barriers and Interventions for Battered Women. *Public Health Reports.* 109 (3): 328-338.

Maher, L. (1997). *Sexed Work: Gender, Race and Resistance in a Brooklyn Drug Market.* Oxford: Claredon Press.

McCauley, Y., Jenckes, M., & Ford, D. (1998). 'Inside Pandora's' Box, Abused Women's Experiences with Clinicians and Health Services. *Archives of Internal Medicine 13*: 549-555.

Miller, E. (1986). *Street Woman.* Philadelphia: Temple University Press.

Minnesota Coalition Against Prostitution (1997). *Dangerous Sexual Predators.* Minneapolis: Minnesota Coalition Against Prostitution.

National Coalition for the Homeless (2002). *Fact Sheet.* Washington, DC, National Coalition for the Homeless.

Nelson, V. (1993). Prostitution: Where Racism and Sexism Intersect. *Michigan Journal of Gender and Law* 1: 81-89.

O'Leary, C., & Howard, O. (2001). *The Prostitution of Women and Girls in Metropolitan Chicago: A Preliminary Report.* Chicago: Center for Impact Research.

Parker, J. (1998). *How Prostitution Works.* Unpublished Paper. Lola Greene Baldwin Foundation P.O. Box 42393 Portland, Oregon 97242.

Parriott, R. (1994). Health Experiences of Twin Cities Women Used in Prostitution. Minneapolis, Unpublished survey initiated by WHISPER.

Pense, E., & Paymor, M. (1993). Duluth Power and Control Wheel. Duluth, Domestic Containment Program.

Playboy Romania (2000). How to Beat Your Wife . . . Without Leaving Marks, April 2000.

Raymond, J.G., Hughes, D., & Gomez, C. (2001). *Sex Trafficking of Women in the United States. Links between International and Domestic Sex Industries.* N. Amherst, MA: Coalition Against Trafficking in Women.

Russell, D. (1993). *Against Pornography: The Evidence of Harm* Berkeley, CA: Russell Publications.

Silbert, M. H. & Pines, A. M. (1981) Child Sexual Abuse as an Antecedent to Prostitution. *Child Abuse & Neglect*, 5: 407-411.

Stark, C., & Leighton, J. (2002). Personal Communication.

Stark, C., & Hanson, M. (1998). Interview on file with author.

Stark, C., & Mitchell, K. (2002). Personal Communication.

Stark, C., & O'Leary, C. (2002). Personal Communication.

Walker, L. E. (2000). Battered Woman Syndrome (2nd ed.). New York: Springer Press.

Prostitution and Trafficking in Nine Countries: An Update on Violence and Posttraumatic Stress Disorder

Melissa Farley
Ann Cotton
Jacqueline Lynne
Sybille Zumbeck
Frida Spiwak
Maria E. Reyes
Dinorah Alvarez
Ufuk Sezgin

SUMMARY. We interviewed 854 people currently or recently in prostitution in 9 countries (Canada, Colombia, Germany, Mexico, South Af-

Melissa Farley, PhD, is at Prostitution Research & Education, Box 16254, San Francisco, CA 94116-0254 USA (Email: mfarley@prostitutionresearch.com).

Ann Cotton, PsyD, is at University of Washington School of Medicine and VA Puget Sound Health Care System, Seattle, WA USA (Email: ann.cotton2@ med.va.gov).

Jacqueline Lynne, MSW, is at Vancouver Coastal Health, Vancouver, Canada.

Sybille Zumbeck, PhD, is at Psychological Institute III, University of Hamburg, Germany.

Frida Spiwak, PhD, is in Bogota, Colombia (Email: f.rotlewicz@worldnet.att.net).

Maria E. Reyes, PhD, is at Instituto Colombiano de Bienestar Familiar (ICBF) in Bogota, Colombia.

Dinorah Alvarez, BA, is at San Francisco State University, CA USA.

Ufuk Sezgin, PhD, is at the Psychiatry Department of Istanbul Medical University, Istanbul, Turkey (Email: usezgin@superonline.com).

The authors express their appreciation to Steven N. Gold, PhD, and to Harvey L. Schwartz, PhD, for their helpful editing suggestions.

Printed with permission.

[Haworth co-indexing entry note]: "Prostitution and Trafficking in Nine Countries: An Update on Violence and Posttraumatic Stress Disorder." Farley et al. Co-published simultaneously in *Journal of Trauma Practice* (The Haworth Maltreatment & Trauma Press, an imprint of The Haworth Press, Inc.) Vol. 2, No. 3/4, 2003, pp. 33-74; and: *Prostitution, Trafficking, and Traumatic Stress* (ed: Melissa Farley) The Haworth Maltreatment & Trauma Press, an imprint of The Haworth Press, Inc., 2003, pp. 33-74. Single or multiple copies of this article are available for a fee from The Haworth Document Delivery Service [1-800-HAWORTH, 9:00 a.m. - 5:00 p.m. (EST). E-mail address: docdelivery@haworthpress.com].

http://www.haworthpress.com/store/product.asp?sku=J189
10.1300/J189v02n03_03

rica, Thailand, Turkey, United States, and Zambia), inquiring about current and lifetime history of sexual and physical violence. We found that prostitution was multitraumatic: 71% were physically assaulted in prostitution; 63% were raped; 89% of these respondents wanted to escape prostitution, but did not have other options for survival. A total of 75% had been homeless at some point in their lives; 68% met criteria for PTSD. Severity of PTSD symptoms was strongly associated with the number of different types of lifetime sexual and physical violence.

Our findings contradict common myths about prostitution: the assumption that street prostitution is the worst type of prostitution, that prostitution of men and boys is different from prostitution of women and girls, that most of those in prostitution freely consent to it, that most people are in prostitution because of drug addiction, that prostitution is qualitatively different from trafficking, and that legalizing or decriminalizing prostitution would decrease its harm.

INTRODUCTION

Commercial sex businesses include street prostitution, massage brothels, escort services, outcall services, strip clubs, lap dancing, phone sex, adult and child pornography (including the sexual assault of children by organized groups of pedophiles as well as non-pedophile rapists), child prostitution, video and Internet pornography, trafficking, and prostitution tourism. Most people who are in prostitution for longer than a few months drift among these various permutations of the commercial sex businesses (Dalla, 2000; Kramer, 2003).

Prostitution dehumanizes, commodifies and fetishizes women, in contrast to non-commercial casual sex where both people act on the basis of sexual desire and both people are free to retract without economic consequence. In prostitution, there is always a power imbalance, where the john[1] has the social and economic power to hire her/him to act like a sexualized puppet. Prostitution excludes any mutuality of privilege or pleasure: its goal is to ensure that one person does *not* use her personal desire to determine which sexual acts do and do not occur–while the other person acts on the basis of his personal desire (Davidson, 1998).

The account of a woman from the United States who prostituted primarily in strip clubs but also in massage, escort, and street prostitution is typical in that it encompasses the following types of violence. In strip club prostitution she was sexually harassed and assaulted. The job required her to tolerate verbal abuse (with a coerced smile), being grabbed and pinched on the legs, buttocks, breasts, and crotch. Sometimes this resulted in bruises and scratches on her thighs and arms and breasts. Her breasts were squeezed until she was in severe pain. She was humiliated by customers ejaculating on her face. She was physically brutalized, and her hair was pulled as a means of control and torture. She was severely bruised from beatings and frequently had black eyes. She was repeatedly beaten on the head with closed fists, sometimes causing concussions and unconsciousness. From these beatings, her jaw was dislocated and her eardrum was damaged. Many years later her jaw is still dislocated. She was cut with knives. She was burned with cigarettes by customers who smoked while raping her. She was gang raped. She was raped individually by at least twenty men at different times in her life. Rapes by johns and pimps sometimes resulted in internal bleeding.

Seventy percent of women in prostitution in San Francisco, California were raped (Silbert & Pines, 1982). A study in Portland, Oregon found that prostituted women were raped on average once a week (Hunter, 1994). Eighty-five percent of women in Minneapolis, Minnesota had been raped in prostitution (Parriott, 1994). Ninety-four percent of those in street prostitution experienced sexual assault and 75% were raped by one or more johns (Miller, 1995). In the Netherlands (where prostitution is legal) 60% of prostituted women suffered physical assaults; 70% experienced verbal threats of assault, 40% experienced sexual violence and 40% were forced into prostitution and/or sexual abuse by acquaintances (Vanwesenbeeck, de Graaf, van Zessen, Straver, & Visser, 1995; Vanwesenbeeck, 1994).

Prolonged and repeated trauma usually precedes entry into prostitution. From 55% to 90% of prostitutes report a childhood sexual abuse history (James & Meyerding, 1977; Silbert & Pines, 1981; Harlan et al., 1981; Silbert & Pines, 1983; Bagley & Young, 1987; Simons & Whitbeck, 1991; Belton, 1992; Farley & Barkan, 1998). Silbert and Pines (1981, 1983) noted that 70% of their interviewees said that childhood sexual abuse had an influence on their entry into prostitution. A conservative estimate of the average age of recruitment into prostitution in U.S.A. is 13-14 years. (Silbert & Pines, 1982; Weisberg, 1985).

Clearly, violence is the norm for women in prostitution. Incest, sexual harassment, verbal abuse, stalking, rape, battering, and torture–are points on a continuum of violence, all of which occur regularly in prostitution. In fact, prostitution itself is a form of sexual violence that results in economic profit for those who sell women, men, and children. Though often denied or minimized, other types of gender violence (while epidemic) are not sources of mass revenue.

Prostituted women are unrecognized victims of intimate partner violence by pimps as well as johns (Stark & Hodgson, 2003). Although there are little research data available, agencies serving prostituted women observe that a majority of prostitution is pimp-controlled.[2] Giobbe described similar methods of coercion and control used by pimps and non-pimp batterers to control women: minimization and denial of physical violence and abuse, economic exploitation, social isolation, verbal abuse, threats, intimidation, physical violence, sexual assault, and captivity (Giobbe, 1991; Giobbe, 1993; Giobbe, Harrigan, Ryan, & Gamache, 1990). The systematic violence of pimps against prostituted women is aimed not only at control, but also emphasizes the victim's powerlessness, worthlessness and invisibility except in her role as prostitute.

A qualitative distinction between prostitution of children and prostitution of adults is arbitrary and it obscures the lengthy and extensive history of trauma that is commonplace in prostitution. For example the 5-year-old incested by her father and used in child prostitution and pornography may become partially amnesic for these traumas and at adolescence may find herself drifting into prostitution and other savage relationships. The 14-year-old in prostitution eventually turns 18 but she has not suddenly made a new "vocational choice." The abuse and reenactment of abuse simply continue. Women who began prostituting as adolescents may have parts of themselves that are dissociatively compartmentalized into a much younger child's time and place.[3]

Posttraumatic stress disorder (PTSD) can result when people have experienced

> ... extreme traumatic stressors involving direct personal experience of an event that involves actual or threatened death or serious injury; threat to one's personal integrity; witnessing an event that involves death, injury or a threat to the physical integrity of another person; learning about unexpected or violent death, serious harm, or threat of death or injury experienced by a family member or other close associate. (American Psychiatric Association, 1994)

In fact most prostitution, most of the time includes these traumatic stressors. In response to these events, the person with PTSD experiences fear and powerlessness, oscillating between emotional numbing and emotional/physiologic hyperarousal. PTSD is likely to be especially severe or long lasting when the stressor is planned and implemented by humans (as in war, rape, incest, battering, torture, or prostitution) rather than being a natural catastrophe.

Exposure to paid or unpaid sexual violence may result in symptoms of PTSD. Symptoms are grouped into three categories: (1) traumatic re-experiencing of events, or flashbacks; (2) avoidance of situations which are reminiscent of the traumatic events, and a protective emotional numbing of responsiveness; and (3) autonomic nervous system hyperarousal (e.g., jittery irritability, being super-alert, insomnia). The symptoms of PTSD may accumulate over one's lifetime. Many studies report a positive correlation between a history of childhood sexual assault and symptoms of PTSD in adult women (Friedman & Schnurr, 1995; Rodriguez, Ryan, Van de Kemp, & Foy, 1997). Since almost all prostituted women have histories of childhood sexual abuse, this undoubtedly contributes to their symptoms of posttraumatic stress. PTSD is not only related to the overall number of traumatic events, but it is also directly related to the severity of that violence (Houskamp & Foy, 1991). The incidence of PTSD has been investigated among battered women and ranges from 45% to as high as 84% (Houskamp and Foy, 1991; Saunders, 1994; Kemp, Rawlings, & Green 1991). The prevalence of PTSD among prostituted women from 5 countries was 67% (Farley, Baral, Kiremire, & Sezgin, 1998), which is in the same range as that of combat veterans (Weathers, Litz, Herman, Huska, & Keane, 1993).

Following publication of an article which discussed the violence preceding and intrinsic to prostitution, and the symptoms of posttraumatic stress disorder resulting from prostitution in 5 countries–(South Africa, Thailand, Turkey, United States, and Zambia)–the authors were contacted by other researchers and advocates from around the world who were interested in collaborating in further study of prostitution. Consequently, the present study expands the original through the inclusion of four additional countries: Canada, Colombia, Germany, and Mexico.

METHODS

Brief structured interviews of people in prostitution were conducted in Vancouver, Canada; Bogota, Colombia; Hamburg, Germany; Mexico City and Puebla, Mexico; San Francisco, CA, U.S.A.; two cities in Thailand; Lusaka, Zambia; Istanbul, Turkey; Johannesburg and Capetown, South Africa. These countries were included in the study because investigators in those states shared a commitment to documenting the experiences of women in prostitution, and in some instances to providing alternatives to prostitution.

Participants

In Canada, we interviewed 100 women prostituting in or near Vancouver's Downtown Eastside, one of the most economically destitute regions in North America. The effects of colonization of First Nations people were evident from their overrepresentation in Canadian prostitution. Fifty-two percent were First Nations (in a community where 1.7-7% are the official estimates of the First Nations population), 38% were white European-Canadian, 5% were African Canadian, and 5% left the question blank. The majority of the 52 First Nations women described themselves as Native. Next most often, they described themselves as Metis, a French word that translates to English as "mixed blood" and is used to describe people who are of both First Nations and European ancestries. The two major colonizers of First Nations of Canada were the British and the French; therefore, the majority of those called Metis were First Nations/French or First Nations/British. The First Nations women also categorized themselves as Native Indian, Cree, Cree Native, First Nations, Cree Metis, Ojibwa, Blackfoot/Cree, Aboriginal, and Interior Salish.

In Mexico, we interviewed 123 women prostituting in street, brothel, stripclub and massage prostitution in Mexico City and in Puebla.

Fifty-four women were interviewed in Hamburg, Germany where prostitution is legal. The German women were from a drop-in shelter for drug addicted women, from a program which offered vocational rehabilitation for those prostituted, and were also referred by peers, and by advertisement in a local newspaper. With respect to country of origin, 82% were German and 11% were trafficked into Germany from Thailand or the former Soviet Union. Seven percent were raised in Germany and described themselves as ethnically Polish, Chilean, or Turkish. Two found the experience of answering questions about traumatic events too painful to continue, and a third woman was too intoxicated to participate.

In San Francisco we interviewed 130 respondents on the street who verbally confirmed that they were prostituting. We interviewed respondents in four different areas in San Francisco where people worked as prostitutes. Thirty-nine percent of the 130 interviewees were white European/American, 33% were African American, 18% were Latina, 6% were Asian or Pacific Islander, and 5% described themselves as of mixed race or left the question blank.

In Thailand we interviewed several of the 110 respondents on the street, but found that pimps did not allow the prostitutes to answer our questions. We interviewed some respondents at a beauty parlor that provided a supportive atmosphere. The majority of the Thai respondents were interviewed at an agency in northern Thailand that offered nonjudgmental support and job training.

We interviewed 68 prostituted people in Johannesburg and Capetown, South Africa in brothels, on the street and at a drop-in center for prostitutes. Respondents were racially diverse: 50% were white European; 29% were African or Black; 12% described themselves as Coloured or Brown or of mixed race; 3% were Indian; and 6% left the question blank.

We interviewed 117 current and former prostitutes at TASINTHA in Lusaka, Zambia. TASINTHA is a non-governmental organization that offered food, vocational training, and community to approximately 600 prostituted women a week.

In Turkey some prostitutes work legally in brothels which are privately owned and controlled by local commissions composed of physicians, police, and others who are "in charge of public morality." We were not permitted to interview women in brothels, so we interviewed 50 prostituted women who were brought to a hospital in Istanbul by police for the purpose of STD control.

In Bogota we interviewed 96 women and children at agencies that offered services to them. Prostitution in Colombia starts at a young age, often by adolescence, and is accompanied by unwanted pregnancy (Spiwak & Reyes, 1999; UNICEF, 2000; UNICEF Colombia, 2001; Rodriguez & Cabrera, 1991; Fundación Renacer, 2000, 2001; ICBF, 1999; Cárdenas and Rivera, 2000; DABS, 2002). Spiwak & Reyes (1999) found that 72% of the women and children prostituting in Colombia were from families that had been internally displaced by political violence. Civil wars and internal displacement are known to be risk factors for sexual exploitation (UNICEF Colombia, 2001; Fundacion Renacer, 2000; 2001; Fundación Esperanza, 1998, 2000; CATW, 2002; U.S. Report of Trafficking in Persons, 2001; NCMEC, 1992; ICBF, 2000; Leech, 2001). Prostitution is legal in Colombia, with thousands of brothels in urban areas, as well as in paramilitary and guerilla-controlled rural regions. It is legal to prostitute a 14-year-old girl or boy (Código Penal de Colombia, 2002), although that act of sexual abuse violates the Convention on the Rights of the Child endorsed by Colombia in 1999 (UNICEF, 2000; UNICEF Colombia, 2001; Seitles, 1997; ICBF-UNESCO, 1997; Motta et al., 1998; Morgan & Buitrago, 1992).

In six of the nine countries, we interviewed women and girls. In South Africa we interviewed 10 men (14% of the South African sample) and one transgendered person. In Thailand we interviewed 28 transgendered people (25% of the Thai sample). In the United States we interviewed 18 men (13%) and 15 transgendered people (12%) in addition to women and girls. Transgendered people represent a significant minority of those in prostitution. A previous study (Farley & Barkan, 1998) found that transgendered people (male-to-female) in prostitution experienced the same frequency of physical assaults and rapes as did women.

Mean age, age ranges and mean age of entry into prostitution, percentages under age 18 at time of entry into prostitution, and mean number of years in prostitution by country are shown in Table 1. Across 9 countries, ages of respondents ranged from 12 to 68 with a mean age of 28 years (N = 779, SD = 8) The average age of entry into prostitution was 19 years (SD = 6). Forty-seven

TABLE 1. Age, Age of Entry, and Length of Time in Prostitution

	9 Country Summary (N = 854)	Canada (n = 100)	Colombia (n = 96)	Germany (n = 54)	Mexico (n = 123)	South Africa (n = 68)	Thailand (n = 166)	Turkey (n = 50)	USA (n = 130)	Zambia (n = 117)
Mean age (SD)	28 (8)	28 (8)	31 (10)	26 (10)	27 (7)	24 (5)	26 (7)	29	31 (9)	27 (7)
Age range	12-68	13-49	14-58	15-68	18-60	17-38	14-46	16-55	14-61	12-53
Mean age entered prostitution (SD)	19 (6)	18 (6)	17 (4)	19 (6)	20 (4)	20 (5)	21 (5)	Unknown	20 (8)	17 (4)
Years in prostitution (SD)	9 (8)	10 (8)	14 (8)	7 (8)	7 (8)	4 (4)	5 (4)	Unknown	11 (9)	10 (7)
Percent younger than age 18 at entry	47% (353)	54% (54)	59% (56)	41% (22)	32% (38)	40% (27)	32% (28)	Unknown	42% (53)	68% (75)

40

percent reported that they were under 18 years of age at the time of entry into prostitution. Based on respondents' current age and age of entry into prostitution we calculated the average length of time in prostitution to be 9 years (SD = 8) across countries. This calculation was based on the assumption that from the age at first prostitution to the time of the interview, there was no period of time during which they did not prostitute. Since people seize the opportunity to interrupt or escape from prostitution, this number probably overestimates the amount of time spent in prostitution.

Measures

The Prostitution Questionnaire inquired about lifetime history of physical and sexual violence and the use of or making of pornography during prostitution. We asked whether respondents wished to leave prostitution and what they needed in order to leave. We asked if they had been homeless; if they had physical health problems; and if they used drugs or alcohol or both. Three questions assessed rape: "Have you been raped?" "Who raped you?" and "How many times have you been raped since you were in prostitution?" Some respondents answered "no" when asked if they were raped, but then identified who had raped them and/or how many times they had been raped. Therefore to assess rape in prostitution, if a respondent identified "pimp" or "customer" in response to "Who raped you?" or if the respondent reported one or more rapes since being in prostitution then that respondent was identified as having been raped in prostitution.

Respondents also completed the PTSD Checklist (PCL), a self-report inventory for assessing the 17 DSM-IV symptoms of PTSD (Weathers, Litz, Herman, Huska, & Keane, 1993; Blanchard, Jones-Alexander, Buckley, & Forneris, 1996). Respondents were asked to rate symptoms of PTSD on a scale with (1 =) not at all; (2 =) a little bit; (3 =) moderately; (4 =) quite a bit; and (5 =) extremely. PCL test-retest reliability was .96. Internal consistency, as measured by an alpha coefficient was .97. Validity of the scale was reflected in its strong correlations with the Mississippi Scale (.93); the PK scale of the MMPI-2 (.77); and the Impact of Events Scale (.90) (Weathers et al., 1993). The PCL has functioned comparably across ethnic subcultures in U.S.A. (Keane et al., 1996).

We measured symptoms of PTSD in two ways. First, using a procedure established by the scale's authors, we generated a measure of overall PTSD symptom severity by summing respondents' ratings across all 17 items. If a respondent filled out less than half of the PCL (more than 8 blank items) it was not included in the analysis. For those omitting one to eight items, the PCL sum was estimated by using the respondent's mean PCL score in place of the blank items.

Second, using Weathers' (1993) scoring suggestion, we considered a score of 3 or above on a given PCL item to be a symptom of PTSD. Using those scores, we then noted whether each respondent met criteria for a diagnosis of PTSD. We report the numbers and percentages of respondents who qualified for a diagnosis of PTSD in each country.

In Canada and United States, we administered a Chronic Health Problem Questionnaire that included items developed from responses to an earlier open-ended item which inquired about health problems of women in prostitution. Unanswered items were considered to indicate the absence of the health problem. Therefore, percentages reported below are percentages of the entire sample endorsing that item.

Procedure

In Canada, Colombia, Mexico, South Africa, and United States, if interviewees indicated that they were prostituting, they were asked to fill out the Prostitution Questionnaire (PQ), the Post Traumatic Stress Disorder Checklist (PCL), and the Chronic Health Problem Questionnaire (CHPQ). We interviewed respondents in street, brothel, strip clubs, and massage prostitution. In Germany and Turkey, respondents were administered interviews in medical clinics. In Zambia and in Thailand, most respondents were interviewed in agencies offering services to women in prostitution. The questionnaires were administered in English, German, Spanish, Thai and Turkish. In Zambia, interviewers translated as needed–most participants spoke some English. The authors either administered or directly supervised the administration of all questionnaires. If respondents could not read, the questions were read to them by the researchers.

RESULTS

A range of sexual and other physical violence was reported by a majority of these prostituted people in all nine countries (see Table 2). Listed in the following tables are the percentages of respondents endorsing each item out of the total number of respondents who answered that item. The number of participants endorsing each item is in parentheses.

Across countries, 59% of these interviewees reported that as children they were beaten by a caregiver to the point of injury. Sixty-three percent were sexually abused as children, with an average of four perpetrators against each

TABLE 2. Violence in Prostitution

	9 Country Summary (N = 854)	Canada (n = 100)	Colombia (n = 96)	Germany (n = 54)	Mexico (n = 123)	South Africa (n = 68)	Thailand (n = 166)	Turkey (n = 50)	USA (n = 130)	Zambia (n = 117)
Threatened with a weapon in prostitution	64% (503)	67% (66)	59% (57)	52% (28)	48% (46)	68% (45)	39% (33)	68% (34)	78% (100)	86% (94)
Physically assaulted in prostitution	73% (595)	91% (91)	70% (67)	61% (33)	59% (72)	66% (45)	56% (50)	80% (40)	82% (106)	82% (91)
Raped in prostitution	57% (483)	76% (76)	47% (45)	63% (34)	46% (57)	56% (38)	38% (45)	50% (25)	73% (95)	79% (93)
(Of those raped) raped more than five times in prostitution	59% (286)	67% (51)	64% (29)	50% (17)	44% (25)	58% (22)	56% (25)	36% (9)	59% (56)	52% (48)
Current or past homelessness	75% (571)	86% (84)	76% (73)	74% (40)	55% (65)	73% (49)	57% (53)	58% (29)	84% (108)	89% (99)
As a child, was hit or beaten by caregiver until injured or bruised	59% (448)	73% (72)	66% (63)	48% (26)	57% (69)	56% (38)	39% (35)	56% (28)	49% (37)	71% (80)
Sexually abused as a child	63% (508)	84% (82)	67% (64)	48% (26)	54% (64)	66% (45)	47% (41)	34% (17)	57% (73)	84% (93)
Mean number of childhood sexual abuse perpetrators	4	5	2	17	2	2	1	unknown	2	6
Median number of childhood sexual abuse perpetrators	1	3	1	4	1	1	0	unknown	1	3

child. As adults in prostitution, 64% of these respondents had been threatened with a weapon, 71% had experienced physical assault, and 63% had been raped. Current or past homelessness averaged 75% across countries and ranged from 55% (Mexico) to 89% (Zambia).

From this range of violent events, we categorized four types of violence in these people's lives: (1) childhood sexual abuse, (2) childhood physical abuse, (3) rape in prostitution as an adult and (4) physical assault in prostitution as an adult. Respondents might have experienced none, one, two, three, or all four types of violence (see Table 3). Fifty-one percent of the interviewees had experienced three or four different types of lifetime violence, 36% reported one to two types of lifetime violence, and only 13% had not experienced any of these types of violence. Since those who left items blank were assumed not to have experienced the violence, this is a conservative estimate of lifetime violence. We asked 315 respondents in Canada, Colombia, and Mexico about their experience of verbal abuse in prostitution. Eighty-eight percent reported having been verbally abused.

The responses of our participants suggest that pornography is integral to prostitution. Table 4 shows rates by country of those in prostitution who reported that they were upset by attempts to coerce them into imitating pornography and who had pornography made of them in prostitution. Across countries, 47% were upset by attempts to make them do what others had seen in pornography and 49% reported pornography was made of them.

Posttraumatic Stress Disorder

To meet criteria for a diagnosis of posttraumatic stress disorder (PTSD) a person must have at least one of five symptoms of intrusive re-experiencing of trauma symptoms (criterion B), at least three of six symptoms of numbing and avoidance of trauma (criterion C), and at least two of four symptoms of physiologic hyperarousal (criterion D). Given the extremely high rates of interpersonal violence reported by these respondents (stressors which meet criterion A), we made the assumption that the 13% of respondents who had not directly experienced violence themselves–had witnessed it. Thus we assumed that all respondents met criterion A for a diagnosis of PTSD. Eight hundred twenty-six of our respondents answered at least 8 of the 17 items on the Post Traumatic Disorder Check List (PCL) and were included in the following analysis. Across 9 countries, 68% of these respondents met criteria for a diagnosis of PTSD (see Table 5).

Mean PCL score was 53.5 (SD = 16.2) across the 9 countries, a reflection of the severity of the symptoms of PTSD in this sample (see Table 6). Mean PTSD severities in the 9 countries ranged from 49 (Mexico) to 58

TABLE 3. Number of Types of Lifetime Violence

Number of Types of Lifetime Violence	9 Country Summary (N = 854)	Canada (n = 100)	Colombia (n = 96)	Germany (n = 54)	Mexico (n = 123)	South Africa (n = 68)	Thailand (n = 166)	Turkey (n = 50)	USA (n = 130)	Zambia (n = 117)
No violence reported	13% (110)	2% (2)	12% (11)	6% (3)	22% (27)	12% (8)	28% (33)	20% (10)	6% (8)	7% (8)
1 Type of violence	16% (133)	12% (12)	16% (15)	17% (9)	15% (19)	19% (13)	28% (33)	24% (12)	12% (15)	4% (5)
2 Types of violence	20% (171)	7% (7)	22% (21)	37% (20)	16% (20)	16% (11)	21% (24)	22% (11)	34% (44)	11% (13)
3 Types of violence	26% (222)	24% (24)	16% (15)	33% (18)	25% (31)	19% (13)	17% (20)	34% (17)	34% (44)	34% (40)
4 Types of violence	25% (218)	55% (55)	35% (34)	7% (4)	21% (26)	34% (23)	5% (6)	0% (0)	15% (19)	44% (51)

45

TABLE 4. Prostitution and Pornography

	9 Country Summary (N = 854)	Canada (n = 100)	Colombia (n = 96)	Germany (n = 54)	Mexico (n = 123)	South Africa (n = 68)	Thailand (n = 166)	Turkey (n = 50)	USA (n = 130)	Zambia (n = 117)
Upset by an attempt to make them do what had been seen in pornography	47% (377)	64% (63)	62% (60)	44% (24)	35% (42)	56% (37)	48% (43)	20% (10)	32% (41)	47% (51)
Pornography made of her in prostitution	49% (371)	67% (64)	50% (48)	52% (28)	44% (53)	40% (26)	45% (39)	N/A	49% (63)	47% (52)

TABLE 5. Posttraumatic Stress Disorder of Prostituted Respondents in 9 Countries

	9 Country Summary (N = 854)	Canada (n = 100)	Colombia (n = 96)	Germany (n = 54)	Mexico (n = 123)	South Africa (n = 68)	Thailand (n = 116)	Turkey (n = 50)	USA (n = 130)	Zambia (n = 117)
PTSD DIAGNOSIS (DSM-IV)	68% (562)	74% (72)	86% (83)	60% (32)	54% (67)	75% (51)	58% (59)	66% (33)	69% (87)	71% (78)

TABLE 6. PTSD Checklist (PCL) Means from Three Studies

	Mean PCLC Sum (SD)
1 Current study	
99 women in prostitution (Canada)	56 (16)
96 women in prostitution (Colombia)	58 (14)
53 women in prostitution (Germany)	51 (16)
123 women in prostitution (Mexico)	49 (18)
68 people in prostitution (South Africa)	55 (16)
111 people in prostitution (Thailand)	51 (18)
50 women in prostitution (Turkey)	53 (16)
128 people in prostitution (USA)	55 (17)
112 women in prostitution (Zambia)	53 (12)
2 Weathers et al. (1993)	
123 Vietnam veterans requesting treatment	51 (20)
1006 Persian Gulf War veterans	35 (16)
3 Farley & Patsalides, (2001)	
(adult women)	
26 controls	24 (7)
25 w/ childhood physical abuse history	31 (10)
27 w/ childhood physical and sexual abuse history	37 (15)

*PTSD sum is an indicator of PTSD severity.

(Columbia). PTSD severity was significantly positively correlated with the number of types of lifetime violence experienced ($r = .33$, $p = .001$). For comparison, Table 6 includes mean PCL scores from two other studies of PTSD severity–Vietnam and Persian Gulf veterans (Weathers et al., 1993) and samples of women from a health maintenance plan who had and had not experienced physical and sexual abuse (Farley & Patsalides, 2001).

We asked interviewees in the 9 countries about their use of drugs and alcohol. Table 7 lists substance use by country. Across countries, 48% of those responding to this item reported drug use, and 52% reported alcohol use. Colombia and Zambia reported the lowest use of drugs. Drugs were probably not available due to the poverty of respondents. We did not inquire specifically about glue sniffing which is common in Colombia. Colombia and Zambia, along with Mexico, had the highest rates of alcohol use (71%-100%). Canada, USA, and Germany reported the highest rates of drug use (70% to 95%).

We asked respondents what they needed by offering them a checklist of options that included an open-ended question for write-in responses (see Table 8). Eighty-nine percent told us that they desired to leave prostitution. A total of 75% needed a home or safe place, 76% needed job training, 61% needed health care, 56% needed individual counseling, 51% needed peer support, 51% needed legal assistance, 47% needed drug/alcohol treatment, 45% wanted self-defense training, 44% needed childcare, 34% wanted prostitution to be legalized, and 23% wanted physical protection from a pimp.

We asked those we interviewed in six countries (Canada, Colombia, Germany, Mexico, South Africa, and Zambia) whether they thought that legalizing prostitution would make them physically safer. Across countries 46% stated that prostitution would be no safer if it were legalized (see Table 9). It is noteworthy that in Germany where brothel prostitution is legal, 59% of respondents told us that they did not think that legal prostitution made them any safer from rape and physical assault.

In Mexico we were able to compare several different types of prostitution: 54 women in strip clubs, 44 women in brothels and massage parlors, and 25 women who were prostituting on the street. We inquired about age of entry into prostitution, length of time in prostitution, PTSD severity, number of types of lifetime violence and whether or not women in these different types of prostitution wanted to escape from it. Age of entry into prostitution differentiated strip club from other types of prostitution. Compared to brothel, massage and street prostitution, significantly more women in strip clubs entered prostitution when they were younger than 18 ($F = 3.5$; $df = 2,113$; $p = .03$). There were no statistically significant differences between brothel/massage, street, and strip club prostitution with respect to PTSD severity, length of time in prostitution, childhood sexual abuse, childhood physical abuse, rape in prostitution, number of types of lifetime violence experienced, and percentages of respondents who told us that they wanted escape from prostitution.

We investigated differences in PTSD associated with gender and gender identity. In U.S. differences in PTSD incidence among women, men and transgendered prostitutes were not statistically significant. In Thailand, differences between women and transgendered prostitutes were not statistically significant. In South Africa, differences between women and men prostitutes were not significant.

Previously, we found that 61% of those in prostitution in 5 countries reported a current physical health problem, 52% reported alcohol use, and 45% reported drug use (Farley et al., 1998). We are now able to report in more detail the acute and chronic health problems experienced by those in prostitution in 7 of the 9 countries (Colombia, Mexico, South Africa, Thailand, Turkey, USA, and Zambia). Half of these people reported symptoms that were associated with violence, overwhelming stress, poverty, and homelessness.

Common medical problems of these 700 people in prostitution included tuberculosis, HIV, diabetes, cancer, arthritis, tachycardia, syphilis, malaria, asthma, anemia, and hepatitis. Twenty-four percent reported reproductive symptoms including sexually transmitted diseases (STD), uterine infections,

TABLE 7. Use of Drugs and Alcohol Among People in Prostitution in 9 Countries

	9 Country Summary (N = 854)	Canada (n = 100)	Colombia (n = 96)	Germany (n = 54)	Mexico (n = 123)	South Africa (n = 68)	Thailand (n = 166)	Turkey (n = 50)	USA (n = 130)	Zambia (n = 117)
Used drugs	48% (383)	95% (94)	4% (3)	70% (38)	34% (40)	49% (33)	39% (40)	46% (23)	75% (94)	16% (18)
Used alcohol	52% (416)	47% (44)	100% (29)	54% (29)	71% (84)	43% (29)	56% (57)	64% (32)	26% (33)	72% (79)

TABLE 8. Responses to "What Do You Need?" Asked of 854 People in Prostitution

Needs	9 Country Summary (N = 854)	Canada (n = 100)	Colombia (n = 96)	Germany (n = 54)	Mexico (n = 123)	South Africa (n = 68)	Thailand (n = 116)	Turkey (n = 50)	USA (n = 130)	Zambia (n = 117)
Leave prostitution	89% (699)	95% (89)	97% (93)	85% (33)	68% (81)	89% (58)	92% (82)	90% (45)	87% (111)	99% (107)
Home or safe place	75% (618)	66% (63)	74% (71)	61% (33)	87% (107)	72% (46)	59% (64)	60% (30)	78% (99)	94% (105)
Job training	76% (600)	67% (64)	57% (55)	63% (34)	92% (113)	75% (48)	56% (61)	46% (23)	73% (93)	97% (109)
Drug/alcohol treatment	47% (356)	82% (78)	15% (14)	48% (26)	38% (47)	46% (29)	44% (33)	6% (3)	67% (85)	37% (41)
Health care	61% (480)	41% (39)	56% (54)	46% (25)	67% (82)	69% (44)	41% (45)	38% (19)	58% (74)	88% (98)
Peer support	51% (393)	41% (38)	41% (39)	65% (35)	36% (44)	58% (37)	49% (53)	24% (12)	50% (64)	63% (71)
Individual counseling	56% (431)	58% (54)	34% (33)	69% (37)	43% (53)	61% (39)	66% (72)	46% (23)	48% (61)	53% (59)
Self-defense training	45% (340)	49% (47)	29% (28)	46% (25)	35% (43)	60% (39)	59% (64)	12% (6)	49% (62)	41% (46)
Legal assistance	51% (366)	33% (31)	43% (41)	37% (20)	50% (61)	58% (37)	57% (62)	Unknown	42% (54)	54% (60)
Legalize prostitution	34% (251)	32% (30)	20% (19)	35% (19)	51% (62)	37% (24)	27% (30)	4% (2)	44% (56)	8% (9)
Child care	44% (335)	12% (11)	49% (47)	7% (4)	36% (44)	48% (31)	44% (48)	20% (10)	34% (43)	87% (97)
Physical protection from pimp	23% (157)	4% (4)	6% (6)	6% (3)	15% (19)	33% (21)	20% (22)	Unknown	28% (36)	41% (46)

TABLE 9. Respondents Who Stated That Prostitution Would Not Be Safer if Legalized

	6 Country Summary (N = 558)	Canada (n = 100)	Colombia (n = 96)	Germany (n = 54)	Mexico (n = 123)	South Africa (n = 68)	Zambia (n = 117)
Prostitution would be no safer if legalized	46% (226)	26% (25)	44% (22)	59% (27)	15% (13)	59% (40)	73% (79)

menstrual problems, ovarian pain, abortion complications, pregnancy, hepatitis B, hepatitis C, infertility, syphilis, and HIV.

Without specific query about mental health, 17% described severe emotional problems: depression, suicidality, flashbacks of child abuse, anxiety and extreme tension, terror regarding relationships with pimps, extremely low self-esteem, and mood swings. Fifteen percent reported gastrointestinal symptoms such as ulcers, chronic stomachache, diarrhea, and colitis. Fifteen percent reported neurological symptoms such as migraine headaches and non-migraine headaches, memory loss, numbness, seizures, and dizziness. Fourteen percent of these women and children in prostitution reported respiratory problems such as asthma, lung disease, bronchitis, and pneumonia. Fourteen percent reported joint pain, including hip pain, bad knees, backache, arthritis, rheumatism, and nonspecific multiple-site joint pain.

Twelve percent of those who described health problems in prostitution reported injuries that were a direct result of violence. For example, a number of women had their ribs broken by the police in Istanbul, a woman in San Francisco broke her hips jumping out of a car when a john was attempting to kidnap her. Many women had their teeth knocked out by pimps and johns. Miller (1995) cited bruises, broken bones, cuts, and abrasions that resulted from beatings and sexual assaults.

Of the 50 Turkish women, 18% reported mental distress, 16% reported joint or other pain, 10% reported gastrointestinal symptoms, 10% reported gynecological symptoms, 6% had respiratory symptoms, and 6% cardiac symptoms. Almost half of the Turkish women had never been examined by a physician.

In Mexico, 52 of 123 women responded affirmatively to an open-ended question regarding health problems. Twenty-one percent of those who responded to this question reported gastrointestinal symptoms, and 16% reported neurological problems. Other physical health problems included joint pain (12%) and cardiovascular symptoms (12%).

In Thailand, 60 of 116 women responded to an open-ended question about health problems. Thirty percent of these women reported poor health in general, and 30% described reproductive system problems. Twenty-five percent described physical injuries from violence in prostitution, 23% reported neurological symptoms, 17% joint pain, and 15% gastrointestinal symptoms. Twenty-eight percent of the Thai women described serious emotional problems; many told us that they had been lied to, kidnapped, or trafficked into prostitution, which contributed to their distress. Equating prostitution with death, one woman stated: "Why commit suicide? I'll work in prostitution instead." Another woman explained that she felt "spiritually assaulted" in prostitution.

TABLE 10. Chronic Health Problems of Women in Prostitution and Women No Longer in Prostitution*

Chronic Health Problems endorsed more frequently when *not yet out of prostitution*	Canadian women (n = 100)	U.S. women out of prostitution for at least 1.5 years (n = 21)
Muscle aches/pains	78% (74)	71% (15)
Trouble concentrating	66% (63)	62% (13)
Colds or flu symptoms	61% (58)	43% (9)
Joint pain	60% (57)	38% (8)
Shortness of breath	60% (57)	57% (12)
Stomach problems	59% (56)	57% (12)
Headaches/migraines	56% (54)	48% (10)
Constipation/diarrhea	52% (50)	43% (9)
Dizziness	44% (42)	38% (8)
Skin problems	43% (41)	38% (8)
Chest Pain	43% (41)	33% (7)
Nausea	41% (39)	14% (3)
Sweaty Hands	40% (38)	14% (3)
Hearing problems	40% (38)	19% (4)
Jaw or throat pain	38% (36)	24% (5)
Muscle weakness/paralysis	38% (36)	24% (5)
Vomiting	37% (35)	0% (0)
Trembling	35% (33)	10% (2)
Asthma	32% (30)	29% (6)
Poor health in general	30% (28)	10% (2)
Difficulty swallowing	27% (26)	10% (2)
Pelvic pain	21% (20)	19% (4)
Chronic health problems endorsed more frequently *after getting out of prostitution*	Canadian women (n = 100)	U.S. women out of prostitution for at least 1.5 years (n = 21)
Injury caused by violence	76% (72)	95% (20)
Memory problems	66% (63)	72% (16)
Head injury	53% (50)	95% (20)
Pain/numbness in hands/feet	50% (47)	52% (11)
Vision problems	45% (43)	57% (12)
Trouble with balance or walking	41% (39)	43% (9)
Allergies	35% (33)	38% (8)
Swelling of arms/hands/legs/feet	33% (31)	43% (9)
Rapid or irregular heart beat	33% (31)	38% (8)
Loss of feeling on skin	25% (24)	33% (7)
Painful menstruation	24% (23)	48% (10)
Vaginal pain	24% (23)	38% (8)
Breast pain	23% (22)	24% (5)

*Items from Chronic Health Problems Questionnaire (CHPQ).

In Colombia, the most frequent health complaints were reproductive, cardiovascular and respiratory symptoms, and joint pain.

From these responses, we developed the Chronic Health Problems Questionnaire (CPHQ) which was subsequently given to 100 currently prostituting Canadian women and to a separate sample of 21 women in the U.S. who were no longer in prostitution (see Table 10). Among the Canadian women currently in prostitution, 76% reported injuries from violence in prostitution, with 53% having suffered traumatic head injuries. Once women were out of prostitution, awareness of the severity of the previous violence seemed to increase. For example, 95% of the women already out of prostitution reported violent injuries resulting from prostitution, including a 95% incidence of head injury. Women who were still in prostitution reported these same injuries at 76% (any violence-caused injury) and 53% (head injury). Approximately half of both samples reported headaches or migraines. Some of the cardiovascular, neurological and joint complaints may have been symptoms of substance abuse or withdrawal.

Fourteen of the chronic symptoms we inquired about were *more prevalent* among the 21 women no longer involved in prostitution than among the currently prostituting Canadian women. These symptoms were: any injury caused by violence, report of any medical diagnosis, memory problems, head injury, pain/numbness in hands or feet, vision problems, trouble with balance or walking, allergies, swelling of arms, hands, legs or feet, rapid or irregular heartbeat, loss of feeling on skin, painful menstruation, vaginal pain, and breast pain (see Table 10.) The Canadian respondents still in prostitution endorsed an average of 14 of 32 (SD = 8) symptoms. The U.S. women no longer in prostitution endorsed an average of 12 of 32 (SD = 7) symptoms. There was no significant difference between the two groups in the total number of symptoms endorsed (ANOVA, $F = 3.3$, df. $= 1,118$, $p = .07$).

In three countries (Canada, Colombia, Mexico) we inquired about verbal abuse in prostitution. Eighty-eight percent of 315 respondents reported having been verbally abused ranging from 84% in Mexico to 91% in Colombia.

DISCUSSION

Our findings from 9 countries on 5 continents indicate that the physical and emotional violence in prostitution is overwhelming. To summarize the findings of this study and other research and clinical literature on different types of prostitution (see Farley & Kelly, 2000; Farley, 2003):

1. 95% of those in prostitution experienced sexual harassment which in the United States would be legally actionable in a different job setting.
2. 65% to 95% of those in prostitution were sexually assaulted as children.
3. 70% to 95% were physically assaulted in prostitution.
4. 60% to 75% were raped in prostitution.[4]
5. 75% of those in prostitution have been homeless at some point in their lives.
6. 89% of 785 people in prostitution from nine countries wanted to escape prostitution.
7. 68% of 827 people in several different types of prostitution in 9 countries met criteria for PTSD. The severity of PTSD symptoms of participants in this study were in the same range as treatment-seeking combat veterans, battered women seeking shelter, rape survivors, and refugees from state-organized torture (Bownes, O'Gormen, & Sayers 1991; Houskamp & Foy, 1991, Kemp et al., 1991; Ramsay, Gorst-Unsworth, & Turner, 1993; Weathers et al., 1993). Severity of symptoms of PTSD was strongly associated with the number of different types of lifetime sexual and physical violence. A Covenant House study of homeless adolescents, many of whom were prostituting, found a similar association between PTSD severity and history of violence (DiPaolo, 1999).
8. 88% of those in prostitution experience verbal abuse and social contempt. Verbal abuse in prostitution has rarely been discussed as one of its harms.

Similar findings suggest that the severity of trauma-related symptoms were related to the intensity of involvement in prostitution. Women who serviced more customers in prostitution reported more severe physical symptoms (Vanwesenbeeck, 1994). The longer women were in prostitution, the more STDs were reported (Parriott, 1994). A number of studies document the greatly increased risk among prostituted women as compared to nonprostituted women, for cervical cancer and chronic hepatitis (Chattopadhyay, Bandyopadhyay, & Duttagupta, 1994; de Sanjose, Palacio, Tafur, Vasquez, Espitia, Vasquez, Roman, Munoz, & Bosch, 1993; Nakashima, Kashiwagi, Hayashi, Urabe, Minami, & Maeda, 1996; Parriott, 1994; Pelzer, Duncan, Tibaux, & Mebari, 1992).

Vanwesenbeeck (1994) noted that poverty and length of time spent in prostitution were each associated with greater violence in prostitution. Like Vanwesenbeeck, we concluded that those women who experienced the most extreme violence in prostitution were not represented in our research. Because of this limitation, it is likely that all of the estimates of violence reported here are conservative, and that the actual incidence of violence is greater than we found.

Traumatized individuals tend to minimize or deny their experiences, especially when they are in the midst of ongoing trauma, such as war combat or prostitution. This leads to a decreased rate of reporting violent events. Based on a review of previous research and clinical reports, we think that our statistic on the prevalence of child sexual abuse among those prostituting in 9 countries (63%) is much lower than the actual incidence of childhood sexual abuse in this population, which we estimate to be closer to 85% (Silbert & Pines, 1981, 1983; Giobbe, 1991; Hunter, 1994).

Describing the complex connections between childhood sexual abuse, revictimization, prostitution, and health problems, one woman made a decision to prostitute after realizing that she had been sexually abused as a child:

> . . . there was no sense of having a life; the only life I knew of was prostituting . . . I thought I couldn't be hurt no more and I felt that I could do what I want and I could have sex with whoever I wanted because *somebody already gone and messed my system up.* (Morse, Suchman, & Frankel, 1997. [Authors' italics]

In prostitution, the sexual exploitation of children and women is often indistinguishable from incest, intimate partner violence, and rape (Gysels, Pool, & Nnulasiba, 2002). Like adult prostitutes, incested children are bribed into sex acts by adults and offered food, money, or protection for their silence. Use of a child for sex by adults may thus be understood as prostitution of the child, whether the act occurs in or out of the family, and whether it is with or without payment. When a child is incestuously assaulted, the perpetrator's objectification of the child victim and his rationalization and denial are similar to the john's in prostitution. The psychological symptoms resulting from incest and prostitution are similar. One woman described a "prostituting mentality" beginning after sexual abuse by neighbors and family members starting at age nine and continuing to adolescence, when she began prostituting (Carroll & Trull, 1999).

Although this study assessed only PTSD as a psychological consequence of prostitution, additional symptoms of emotional distress are common among prostituted women, including other anxiety disorders, dissociative disorders (Ross, Farley, & Schwartz, 2003), substance abuse, personality disorders, and depression. Depression is almost universal among prostituted women. For example, Raymond, Hughes and Gomez (2001) found that 86% of domestically trafficked and 85% of internationally trafficked women experienced depression.

Another psychological consequence of longterm prostitution is complex PTSD (CPTSD) which results from chronic traumatic stress, captivity, and totalitarian control. Symptoms of CPTSD include difficulty regulating emotions, altered self-perception (in prostitution: a subordinated sexual self), changes in relations with others (a boyfriend may be gradually seen as another john), and shifts in beliefs about the nature of the world (Herman, 1992; Van der Kolk, Pelcovitz, Roth, Mandel, McFarlane, & Herman 1996). In CPTSD, and in some Axis II personality disorders, the objectification and contempt aimed at those in prostitution can become internalized and solidified, resulting in self-loathing that is long-lasting and resistant to change (Schwartz, 2000). Existing in a state of social death, the prostitute is an outsider who is seen as having no honor or public worth; (Patterson, 1982; Farley, 1997). Those in prostitution, like slaves and concentration camp prisoners, may lose their identities as individuals, becoming primarily what masters, Nazis or customers want them to be. As one woman said about prostitution: "It is internally damaging. You become in your own mind what these people do and say with you" (M. Farley, unpublished interview, 1999).

Sex inequality sets the stage for sexual coercion, intimate partner violence and prostitution, thus contributing to women's likelihood of becoming HIV-infected. Sexual violence has now been recognized as a primary risk factor for HIV in women (Romero-Daza, Weeks, & Singer, 1998). Kalichman and colleagues noted the coincidence of domestic violence and the HIV epidemic in Russia, Rwanda, and in the USA (Kalichman, Kelly, Shaboltas, & Granskaya, 2000; Kalichman, Williams, Cheery, Belcher, & Nachimson, 1998).

Half of new AIDS cases are under age 25, and girls are likely to become infected at a much younger age than boys, in part because of the tolerance of violence against girls and women in most cultures (Piot, 1999). In Africa and Asia, there is still a widespread belief that sex with a girl child cures HIV. In their attempts to escape lives of hunger and poverty, young girls in Africa cannot refuse the sexual assaults of older male teachers who control their educational future (Reilly, 2001). In a review of a number of studies, Sanders-Phillips (2002) observed that prostitution and intravenous drug use are the most common routes of HIV exposure among women of color in the United States. She suggests as does Worth (1989), that women's lack of sexual safety is caused by their subordination by men and by specific other factors that increase their vulnerability such as race/ethnic discrimination and poverty. Aral and Mann (1998) emphasized the importance of addressing human rights issues in conjunction with STDs. They noted that since most women enter prostitution as a result of poverty, rape, infertility, or divorce–public health programs must address the social factors which contribute to STD/HIV. We agree that it is essential to address the root causes of prostitution: sex inequality, racism and colonialism, poverty, tourism, and economic development that destroys traditional ways of living.

In addition to STD and HIV, prostitution causes a multitude of other physical symptoms. Physical health problems result from physical abuse and neglect in childhood (Radomsky, 1995), from sexual assault (Golding, 1994), battering (Crowell & Burgess, 1996), untreated health problems, overwhelming stress, and violence (Friedman & Yehuda, 1995; Koss & Heslet, 1992; Southwick et al., 1995). Prostituted women frequently suffer from all of the foregoing. Intimate partner violence, especially sexual violence, has been shown to increase gynecological, central nervous system, and stress-related problems by 50% to 70% (Campbell, Jones, Dienemann, Kub, Schollenberger, O'Campo, Gielen & Wynne, 2002; McNutt, Carlson, Persaud, & Posmus, 2002). Among our interviewees in 9 countries, we found many health problems which were the direct result of violence in prostitution, and probably also the result of chronic and overwhelming stress.

For example, 75% of the Canadian women we interviewed suffered injuries from violence that occurred during prostitution. These included stabbings and beatings, concussions, broken bones (broken jaws, ribs, collar bones, fingers, spines, skulls). Half of the Canadian women suffered traumatic head injuries as a result of violent assaults with baseball bats, crowbars or from having their heads slammed against walls or against car dashboards. Not surprisingly, they experienced memory problems, trouble concentrating, headaches, vision problems, dizziness, and trouble with balance or walking. These neurological symptoms are sometimes attributed solely to drug or alcohol toxicity, to PTSD or to personality disorders. However, they may also result from traumatic brain injury (TBI). In one study of prostituted women from three countries, 30% of Filipino women, 33% of Russian women, and 77% of US women reported head injuries (Raymond, D'Cunha, Dzuhaytin, Hynes, Rodriguez, & Santos, 2002).

Unfortunately, physical and psychological symptoms often did not disappear when women escaped prostitution. Instead 38% of the physical problems we inquired about were *more frequently* endorsed by women who no longer prostituted as compared to those who were still prostituting (for example, pain/numbness in hands or feet, vision problems, problems with balance, allergies, irregular heartbeat, and reproductive symptoms). Psychological distress is also persistent. Comparing women who were still prostituting with those who were not, a Canadian study found that "exited respondents were only slightly less likely to experience depression, and more likely to experience anxiety attacks and emotional trauma when compared to their counterparts who were still [in prostitution]" (Benoit & Millar, 2001, p. 71).

More than three-quarters of these people in prostitution from 9 countries stated that they needed secure housing and job training. More than half expressed a need for health care in general and half specifically mentioned a need for individual counseling. These findings are consistent with a study in which prostituting respondents emphasized a need for mental health care, specifically requesting drop-in centers, crisis centers, and a phone hotline (Butters & Erickson, 2003).

CONCLUSION

A Canadian woman told us: "What rape is to others, is normal to us." A Thai woman said, "I hate that I have to have sex with someone I don't like or love." For the vast majority of the world's prostituted women, prostitution and trafficking are experiences of being hunted down, dominated, sexually harassed, and assaulted. Women in prostitution are treated like commodities into which men masturbate, causing immense psychological harm to the person acting as receptacle (Hoigard & Finstad, 1986).

There is widespread misinformation about prostitution, based on propaganda that neutralizes the harms described above and which is disseminated by organizations that present prostitution as legitimate, if unpleasant, labor ("sex work"). We address below myths that: street prostitution is the worst type of prostitution, that prostitution of men and boys is significantly different than prostitution of women and girls, that most of those in prostitution freely consent to it, that most people are in prostitution because of a previous drug addiction, that prostitution is qualitatively different from trafficking, and that legalizing prostitution would decrease its harm.

Prostitution is multitraumatic whether its physical location is in clubs, brothels, hotels/motels/john's homes (also called escort prostitution or high class call girl prostitution), motor vehicles or the streets. Women have told us that they felt safer in street prostitution compared to (legal) Nevada brothels, where they were not permitted to reject any customer. Others commented that on the street they could refuse dangerous-appearing or intoxicated customers and that often a friend would make a show of writing down the john's car license plate number, which they considered a deterrent to violence. Raphael and Shapiro (2002) found that women in Chicago reported the same frequency of rape in escort and in street prostitution. In a previous study, although we found more physical violence in street compared to brothel prostitution in South Africa—we found no difference in the incidence of PTSD in these two types of prostitution, suggesting the intrinsically traumatizing nature of prostitution (Farley et al., 1998).

Ross, Anderson, Heber, and Norton (1990) found that women prostituting in stripclubs had significantly *higher* rates of dissociative and other psychiatric symptoms than those in street prostitution. In the present study we compared stripclub/massage, brothel, and street prostitution in Mexico and found no differences in the incidence of physical assault and rape in prostitution, childhood sexual abuse, or symptoms of PTSD. We also found no differences in the percentages of women in brothel, street, or stripclub/massage prostitution who wanted to escape prostitution.

Comparable findings have been reported in the Netherlands, where, although prostitution is legal, it continues to inflict harm on those in it. For example: 90% of women prostituting mainly in clubs, brothels and windows reported extreme nervousness, a symptom which may reflect the physiologic hyperarousal diagnostic of PTSD. In addition, 75% to 80% of the Dutch women reported distrust, symptoms of depression, irritability, and chronic physical discomfort (Vanwesenbeeck, 1994).

Since the 1980s, the line between prostitution and stripping has been increasingly blurred, and the amount of physical contact between exotic dancers and customers has increased, along with verbal sexual harassment and physical assault of women in strip club prostitution.[2] In most strip clubs, customers can now buy a lap dance where the dancer sits on the customer's lap while she wears few or no clothes and grinds her genitals against his. Although he is clothed, he usually expects ejaculation (Lewis, 1998). Touching, grabbing, pinching, and fingering of dancers removes any boundary which previously existed between dancing, stripping, and prostitution. As in other kinds of prostitution, the verbal, physical, and sexual abuse experienced by women in strip club prostitution includes being grabbed on the breasts, buttocks, and genitals, as well as being kicked, bitten, slapped, spit on, and penetrated vaginally and anally during lap dancing (Holsopple, 1998).

Proponents of prostitution argue that most of the violence and trauma-related symptoms among prostitutes result from street violence or from a drug-related lifestyle rather than from prostitution itself. The following comparisons will hopefully set aside that myth. A study of the health of women street vendors in Johannesburg permits a comparison of the violence against them to violence against our South African respondents. The street vendors were similarly situated women who spent much of their lives on the street in the same dangerous neighborhoods as the women we studied but who were not prostituting (Pick, Ross, & Dada, 2002). The average age of the prostituted women we interviewed was several years younger (24 years) than the street vendors (30 years). Seven percent of the South African street vendors experienced a verbal or physical threat, compared to 68% of the South African prostituted women who had been threatened with a weapon. Six percent of the women street vendors had been physically assaulted, compared to 66% of the prostituted women.

Seven percent of the street vendors reported physical sexual harassment, in contrast to the 56% of our South African interviewees who had been raped in prostitution. Prostitutes thus suffered much greater interpersonal violence than street vendors in the same neighborhood in Johannesburg, South Africa. Since the poverty, proximity to drug dealers, experience of street life and civil war were the same for both the street vendors and prostitutes, the large differences in their experiences of sexual and physical violence can be attributed to the nature of prostitution itself.

A Toronto survey of homeless people can be compared to our Canadian sample of women in prostitution. Crowe and Hardill (1993) found that 40% of homeless people had been assaulted in contrast to the 91% of our Canadian respondents in prostitution who had been assaulted. Although homelessness is associated with violence, prostitution is associated with a greater prevalence of violence.

Several researchers have studied the development of men's attitudes toward prostitution. Investigating men's behavior with prostitutes, Scandinavian researchers suggested that prostitution is an expression of men's sexuality but not women's (Mansson, 2001). Like rape myths, prostitution myths (misperceptions about the nature of prostitution as harmless) are a component of a cluster of attitudes that consider sexual violence to be normal. We found that college students' acceptance of prostitution myths was highly correlated with acceptance of rape myths (Cotton, Farley, & Baron, 2002). Furthermore, the college men who were most accepting of prostitution tended to be those who reported having subjected their partners to coercive sexual behaviors (Schmidt, Cotton, & Farley, 2000).

Although it has sometimes been assumed that prostitution of males is qualitatively different from prostitution of females, we did not find this to be the case (Kendall & Funk, 2003). In USA, South Africa, and in Thailand, we compared women, men, and transgendered prostitutes and found no differences in PTSD. A similar study found that 76% of 100 women, men and transgendered prostitutes in Washington, DC stated that they wanted to leave the sex industry. Ninety-one percent of the male prostitutes wanted to escape prostitution (Valera, Sawyer, & Schiraldi, 2001). These findings are consistent with those of the present study. For men, boys, and the transgendered, the experience of being prostituted is similar to that of women and girls.

Another misconception about prostitution is that a large majority of prostitutes are drug-abusing women who entered prostitution to pay for a drug habit. A number of studies have shown that women increase recreational drug use to the point of addiction *after* entry into prostitution (Dalla, 2002). Lange, Ball, Pfeiffer, Snyder, and Cone (1989) found that 8% of women receiving treatment for addiction reported that their drug abuse preceded prostitution, whereas 39% reported that prostitution preceded drug abuse. In another study, 60% of a group of Venezuelan women in prostitution began abusing drugs and alcohol only after entry into prostitution (Raymond et al., 2002). Kramer (2003), and Gossop, Powis, Griffiths, and Stang (1994) discuss women's use of drugs and alcohol to deal with the overwhelming emotions experienced while turning tricks. Medrano, Hatch, Zule and Desmond (2003) found that substance abusing African-American women who had a greater severity of childhood emotional abuse, emotional neglect, or physical neglect were at higher risk of prostituting than women who were less severely abused or neglected in childhood. Medrano et al. noted that this association between childhood abuse and prostitution was *unrelated to crack cocaine use.*

A common tactic used by pimps and traffickers to control prostitutes is to coercively addict them to drugs. In a similar way, perpetrators of sexual abuse against children are known to drug children in order to facilitate sexual attacks or to disorient and silence them (Carroll & Trull, 1999; Schwartz, 2000).

Although it is sometimes assumed that legalization would decrease the violence of prostitution, many of our respondents did not feel that they would be safe from physical and sexual assault if prostitution were legal. We found that 46% of people in prostitution in 6 countries felt that they were no safer from physical and sexual assault if prostitution were legal. Fifty percent of 100 prostituting respondents in a separate study in Washington, DC expressed the same views (Valera, Sawyer, & Schiraldi, 2000). In an indictment of legal prostitution, more than half of our German respondents told us that they would be no safer in legal as compared to illegal prostitution.

The triple force of race, sex and class inequality disparately impact indigenous women. Prostitution of Aboriginal women occurs globally, in epidemic numbers, with indigenous women at the bottom of racialized sexual hierarchies in prostitution itself (Scully, 2001). The toxic legacy of colonialism and generations of community trauma are critical factors contributing to the prostitution of indigenous women (Farley & Lynne, 2003). The overrepresentation of First Nations women in prostitution was reflected in the Canadian results reported here. These findings are a consequence of their marginalized and devalued status in Canada, with a concomitant lack of options for economic survival.

Indigenous women are almost always trafficked from rural communities (sometimes reservations) to urban areas. In the process of trafficking—women, men, and children are transported to markets for the purpose of prostitution or they are sold for sweatshop labor, domestic servitude, or servile marriages (also called mail-order brides).[5] Trafficking may occur within or across international borders, thus a person may be either domestically or internationally trafficked. The harm of prostitution itself is similar whether she crosses an international legal boundary or whether she is moved from, for example, Chiapas to Mexico City, or from Saskatoon to Vancouver. The experience of being uprooted from one's home or community causes distress. Migration itself is frequently a consequence of circumstances of degradation, violence, and dehumanization (deJong, 2000). Migration may also reduce the social support women count on to protect them from sexual violence (Lyons, 1999).

Trafficking cannot occur without an acceptance of prostitution in the receiving country. Governments protect prostitution/trafficking because of the monstrous profits from the business of sexual exploitation. In 1999, Thailand, Vietnam, China, Mexico, Russia, Ukraine, and the Czech Republic were primary source countries for trafficking of women into the United States (Richard, 2000). Source countries vary according to the economic desperation of women, culturally-based gender inequality, the promotion of prostitution and trafficking by corrupt government officials who issue passports and visas, and criminal connections in both the sending and the receiving country such as gang-controlled massage parlors, and the lack of laws to protect immigrating women.

Salgado (2002) described what could be appropriately termed a *trafficking syndrome* resulting from repeated harm and humiliation against a person who is kept isolated and living in prisoner-of-war-like conditions. As in prostitution and domestic trafficking, international trafficking is extremely likely to result in PTSD. Like women domestically trafficked into prostitution, internationally trafficked women experience extreme fear, guilt regarding behaviors which run counter to their religious or cultural beliefs, self-blame, and a sense of betrayal, not only by family and pimps-but by traffickers and governments. In addition, women may fear loss of immigration status if they attempt to leave violent husbands or pimps and they may not know how to access legal or social services. Additional barriers confronted by trafficked immigrant women are absence of services in the language of newcomer groups, discrimination and racism, and models of healthcare that are culturally irrelevant.

In the five years since data from the first five countries of this study were collected (Farley et al., 1998), prostitution has been increasingly normalized in many cultures where, whether legal or not, it is promoted or tolerated as a reasonable job for women. Internet technology has expanded the global reach of sex businesses, which have sometimes been adopted as governments' development strategies. For example, the International Labor Organization (ILO) promoted prostitution as the "sex sector" of Asian economies despite also citing their own surveys which indicated that in Indonesia, for example, 96% of those interviewed wanted to leave prostitution (Lim, 1998). Although they are clear regarding their desire to get out of prostitution, the voices of these women in the "sex sector" are ignored. The economic motivation for this failure to listen to those in prostitution is evident: 2.4% of the gross domestic product of Indonesia (US $3.3 billion per year) and 14% of the gross domestic product of Thailand (US $27 billion per year) was supplied by legal sex businesses (Lim, 1998).

A woman in Thailand told us, "I want the world to understand that prostitution is not a good job–so that there are other jobs for women. I want the government to look into what's going on." Instead of the question, "Did she voluntarily consent to prostitution?" the more relevant question would be: "Did she have real alternatives to prostitution for survival?" The incidence of homelessness (75%) among our respondents in 9 countries, and their desire to get out of prostitution (89%) reflect their lack of options for escape. It is a clinical, as well as a statistical error, to assume that most women in prostitution consent to it. In prostitution, the conditions which make genuine consent possible are absent: physical safety, equal power with customers, and real alternatives (MacKinnon, 1993; Hernandez, 2001). Until it is understood that prostitution and trafficking can *appear voluntary* but are not in reality a free choice made from a range of options, it will be difficult to garner adequate support to assist the women and children in prostitution who wish to escape but have no other economic choices.

> I feel like I imagine people who were in concentration camps feel when they get out . . . It's a real deep pain, an assault to my mind, my body, my dignity as a human being. I feel like what was taken away from me in prostitution is irretrievable. (Giobbe, 1991, cited by Jeffreys, 1997)

We can no longer assume that the harm perpetrated against prostitutes is in any way accidental. The institution of prostitution is carefully constructed and promoted. Those of us concerned with global human rights must address the social invisibility of prostitution, the massive denial regarding its harms, its normalization as an inevitable social evil that can be moved far from the neighborhoods of nice people, and the failure to educate students of law, psychology, public health, and criminal justice. Prostitution and trafficking can only exist in an atmosphere of public, professional, and academic indifference.

NOTES

1. We use the term "john" throughout to refer to customers of those in prostitution, because that US English terminology is most commonly used by those in prostitution themselves. Women in the US also refer to customers as "tricks" or "dates." The word

"trick" comes from customers' practices of tricking women into doing more than they pay for; the word "date" suggests that prostitution as a normal part of male-female relationships. There are many different words those in prostitution use to describe customers. Women in Johannesburg, for example, called customers "steamers," referring to the steamed-up windows of cars of Dutch settlers who drove into the city from their farms to buy African girls in prostitution.

2. A pimp is the man or woman who procures the prostitute, promotes, and sells her, and profits from prostitution. By this definition, pimps are not only the men on the street, pimps are also strip club owners, bar owners, disc jockeys, taxi drivers, concierges, motel managers, etc.

3. One group of women (over the age of eighteen) who worked in a brothel in Nevada had stuffed "kitties and puppies" in their cubicles, and their favorite foods were Captain Crunch cereal, and Nestle's Quik (Rubenstein, 1998). Similarly, Winick and Kinsie (1971, p. 146) wrote that adult prostitutes' leisure activities included roller skating and playing with dolls. We suggest that these are dissociated child parts of young women who alternate between reenacting abuse in prostitution and seeking soothing and safety in children's food and activities.

4. Many women are confused about the definition of rape. If rape is any unwanted sex act or coerced, then the statistic would be a much higher percentage. Some women in prostitution assume there is no difference between prostitution and rape, and they only call it rape if they were not paid, regardless of the violence of the act. Additionally, many studies, including our own, interviewed women who were currently prostituting. Asking them about rape is like asking someone in a combat zone if they are under fire. The responses to inquiries about rape in prostitution must make the clinical as well as the statistical assumption that a significant percentage of women currently prostituting deny rape and other violence because it would be too stressful to acknowledge the extreme danger posed by johns and pimps.

5. Sweatshop labor, domestic servitude, and servile marriage frequently involve sexual exploitation or prostitution in addition to labor exploitation.

REFERENCES

American Psychiatric Association. (1994). *Diagnostic and statistical manual of mental disorders. (4th ed.).* Washington, DC: American Psychiatric Press.

Aral, S. O., & Mann, J.M. (1998). Commercial Sex Work and STD: The Need for Policy Interventions to Change Social Patterns. *Sexually Transmitted Diseases* 25: 455-456.

Bagley, C., & Young, L. (1987) Juvenile prostitution and child sexual abuse: A controlled study. *Canadian Journal of Community Mental Health 6: 5-26.*

Belton, R. (1992). Prostitution as Traumatic Reenactment. Paper presented at 8th Annual Meeting of International Society for Traumatic Stress Studies, Los Angeles, CA. October 22.

Benoit, C., & Millar, A. (2001). Dispelling Myths and Understanding Realities: Working Conditions, Health Status and Exiting Experiences of Sex Workers. *http://web.uvic.ca/~cbenoit/papers/DispMyths.pdf.* Accessed July 17, 2002.

Blanchard, E.G., Jones-Alexander, J., Buckley, T.C., & Forneris, C.A. (1996) Psychometric Properties of the PTSD Checklist (PCL) *Behav. Res Ther.* 34 (8): 669-673.

Bownes, I.T., O'Gorman, E.C., & Sayers, A. (1991). Assault characteristics and post-traumatic stress disorder in rape victims, *Acta Psychiatric Scandinavica*, 83: 27-30.

Bullough, B., & Bullough, V. (1996). Female Prostitution: Current Research and Changing Interpretations. *Annual Review of Sex Research* 7: 158-180.

Butters, J., & Erickson, P.G. (2003). Meeting the Health Care Needs of Female Crack Users: A Canadian Example. *Women & Health* 37(3): 1-17.

Campbell, J., Jones, A.S., Dienemann, J., Kub, J., Schollenberger, J., O'Campo, P., Gielen, A.C., & Wynne, C. (2002). Intimate Partner Violence and Physical Health Consequences. *Arch Intern Med.* 162: 1157-1162. May 27, 2002.

Canada. Royal Commission on Aboriginal Peoples. (1996). *Report of the Royal Commission on Aboriginal Peoples.* Ottawa: Minister of Supply and Services Canada.

Cardenas, S., & Rivera, N. (2000). Renacer: una propuesta para volver a nacer. Bogotá: Fundacion Renacer-UNICEF Colombia.

Carroll, J.J., & Trull, L. A. (1999). Homeless African American Women's Interpretations of Child Abuse as an Antecedent of Chemical Dependence. *Early Child Development and Care* 1565: 1-16.

CATW (2002). Coalition Against Trafficking in Women. *http://www.catwinternational. org* Accessed May 7, 2002.

Chattopadhyay, M., Bandyopadhyay, S., & Duttagupta, C. (1994). Biosocial Factors Influencing Women to Become Prostitutes in India. *Social Biology* 41: 252-259.

Codigo Penal y de Procedimiento Penal (2002). Ley 599,600 de 2000. Anotado. Mario Arboleda Vallejo. Editorial Leyer.

Cotton, A., Farley, M., & Baron, R. (2002). Attitudes toward Prostitution and Acceptance of Rape Myths. *Journal of Applied Social Psychology* 32 (9): 1790-1796.

Crowe, C., & Hardill, K. (1993). Nursing research and political change: The street health report. *Canadian Nurse* 89: 2 1-24.

Crowell, N.A., & Burgess, A.W. (eds.) (1996). *Understanding Violence Against Women.* Washington, D.C.: National Academy Press.

DABS (2002). Departamento Administrativo de Bienestar Social. La Prostitucion en Escena. Bogotá: Impresos El Verbo.

Dalla, R.L. (2000). Exposing the "Pretty Woman" Myth: A Qualitative Examination of the Lives of Female Streetwalking Prostitutes. *Journal of Sex Research* 37: 344-353.

Davidson, J.O. (1998). *Prostitution, Power, and Freedom.* University of Michigan Press, Ann Arbor.

deJong, J. (2000). Inability to Work: Impact of Crisis on Refugees and Internally Displaced Persons. Presentation at Emerging Issues in Mental Health and Work, United Nations, New York, October 12, 2000.

de Sanjose, S., Palacio, V., Tafur, L., Vazquez, S., Espitia,V., Vazquez, F., Roman, G., Munoz, N., & Bosch, F. (1993). Prostitution, HIV, and Cervical Neoplasia: A Survey in Spain and Colombia. *Cancer Epidemiology, Biomarkers and Prevention* 2: 53 1-535.

DiPaolo, M. (1999). *The Impact of Multiple Childhood Trauma on Homeless Runaway Adolescents.* New York: Garland.

Dworkin, A. (1997). Prostitution and Male Supremacy in *Life and Death,* pp. 139-151. New York: Free Press.

Ekberg, G.S. (2001). Prostitution and Trafficking: The Legal Situation in Sweden. Paper presented at Journées de formation sur la mondialisation de la prostitution et du trafic sexuel, Association québécoise des organismes de coopération internationale, Montréal, Québec, Canada. March 15, 2001.

Farley, M. (2003). Prostitution and the Invisibility of Harm. *Women & Therapy,* 26 (3/4).

Farley, M. (1997). Prostitution, Slavery, and Complex PTSD. Paper presented at 13th Annual Meeting of the International Society for Traumatic Stress Studies. Montreal, November 8, 1997.

Farley, M., Baral, I., Kiremire, M., & Sezgin, U. (1998). Prostitution in Five Countries: Violence and Posttraumatic Stress Disorder. *Feminism & Psychology* 8 (4): 415-426.

Farley, M., & Barkan, H. (1998). Prostitution, violence and posttraumatic stress disorder. *Women & Health,* 27 (3): 37-49.

Farley, M., & Kelly, V. (2000). Prostitution: A critical review of the medical and social sciences literature. *Women & Criminal Justice,* 11 (4): 29-64.

Farley, M., & Lynne, J. (2003). Prostitution in Vancouver: Violence and the Colonization of First Nations Women. Fourth World Journal. Available online at http://www.cwis.org/fwj/index.htm.

Farley, M., & Patsalides, B. (2001). Physical symptoms, Posttraumatic Stress Disorder, and Healthcare Utilization of Women with and without Childhood Physical and Sexual Abuse. *Psychological Reports* 89: 595-606.

Friedman, M. J., & Yehuda, R. (1995). Post-Traumatic Stress Disorder and Comorbidity: Psychobiological Approaches to Differential Diagnosis. In M. J. Friedman, D. Charney, A. Deutch (Eds.) *Neurobiological and Clinical Consequences of Stress: From Normal Adaptation to Posttraumatic Stress Disorder.* Philadelphia: Lippincott-Raven. pp. 429-445.

Friedman, M.J., & Schnurr, P.P. (1995). The relationship between trauma, post-traumatic stress disorder, and physical health. In M. J. Friedman, D.S. Charney, & A.Y. Deutsch (eds.) *Neurobiological and clinical consequences of stress: From normal adaptation to PTSD.* Philadelphia: Lippincott-Raven.

Fundacion Esperanza. (2000). Trafico de niñas. Accessed April 2002 at http//www.fundacion esperanza.org.com

Fundacion Esperanza (1998). Trafico de Mujeres en Colombia. Bogota, Colombia.

Fundacion Renacer (2000). Entrevista personal con el Doctor Wilson Montano. Director Renacer, Cartagena.

Fundación Renacer (2001). Explotación Sexual Infantil en Colombia. Accessed March 2002 at *http://www.fundacionrenacer.org/fundacion-apoyo.*

Giobbe, E. (1991). Prostitution, Buying the Right to Rape, in Ann W. Burgess, (ed.) *Rape and Sexual Assault III: A Research Handbook.* New York: Garland Press p. 143-160.

Giobbe, E. (1993). An Analysis of Individual, Institutional and Cultural Pimping, *Michigan Journal of Gender & Law* 1: 33-57.

Giobbe, E., Harrigan, M., Ryan, J., & Gamache, D. (1990). Prostitution: A Matter of Violence against Women. WHISPER, Minneapolis, MN.

Golding, J. (1994). Sexual Assault History and Physical Health in Randomly Selected Los Angeles Women. *Health Promotion* 13:130-138.

Gossop, M., Powis, B., Griffiths, P., & Stang, J. (1994). Sexual behavior and its relationship to drug-taking among prostitutes in south London. *Addiction* 8: 961-970.

Gysels, M., Pool., R., & Nnulasiba, B. (2002). Women who sell sex in a Ugandan trading town: Life histories, survival strategies and risk. *Social Science & Medicine* 54: 179-192.

Herman, J.L. (1992). *Trauma and Recovery.* New York: Basic Books.

Hernandez, T. K. (2001). Sexual harassment and racial disparity: The mutual construction of gender and race. *U. Iowa Journal of Gender, Race & Justice,* 4: 183-224.

Hoigard, C., & Finstad, L. (1986). *Backstreets: Prostitution, Money and Love.* Pennsylvania State University Press, University Park, PA.

Holsopple, K. (1998). Strip Clubs According to Strippers: Exposing Workplace Sexual Violence. Unpublished paper, available online at *http://www.catwinternational. org/stripc1.htm.*

Houskamp, B. M., & Foy, D.W. (1991). The assessment of posttraumatic stress disorder in battered women. *Journal of Interpersonal Violence,* 6, 367-375.

Hunter, S. K. (1994). Prostitution is cruelty and abuse to women and children. *Michigan Journal of Gender and Law* 1: 1-14.

ICBF. Instituto Colombiano de Bienestar Familiar (2000). Sistema de Información ICBF. Accessed April 2002 at http://www.icbf.gov.co/espanol/estadisticas.asp.

ICBF-UNESCO & Universidad Externado (1997). Plan de acción en Favor de los Derechos de la Infancia Explotada Sexualmente y Contra la Explotacion Sexual. Bogotá.

James, J., & Meyerding, J. (1977) Early sexual experience and prostitution. *American Journal of Psychiatry* 134: 1381-1385.

Jeffreys, S. (1997). *The Idea of Prostitution.* North Melbourne, Victoria: Spinifex Press.

Kalichman, S.C., Kelly, J.A., Shaboltas, A., & Granskaya, J. (2000). Violence Against Women and the Impending AIDS Crisis in Russia. *American Psychologist* 55: 279-280.

Kalichman, S.C., Williams, E.A., Cheery, C., Beicher, L., & Nachimson, D. (1998). Sexual Coercion, Domestic Violence, and Negotiating Condom Use Among Low-Income African American Women. *Journal of Women's Health* 7: 371-378.

Keane, T. M., Kaloupek, D. G., & Weathers, F. W. (1996). Ethnocultural Considerations in the Assessment of PTSD. In A. J. Marsella, M. J. Friedman, E. T. Gerrity, & R. M. Scurfield (eds.) *Ethnocultural Aspects of Posttraumatic Stress Disorder: Issues, Research, and Clinical Applications.* Washington, DC: American Psychological Association. 183-205.

Kemp, A., Rawlings, E., & Green, B. (1991). Post-traumatic stress disorder (PTSD) in battered women: A shelter sample. *Journal of Traumatic Stress,* 4, 137-147.

Kendall, C.N., & Funk, R. E. (2003). Gay Male Pornography's "Actors": When "Fantasy" Isn't. In M. Farley (ed.) *Prostitution, Trafficking, and Traumatic Stress.* Binghamton, NY: Haworth.

Koss, M., & Heslet, L. (1992). Somatic Consequences of Violence Against Women. *Archives of Family Medicine* 1: 53-59.

Kramer, L. (2003). Emotional Experiences of Performing Prostitution. In M. Farley (ed.) *Prostitution, Trafficking, and Traumatic Stress.* Binghamton, NY: Haworth.

Lange, W.R., Ball, J.C., Pfeiffer, M.B., Snyder, F.R., & Cone, E.J. (1989). The Lexington addicts, 1971-1972: Demographic characteristics, drug use patterns, and selected infectious disease experience. *The International Journal of the Addictions*, 24(7): 609-626.

Leech, G.M. (2001). Young Women Struggle to survive in War-torn Colombia. Colombia Report, Jun 11, 2001.

Lewis, J. (1998). "Lap Dancing: Personal and Legal Implications for Exotic Dancers" in Elias, J.A., Bullough, V.L., Elias, V., Brewer, G. (1998). (editors) *Prostitution: On Whores, Hustlers, and Johns*. p. 376-389. Amherst, NY: Prometheus Books.

Lim, L.L. (ed.) (1998). *The Sex Sector: The economic and social bases of prostitution in Southeast Asia*. Geneva: International Labor Organization.

Lyons, H. (1999). Foreward. Counts, D., Brown, J., & Campbell, J. (eds.) *To Have and To Hit: Cultural Perspectives on Wife Beating*. pp. vii-xii. Chicago: University of Illinois Press.

MacKinnon, C.A. (1993). Prostitution and Civil Rights. *Michigan Journal of Gender & Law* 1:13-31.

Mansson, S.A. (2001). Men's Practices in Prostitution: The case of Sweden. In B. Pease & K. Pringle (eds.) *A Man's World? Changing Men's Practices in a Globalized World*. pp. 135-149. New York: Zed Books.

Marsella, A.J. (1997). Migration, poverty, and ethnocultural diversity: A global perspective on immigrant and refugee adaptation. *Scandinavian Journal of Work, Health, and Environment*, 23, 28-46.

McNutt, L.A., Carlson, B.E., Persaud, M., & Posmus, J. (2002). Cumulative Abuse Experiences, Physical Health, and Health Behaviors. *Ann Epidemiol* 12: 123-130.

Medrano, M.A., Hatch, J.P., Zule, W.A., & Desmond, D.P. (2003). Childhood Trauma and Adult Prostitution Behavior in a Multiethnic Heterosexual Drug-Using Population. *American Journal of Drug and Alcohol Abuse* 29(2): 463-486.

Miller, J. (1995). Gender and Power on the Streets: Street Prostitution in the Era of Crack Cocaine. *Journal of Contemporary Ethnography* 23(4): 427-452.

Ministry of Labour in cooperation with the Ministry of Justice and the Ministry of Health and Social Affairs, Government of Sweden. (1998). Fact Sheet. Secretariat for Information and Communication, Ministry of Labour. Tel +46-8-405 11 55, Fax +46-8-405 12 98 Artiklnr, A98.004 page 3-4. Available at *http://www.prostitutionresearch.com/swedish.html*.

Morgan, M., & Buitrago, M.M.A. (1992). Constitution-making in a time of cholera: Women in the 1991 Colombian constitution. *Yale Journal of Law and Feminism*, 4: 353-413.

Morse, D.S., Suchman, A.L., & Frankel, R.M. (1997). The Meaning of Symptoms in 10 Women with Somatization Disorder and a History of Childhood Abuse. *Arch Fam Med*: 6: 468-476.

Motta, C., Jaramillo, C., Perafan, B., & Roa, M. (1998). Observatorio Legal de la Mujer: El Legado de la Constitucion. Bogotá: Estudios Ocasionales. CIJUS.

Nakashima, K., Kashiwagi, S., Hayashi, J., Urabe, K., Minami, K., & Maeda, Y. (1996). Prevalence of Hepatitis C Virus Infection among Female Prostitutes in Fukuoka, Japan. *Journal of Gastoenterology* 31: 664-448.

NCMEC (1992). National Center for Missing and Exploited Children & Office of Juvenile Justice and Delinquency Prevention. Female Juvenile Prostitution: Problem and Response. Washington, DC: US Dept. of Justice.

Parriott, R. (1994). *Health Experiences of Twin Cities Women Used In Prostitution.* Unpublished survey initiated by WHISPER, Minneapolis, MN.

Patterson, O. (1982). *Slavery and Social Death.* Cambridge: Harvard University Press.

Pelzer, A., Duncan, M., Tibaux, G., & Mehari, L. (1992). A Study of Cervical Cancer in Ethiopian Women. *Cytopathology* 3(3): 139-148.

Pick, W.M., Ross, M.H., & Dada, Y. (2002). The reproductive and occupational health of women street vendors in Johannesburg, South Africa. *Social Science & Medicine* 54: 193-204.

Piot, P. (1999). Remarks at United Nations Commission on the Status of Women. New York: United Nations Press Release. March 3, 1999.

Radomsky, N.A. (1995). *Lost Voices: Women, Chronic Pain, and Abuse.* New York: Harrington Park Press.

Ramsay, R., Gorst-Unsworth, C., & Turner, S. (1993). Psychiatric morbidity in survivors of organized state violence including torture. A retrospective series. *British Journal of Psychiatry*, 162: 55-59.

Raphael, J., & Shapiro, D.L. (2002). Sisters Speak Out: The Lives and Needs of Prostituted Women in Chicago. Chicago, Illinois: Center for Impact Research.

Raymond, J., Hughes, D., & Gomez, C. (2001). *Sex Trafficking of Women in the United States: Links Between International and Domestic Sex Industries.* N. Amherst, MA: Coalition Against Trafficking in Women. Available at *www.catwinternational.org*

Raymond, J.G., Hughes, D.M., & Gomez, C.J. (2001). *Sex Trafficking of Women in the United States: International and Domestic Trends.* Coalition Against Trafficking in Women, Amherst, MA.

Raymond, J.G., D'Cunha, J., Dzuhayatin, S.R., Hynes, H.P., Rodriguez, Z.R., & Santos, A. (2002). *A Comparative Study of Women Trafficked in the Migration Process.* Amherst, MA. Coalition Against Trafficking in Women.

Reilly, C. (2001). Girl power is Africa's own vaccine for HIV: Special report: AIDS. *The Guardian.* London Tuesday June 26, 2001.

Richard, A. O. (2000). *International Trafficking in Women to the United States: A Contemporary Manifestation of Slavery and Organized Crime.* DCI Report: United States Department of State.

Rodriguez, L.F., & Cabrera, O. (1991). La Prostitución en el centro de Bogotá: Censo de establecimientos y personas, analisis socioeconomico. Bogotá: Cámara de Comercio.

Rodriguez, N., Ryan, S.W., Van de Kemp, H., & Foy, D.W. (1997). Post-Traumatic Stress Disorder in Adult Female Survivors of Childhood Sexual Abuse: A Comparison Study. *Journal of Consulting and Clinical Psychology* 65: 53-59.

Romero-Daza, N., Weeks, M., Singer, M. (1998). Much More Than HIV! The Reality of Life on the Streets for Drug-using Sex Workers in Inner City Hartford. *International Quarterly of Community Health Education* 18: 107-118.

Ross, C.A., Anderson, G., Heber, S., & Norton, G.R. (1990). Dissociation and Abuse Among Multiple Personality Patients, Prostitutes and Exotic Dancers. *Hospital & Community Psychiatry* 41: 328-330.

Ross, C.A., Farley, M., and Schwartz, H.L. (2003). Dissociation Among Women in Prostitution. In M. Farley (ed.) *Prostitution, Trafficking, & Traumatic Stress.* Binghamton, NY: The Haworth Press, Inc.

Rubenstein, S. (1998). Viagra and the Working Girl: At Nevada's Mustang Ranch It's Been Pleasure As Usual. *San Francisco Chronicle.* July 14, 1998.

Ryser, R. (1995). Collapsing States and Re-emerging Nations: the Rise of State Terror; Terrorism, and Crime as Politics. In *Fourth World Geopolitical Reader I: International Relations and Political Geography between Nations and States.* R.C. Ryser & R.A. Griggs (eds.) Center for World Indigenous Studies p. 1-8. Olympia, WA: DayKeeper Press.

Salgado, X. (2002). "Victim Assistance & Sexual Assault Program," Montgomery County, Maryland, VASAP. Presentation at Seminar on Human Trafficking, Jan 11 2002, Falls Church Virginia.

Sanders-Phillips, K. (2002). Factors Influencing HIV/AIDS in Women of Color. *Public Health Reports.* 117(S1): S151-S156.

Saunders, D.G. (1994) Post-traumatic Stress Symptom Profiles of Battered Women: A Comparison of Survivors in Two Settings. *Violence & Victims* 9: 31-44.

Schmidt, M., Cotton, A., & Farley, M. (2000). Attitudes toward prostitution and self-reported sexual violence. Presentation at the 16th Annual Meeting of the International Society for Traumatic Stress Studies, San Antonio, Texas, November 18, 2000.

Schwartz, H. (2000). *Dialogues with forgotten voices: Relational perspectives on child abuse trauma and treatment of dissociative disorders.* New York: Basic Books.

Scully, E. (2001). Pre-Cold War Traffic in Sexual Labor and Its Foes: Some Contemporary Lessons 74-106. In D. Kyle & R. Koslowski (eds.) *Global Human Smuggling: Comparative Perspectives.* Baltimore: Johns Hopkins University Press.

Seitles, M.D. (1997). Effect of the convention on the rights of the child upon street children in Latin America: A study of Brazil, Colombia and Guatemala. *In the Public Interest* 16: 159-193.

Silbert, M.H., & Pines, A.M. (1981). Sexual child abuse as an antecedent to prostitution. *Child Abuse and Neglect* 5: 407-411.

Silbert, M.H., & Pines, A.M. (1983). Early sexual exploitation as an influence in prostitution. *Social Work* 28: 285-289.

Silbert, M.H., & Pines, A.M. (1984). Pornography and sexual abuse of women. *Sex Roles* 10: 857-868.

Silbert, M.H., & Pines, A.M. (1982). Victimization of street prostitutes. *Victimology* 7 (1-4): 122-133.

Simons, R.L., & Whitbeck, L.B. (1991). Sexual Abuse as a Precursor to Prostitution and Victimization Among Adolescent and Adult Homeless Women. *Journal of Family Issues* 12(3): 361-379.

South African Press Association online, Accessed August 13 2001 *http://news.24.com/News24/Health/Aids_Focus/0,1113,2-14-659_1065314,00.html.*

Southwick, S., Yehuda, R., & Morgan, C. (1995). Clinical Studies of Neurotransmitter Alterations in Post-Traumatic Stress Disorder. In M.J. Friedman, D. Charney, A.

Deutch (eds.) Neurobiological and Clinical Consequences of Stress: From Normal Adaptation to Posfraumatic Stress Disorder. Philadelphia: Lippincott-Raven.

Spiwak, F., & Reyes, M.E. (1999). Estudio sobre Prostitución en Colombia: Trauma Tortura y Cautiverio. Unpublished manuscript.

Stark, C., & Hodgson, C. (2003). Sister Oppressions: A Comparison of Wife Battering and Prostitution. In M. Farley (ed.) *Prostitution, Trafficking, and Traumatic Stress.* Binghamton, NY: The Haworth Press, Inc.

UNICEF. (2000). United Nations Reports on Abuses of Children in Columbia.

UNICEF Columbia (2001). Columbia-Children Unicef: Up to 35.000 Children Practice Prostitution in Columbia. EFE News Service, Jan 27, 2001.

UNICEF. (2001). The convention on the rights of the child.

US Report of trafficking in persons. Embajada de los Estados Unidos. (2001). Trafico de Personas en Colombia. *http://www.usembassy.state.gov/colombia.*

Valera, R.J., Sawyer, R.G., & Schiraldi, G.R. (2001). Perceived Health Needs of Inner-City Street Prostitutes: A preliminary study. *Am J Health Behavior* 25: 50-59.

Van der Kolk, B.A., MacFarlane, A.C., & Weisaeth, L. (1996). *Traumatic stress: The effects of overwhelming experience on mind, body, and society.* New York: Guilford Press.

van der Kolk B.A., Pelcovitz, D., Roth, S., Mandel, F., McFarlane, A., & Herman, J.L. (1996). Dissociation, Affect Dysregulation and Somatization: The Complexity of Adaptation to Trauma. *American Journal of Psychiatry 153:* 83-93.

Vancouver/Richmond Health Board (1999). *Healing Ways Aboriginal Health and Service Review.* Vancouver: Vancouver Richmond Health Board.

Vanwesenbeeck, I. (1994). *Prostitutes' Well-Being and Risk.* Amsterdam: VU University Press.

Vanwesenbeeck, I., de Graaf, R., van Zessen, G., Straver, C.J., & Visser, J.H. (1995). Professional HIV risk taking, levels of victimization, and well-being in female prostitutes in the Netherlands. *Archives of Sexual Behavior* 24(5): 503-515.

Weathers, F.W., Litz, B.T., Herman, D.S., Huska, J.A., & Keane, T. M. (1993). The PTSD Checklist (PCL): Reliability, validity, and diagnostic utility. Paper presented at the 9th *Annual Meeting of the International Society for Traumatic Stress Studies,* October 24-27, 1993, San Antonio, Texas.

Weisberg, D. K. *(1985). Children of the Night: A Study of Adolescent Prostitution.* Lexington: Lexington Books.

White, J.W., & Koss, M.P. (1993). Adolescent sexual aggression within heterosexual relationships: Prevalence, characteristics, and causes. In H.E. Barbaree, W.L. Marshall & D. R. Laws. (eds.) *The Juvenile Sex Offender.* Guilford Press, New York.

Winick, C., & Kinsie, P. (1971). *The Lively Commerce: Prostitution in the United States,* Quadrangle books, Chicago.

World Health Organization (1998). Report on the global HIV/AIDS Epidemic June 1998, WHO online website http://www.who.org.

Worth, D. (1989). Sexual decision-making and AIDS: Why condom promotion among vulnerable women is likely to fail. *Studies in Family Planning.* 20: 297-307.

Zessen, G., Straver, C.J., & Visser, J.H. (1995). Professional HIV risk taking, levels of victimization, and well-being in female prostitutes in the Netherlands. *Archives of Sexual Behavior* 24(5): 503-515.

Zumbeck, S., Teegen, F., Dahme, B., & Farley, M. (2003). Posttraumatische Belastungsstörung bei Prostituierten-Ergebnisse einer Hamburger Studie im Rahmen eines internationalen Projektes. *Zeitschrift für Klinische Psychologie Psychiatrie und Psychotherapie* 51 (2): 121-136.

Prostitution and Trauma in U.S. Rape Law

Michelle J. Anderson

SUMMARY. Although the rapes that prostitutes suffer are especially frequent and violent, prostitutes rarely report having been attacked to police and, when they do, those reports rarely end in convictions of their attackers. One reason for this low conviction rate is the admission of evidence of the complainant's prior prostitution at trial to prove that she consented to the sexual intercourse alleged to have been rape. Some courts hold that such evidence is admissible when the defendant claims that what happened on the instance in question was an act of prostitution. Other courts hold that it is inadmissible unless it proves the complainant's bias or a motive to fabricate a claim of rape. Still other courts hold that it is inadmissible unless it reveals prior threats to retaliate against a customer.

INTRODUCTION

This article focuses on United States appellate court decisions in rape cases involving complainants who have formerly prostituted for money or drugs.

Michelle J. Anderson is Professor of Law at Villanova University School of Law. Her specialty is rape law.

Address correspondence to: Professor Michelle Anderson, Villanova University School of Law, 299 North Spring Mill Road, Villanova, PA 19085 (E-mail: anderson@ law.villanova.edu).

The author would like to thank those who assisted with the preparation of this manuscript: Elizabeth Cameron, Ned Nurick, Nazareth Pantaloni, and Samantha Pitts-Kiefer.

Printed with permission.

[Haworth co-indexing entry note]: "Prostitution and Trauma in U.S. Rape Law." Anderson, Michelle J. Co-published simultaneously in *Journal of Trauma Practice* (The Haworth Maltreatment & Trauma Press, an imprint of The Haworth Press, Inc.) Vol. 2, No. 3/4, 2003, pp. 75-92; and: *Prostitution, Trafficking, and Traumatic Stress* (ed: Melissa Farley) The Haworth Maltreatment & Trauma Press, an imprint of The Haworth Press, Inc., 2003, pp. 75-92. Single or multiple copies of this article are available for a fee from The Haworth Document Delivery Service [1-800-HAWORTH, 9:00 a.m. - 5:00 p.m. (EST). E-mail address: docdelivery@haworthpress.com].

http://www.haworthpress.com/store/product.asp?sku=J189
10.1300/J189v02n03_04

The law is both insignificant and significant to prostituted women who are raped in this country. The law is insignificant because few prostitutes can obtain justice through it. In general, women who are raped seldom report their rapes to the police, and when they do, the law seldom offers the victims vindication. The details of the law do not matter to most women who are raped. To most prostitutes who are raped, the law is even less helpful. Prostitutes fear the criminal justice system because it threatens to incarcerate them for engaging in prostitution.

But the fact that few prostituted women realize the law's promise of justice with regard to the sexual violence they suffer should not prevent one from recognizing how the law is also significant in their lives. Law is the formal construction by which society evaluates what has happened to prostitutes who are raped. By holding itself out as the arbiter of truth, the law embodies the social norms against which a raped prostitute will be judged and against which she will often be found deficient.

Public health practitioners know that survivors of sexual trauma frequently blame themselves for having been attacked (Katz & Burt, 1988). This self-blame, and the trauma of the rape itself, may lead some women to experience psychological problems, including posttraumatic stress disorder (Valentiner, Foa, Riggs, & Gershuny, 1996). Nearly one-third of rape victims develop posttraumatic stress disorder and 13% of rape victims attempt suicide (Kilpatrick, Edmunds, & Seymour, 1992). What public health practitioners may not know is how the law itself contributes to the negative sequelae that the victims of sexual trauma experience. Negative psychological reactions such as self-blame are a victim's natural responses to a society that insists that the sexual abuse women suffer is largely their own fault. The law of rape is one of the formal mechanisms by which society transmits the blame of rape victims from one generation to the next.

Section One of this article discusses the prevalence of rape in both the general population of women in the United States and also among prostitutes. It explains why prostitutes are particularly vulnerable to sexual abuse. Section Two traces prostitution's importance in the law of rape. Historically, rape law maintained that the sexual chastity or promiscuity of a rape complainant was of paramount importance not only to reveal her propensity to have consented to sex with the defendant, but also to reveal her propensity to lie as a witness on the stand. For women deemed unchaste, such as prostitutes, evidence of their sexual histories diminished their opportunity for legal relief.

Section Three analyzes the three major ways that courts currently grapple with the admissibility of evidence of a rape complainant's prior prostitution. First, some courts have held that, when a rape defendant alleges that what happened on the instance in question was an act of prostitution, evidence of the complainant's prior prostitution is relevant and admissible. Second, and by contrast, other courts have held that, when a rape defendant alleges that what happened on the instance in question was an act of prostitution, evidence of the complainant's prior prostitution is inadmissible unless such evidence provides a basis for proving the her bias or motive to fabricate, such as an allegation that she falsely claimed she was raped in order to avoid an arrest for prostitution. Third, other courts have agreed that evidence of the complainant's prior prostitution is admissible evidence when it provides a basis for proving the complainant's bias or motive to fabricate; however, they have held that such evidence must involve prior threats to report a false rape or to take other revenge against a customer for failure to pay.

Section Four highlights the increasingly common circumstance in which the complainant's prior sexual behavior was prostitution in exchange for drugs instead of money or other compensation. It demonstrates how this circumstance may pose additional credibility problems for the victim. Section Five analyzes the ways that some courts misunderstand the reality of prostitution and the impact that misunderstanding has in circumstances in which a complainant's record of prostitution is at issue.

I. RAPE OF PROSTITUTES

Rape is an enormous legal and public health problem for all women. The Centers for Disease Control and Prevention's National Violence Against Women Survey of 8000 women indicates that 18% of women in the general population have experienced an attempted or completed rape (Tjaden & Thoennes, 2000). Women who are prostituted are especially vulnerable to sexual abuse. The threat of such assault is greater for prostitutes than for women working in other fields (Miller & Jayasundara, 2001). For example, Silbert and Pines (1982) interviewed 200 prostitutes and found that 73% of them had been raped under circumstances unrelated to their work as prostitutes. Another study found that 94% of 16 street prostitutes interviewed had experienced sexual assault, 75% had been raped by one or more customers, and 63% had been raped in contexts unrelated to their work as prostitutes (Miller & Schwartz, 1995). Farley and Barkan (1998, Farley, Cotton, Lynne, Zumbeck, Spiwak, Reyes, Alvarez, & Sezgin, 2003) surveyed 130 street prostitutes and found that 73% of them had been raped while working as prostitutes. They also found that 59% of those who had been raped while working as prostitutes experienced rape more than five times.

The words of some of the women who have been interviewed for this research shed light on the frequency of the violence prostitutes suffer. In response to the question of how often she had been beaten, kicked, or raped, one woman in Miller and Schwartz's (1995) study said, "All of the time, all of the time. It happens to us girls all the time . . . I could tell you, we could sit here all day and talk about it. Like I said, it happens so much" (p. 8). Another woman said she had been raped or robbed, "at least once a week–once a week, twice a week" (p. 8). She continued, "That's just part of the business. That's just part of working; that's just what happens" (p. 8). A third woman emphasized the sexual violence she suffered: "You know, this happens so many times, um, it's just, a lot of times men just grab you, like I said, grab your hair or whatever, and make you do shit. You can't get away from 'em" (p. 8).

According to the Bureau of Justice Statistics, although approximately 40% of rapes of women in the general population involve some extrinsic injury beyond the rape itself, only 5% of those rapes involve serious, extrinsic injuries, such as broken bones or teeth, loss of consciousness, severe lacerations, or wounds that require hospitalization (Greenfeld, 1997). The rapes prostitutes suffer, however, appear to involve substantially more serious, extrinsic injury. For example, two-thirds of the raped street prostitutes in one study suffered serious extrinsic injury–broken bones, lacerations, or bruises requiring medical attention, etc.–as a result of having been raped (Silbert, Pines, & Lynch, 1980). Additionally, some rapists, including serial rapists, target prostitutes because they are particularly vulnerable to sexual abuse and frequently unable to obtain legal redress. In *State v. King* (1996), defendant King admitted to committing approximately 50 rapes. In what the Washington court identified as a "move calculated to avoid detection," he chose to prey "largely on hitchhikers and prostitutes" (p. 619). The court also recounted: "King committed his first rape after reading a newspaper article that implied that many rape victims failed to report the crimes because they felt ashamed, dehumanized, and humiliated by the experience" (p. 619). The negative psychological reactions victims suffer, as this rapist knew, are tied to their decisions not to report to police.

Studies that attempt to estimate the percentage of raped women in the general population who report their rapes to the police have limitations. In the better studies, involving random sample surveys of large numbers of women, estimates range from 16% (Kilpatrick, Edmunds, & Seymour, 1992) to 36% (Bureau of Justice Statistics, 1997). Women in the general population who are raped, then, tend not to report the violence they suffer to police. Because interacting with law enforcement officials can create further trauma for a rape victim, going through the process of reporting to police subjects a sexual assault victim to what has been called a "second rape" (Madigan & Gamble, 1991). It is not surprising, then, that rape is the violent crime least likely to be reported to the police (Kilpatrick, Edmunds, & Seymour, 1992). Unlike other crime victims, rape victims tend to anticipate how they will be treated and the likely legal outcome of the case before they decide whether to report having been raped to the police (Lizotte, 1985). As a result, rape victims "tend to report to the police only when the probability of conviction is high. And, of course, they tend not to report when it is low" (p. 185).

Prostitutes know they do not have a high probability of obtaining convictions against their rapists. Even though the rapes they suffer are more violent than rapes in the general population, and they likely sustain more serious extrinsic injuries, studies suggest that the rate of rape reporting by prostitutes remains low (Miller & Jayasundara, 2001; Silbert, Pines, & Lynch, 1980). In order to understand the disconnect between the frequency and severity of the rapes that prostitutes suffer on the one hand and the reticence of prostitutes to report to the police on the other hand, one must understand the law of rape and the importance of prostitution within it.

II. PROSTITUTION'S IMPORTANCE IN RAPE LAW

Historically, a rape complainant's reputation for lack of chastity was admissible evidence at trial to prove that she was more likely to have consented to the sexual act, less likely to have been forced into it by the defendant, and more likely to have fabricated an allegation of rape (Anderson, 2002). Cases focused not just on evidence of prostitution, but also on evidence of the complainant's sexual promiscuity. The assumption that unchaste women were likely to consent to sexual intercourse and lie about it on the stand meted out particularly harsh results to prostitutes who were raped. Courts sometimes remarked upon the issue in colorful language, as did the New York court in *People v. Abbot* (1838):

> [A]re we to be told that previous prostitution shall not make one among those circumstances which raise a doubt of assent?–that the triers should make no distinction in their minds between the virgin and the tenant of the stew?–between one who would prefer death to pollution, and another who, incited by lust and lucre, daily offers her person to the indiscriminate embrace of the other sex? . . . [N]o court can override the law of human nature, which declares that one who has already started on the road of prostitution, would be less reluctant to pursue her way than another who remains at her home of innocence and looks upon such a career with horror. (pp. 195-196)

As this court's analysis makes clear, judges were distrustful of both prostitutes and other women with prior sexual experience who reported having been raped.

In the 1900s, courts in rape cases began to emphasize that it was possible, in theory, to rape a prostitute, but that it was unlikely. The Iowa Supreme Court stated:

> That the prosecutrix was a common prostitute surely should be considered as bearing on her credibility as a witness . . . Of course, a common prostitute may be raped, and one may rape a woman, although she be his mistress; but it is not so likely that his act was by force and against her will. (*State v. Johnson*, p. 116, 1911)

A few years later, the Tennessee Supreme Court concurred: "Although the body of a harlot may, in law, no more be ravished than the person of a chaste woman, nevertheless it is true that the former is more likely than the latter voluntarily to have yielded" (*Lee v. State*, p. 146, 1915).

In the late 1970s and early 1980s, legislatures began to question whether evidence of a complainant's prior sexual behavior in rape cases should be admissible. They passed what are known as "rape shield laws" to decrease the defendant's ability to admit evidence of a complainant's prior sexual history. Today, rape shield laws in most jurisdictions limit the kind of prior sexual history evidence that defendants are allowed to have admitted at trial to prove that the complainant consented without force. Rape shield laws often contain legislated exceptions to what would otherwise be blanket prohibitions on the admission of a complainant's prior sexual history (Anderson, 2002).

Prostitution is an important kind of prior sexual history under rape shield laws. In at least one state, however, there is an explicit, legislated exception to the general prohibition on prior sexual history evidence for a complainant's prior sexual conduct involving prostitution. A complainant's prior convictions for prostitution within three years of the act alleged to have been rape are admissible in rape trials in New York (N.Y. CRIM. PROC. LAW § 60.42 (McKinney, 1992)). Although evidence of prostitution is formally excluded under many rape shield laws in other jurisdictions, rape defendants continue to try to have such evidence admitted at trial. Some judges have admitted such prior prostitution evidence, despite the fact that their legislatures did not explicitly authorize its admission.

III. PRIOR PROSTITUTION TO PROVE CONSENT AND BIAS

Today, courts often declare that evidence of a complainant's prior prostitution is not *always* admissible in a rape case and that it is *possible* to rape a prostitute. These declarations echo remarks courts have made for generations regarding these matters. Despite applicable rape shield laws, courts today continue to carve out various circumstances in which evidence of prior prostitution is admissible. Most cases addressing the admissibility of evidence of a complainant's prior prostitution involve a rape defendant who claims to have hired a woman as a prostitute, engaged in consensual sex, but then tricked her out of the money owed or the other negotiated compensation. Then, according to the defendant, she falsely reported having been raped to the police in order to exact revenge upon him. This scenario seems possible but improbable. On the one hand, if a prostitute were trying to encourage a recalcitrant customer to pay compensation owed, this strategy seems an unlikely way to extort cooperation because prostitutes know that the chance of police taking their rapes seriously is relatively low. On the other hand, if a man were to prey sexually on prostitutes because they are particularly vulnerable victims, this narrative is the story one would expect him to advance if one of his victims went to the police to report that she was raped.

Courts tend to analyze the admissibility of evidence of the complainant's prior prostitution in one of three different ways. First, some courts have held that, whenever a defendant alleges that what happened on the instance in question was an act of prostitution, evidence of the complainant's prior prostitution is generally admissible. Second, other courts have held that a defendant cannot ordinarily admit evidence of the complainant's prior prostitution unless such evidence provides a basis for proving her bias or motive to fabricate. Third, still other courts have held that, when a defendant alleges that what happened on the instance in question was an act of prostitution, a defendant cannot admit evidence of her prior prostitution to show bias or motive to fabricate unless such evidence involves prior extortionate threats to report a false rape or to take other revenge against a customer.

A. Evidence of Prior Prostitution Generally Admissible

First, some courts have held that, when a defendant alleges that what happened on the instance in question was an act of prostitution, evidence of the complainant's prior prostitution is generally admissible. In some of these jurisdictions, if the defendant claims that the instance in question was simply consensual intercourse and not an act of prostitution, he cannot admit evidence of the complainant's prior prostitution.

United States v. Harris (1995) involved the question of whether the trial judge had "abused his discretion when he excluded evidence of the victim's prior misdemeanor conviction for solicitation for the purpose of prostitution" (p. 891). The appellate court recounted the defense theory: The complainant had "agreed to sexual intercourse in expectation of receiving enough money for a bus ticket to Cleveland, Ohio, and was subsequently motivated to retaliate against appellant by falsely alleging rape when he refused to pay her for sexual services and then called her a 'scank [sic] bitch'" (p. 891). The court held that her seven-year-old conviction for prostitution was "relevant because of its strong tendency to prove the appellant's defense of consent" and that this value outweighed the danger that it might prejudice the jury (pp. 893-894).

Some courts even admit evidence of the complainant's prior prostitution when she suffered considerable extrinsic injury on the instance in question. In *State v. Slovinski* (1988), the complainant testified that Slovinski picked her up in his van, drove her to the woods, hit her on the head, and she passed out. When she regained consciousness, he was raping her. He then hit her on the face for about 20 minutes, kicked her in the face, drove away from the area, and threw her out of the van. He then followed her to the ground and continued to hit her until a truck pulled up, at which point he fled. The truck driver summoned an ambulance and the victim was hospitalized. Despite the exceptional level of violence Slovinski employed, the Court of Appeals in Michigan held that the evidence of the complainant's prior prostitution was admissible to prove Slovinski's defense of consent because, "It has a tendency to make it more probable that the complainant entered into a financial arrangement with the defendant for sexual acts" (pp. 153-154).

Other courts, by contrast, have agreed that a defendant may ordinarily admit evidence of the complainant's prior prostitution when he alleges that what happened on the instance in question was an act of prostitution; however, such evidence may still be excluded if there is evidence that the rape was particularly violent. These cases try to avoid the potential injustice of admitting evidence of the complainant's prior prostitution when she suffered substantial extrinsic brutality that is corroborated by other evidence.

In the Florida appeal of *Robinson v. State* (1991), for example, the complainant testified that Robinson attacked her, beat her with his fists, and raped her. She suffered bruises over her right eye, left cheek, and right upper lip and she also suffered a loose tooth. Robinson himself testified that the complainant had oral sex with him on an earlier occasion for $3 and agreed to have oral sex with him on the instance in question for $5, but that he refused to pay her. The trial court allowed Robinson to testify as to his story but would not allow him to introduce evidence of the complainant's general reputation as a prostitute. Robinson was convicted of sexual battery and aggravated assault. When Robinson challenged the trial court's ruling excluding the complainant's reputation for prostitution on appeal, the Florida appellate court stated,

> Evidence of prostitution may well have a bearing on the issue of consent where the defendant's defense is that the sexual encounter which he had with the victim was in connection with an act of prostitution. (p. 702)

The court, however, refused to overturn Robinson's conviction, noting,

> the level of violence against the victim made apparent from the evidence
> in this case weighs heavily against appellant's contention that the vic-
> tim's reputation [as a prostitute] would have any significant bearing on
> the issue of consent. (p. 703)

In jurisdictions in which courts follow this type of analysis, women who suffer severe extrinsic violence when they are raped may be able to keep evidence of their prior prostitution from the jury but those who suffer less severe extrinsic violence will not have that chance.

B. Evidence of Prior Prostitution Generally Inadmissible Unless It Proves Motive to Fabricate

Second, and by contrast, some other courts have disagreed that evidence of a complainant's prior prostitution is routinely admissible when a defendant claims that what happened was an act of prostitution. Instead, these courts have held that a defendant cannot admit evidence of the complainant's prior prostitution unless it provides a basis for proving her bias or motive to fabricate. In these jurisdictions, the circumstances that prove bias or motive to fabricate usually involve the defendant's allegation that the complainant claimed she was raped in order to avoid a charge of prostitution on the instance in question. In *Commonwealth v. Joyce* (1981), for example, the Massachusetts Supreme Court reversed Joyce's rape conviction because the trial judge did not admit evidence of the complainant's prior convictions for prostitution to prove she consented on the instance in question. Joyce picked up the complainant off the street at 3 a.m. when she was hitchhiking. The complainant testified that she asked to be taken to her boyfriend's house, but instead, Joyce drove her to a church parking lot and forced her to engage in oral sex and to have sexual intercourse twice. She tried to escape from the car twice and screamed loudly. Joyce punched her repeatedly to gain her compliance. When the headlights of an approaching car came toward them, she jumped out of the car, naked, screaming, and bleeding and ran toward it waving her arms. The approaching car happened to be a police cruiser investigating her reported screams.

Joyce's defense at trial was that the complainant consented to sex. He testified that her mouth was already bloody when he picked her up, they went to the church parking lot to take drugs together, and they engaged in sexual acts at her suggestion. As the police car approached, Joyce warned her to get dressed and she instead jumped out of the car and accused him of rape. Although Joyce did not claim that what occurred was an act of prostitution, he nevertheless sought to introduce evidence that the complainant had been pre-viously charged with prostitution twice. According to the court:

> The defendant intended to show that the complainant, having been found in a similar situation on two prior occasions, had been arrested on each occasion and charged with prostitution. We cannot say that this evidence has no rational tendency to prove that the complainant was motivated falsely to accuse the defendant of rape by a desire to avoid further prose-cution. (p. 187)

The court therefore held that the evidence was admissible, not to show that the complainant was a prostitute and therefore more likely to consent to sex, but rather to show that the complainant's allegations might have been motivated by a desire to avoid prosecution for prostitution. Despite the corroborated evi-dence of considerable extrinsic violence, the court held that evidence of the complainant's prior prostitution was admissible (*Commonwealth v. Joyce*, 1981).

In *Commonwealth v. Houston* (2000), the Supreme Court of Massachusetts narrowed the potential scope of the *Joyce* analysis. The complainant testified that Houston abducted her from a street, showed her a gun, threatened to kill her, vaginally and anally raped her repeatedly, and told her that he "owned" her. Afterward, police picked up the complainant, who was bruised, crying, confused, and incoherent. Houston testified that what had occurred was an act of prostitution. After engaging in sex, he said he told the complainant to get out of the car and refused to give her a ride home. He claimed: "Before driving off, he pretended to give her $30, but in fact gave her only three dollars" (p. 944). Therefore, he testified, she sought to punish him with a false claim of rape. The trial court prohibited Houston from introducing evidence of the complainant's five prior convictions for prostitution. The Massachusetts Supreme Court held that the prior convictions in this case were distinct from the *Joyce* convictions because:

> When the police arrived, the victim was clothed and alone; she was not discovered in a compromising position. There is also no suggestion that the victim feared she might be arrested for prostitution if she did not fab-ricate a rape complaint. (p. 946)

The *Houston* analysis may restrict the *Joyce* decision to circumstances in which the police discover the two people in a "compromising position." The fact that *Houston* is a case involving considerable extrinsic violence may also have driven the court to decide the issue in the way that it did.

C. Evidence of Prior Prostitution Generally Inadmissible Unless It Proves Prior Extortion or False Rape Charge

Third, other courts have agreed with preceding legal decisions that evidence of a complainant's prior prostitution may be admitted if it provides support for a claim of bias or motive to fabricate; however, they have narrowed in a different and fairer way the circumstances in which such evidence will be sufficient to show bias or motive to fabricate. These courts have held that, when a defendant alleges that what happened on the instance in question was an act of prostitution, a defendant cannot admit evidence of the complainant's prior prostitution to show bias or motive to fabricate unless such evidence involves prior threats to report a false rape or to take other revenge against a customer.

In *State v. Johnson* (1997), for example, the complainant testified that Johnson enticed her into his car, drove her to a secluded area, and raped her. Another woman also testified that, on a different date, Johnson offered her a ride, drove her to a secluded area, and raped her. Johnson claimed that what occurred with both women was consensual prostitution but that, during the course of those acts, he annoyed, angered, or frightened the women so that they sought revenge on him with false claims of rape. In support of his position, he sought to admit evidence of the complainants' prior prostitution with third parties. In analyzing this case, the Supreme Court of New Mexico described the impermissible assumption that, because a woman said *yes* to certain sexual acts before, she would say *yes* again (called the "yes/yes" inference) (p. 879). The court explained, "[t]he evidence offered should be relevant to a defense theory other than a theory based on propensity [to prostitute]" (p. 879).

According to the court, "a distinctive pattern of past sexual conduct, involving the extortion of money by threat after acts of prostitution" (p. 879) would be relevant to the defendant's theory of revenge and therefore admissible. Prior false claims of rape or threats of false claims would be appropriately admitted. However, the court held, "Simply showing that the victim engaged in an act or acts of prostitution is not sufficient to show motive to fabricate" (p. 879). In applying the law to the facts of the case, the *Johnson* court decided:

> The possibility that [the two victims] had engaged in prostitution either before or after the incidents in question does not support an inference that they had a reason to fabricate an accusation of rape. Defendant sought to introduce testimony that [one victim] had admitted to the police that she had occasionally sold sex for money to pay the rent. Defendant also sought to introduce evidence that [the other victim] had been

arrested on a prostitution charge subsequent to his arrest for sexual assault. This evidence does not show that either would retaliate against those who failed to pay by fabricating false charges. (p. 880)

Therefore, the New Mexico Supreme Court acknowledged that fabrication is an appropriate theory upon which evidence of a complainant's prior prostitution might be admissible. But prior acts of prostitution that did *not* involve false charges or extortion are irrelevant to the question of whether the complainant would consent to sexual intercourse with the defendant and then lodge a false charge against him.

Sometimes cases with the kind of evidence necessary in *Johnson* arise. For example, in *Winfield v. Commonwealth* (1983), Winfield sought to admit the testimony of a third party that the complainant "agreed to have sexual intercourse with him on the condition that he pay her twenty dollars; that he had sexual intercourse with [her]; that he did not pay her twenty dollars; that [she] stated that if he did not pay her the twenty dollars that she would tell his wife" (p. 17). The Supreme Court of Virginia held that "evidence tending to show a distinctive pattern of past sexual conduct, involving extortion of money by threats after acts of prostitution, of which her alleged conduct in this case was but an example, is relevant, probative, and admissible in his defense" (p. 19).

In sum, a number of jurisdictions continue to admit evidence of prior prostitution whenever the defendant claims that what occurred on the instance in question was an act of prostitution. Others refuse to allow evidence of prostitution when the rape was particularly brutal, but that rule does not help those rape victims who suffer great intrinsic harm but little extrinsic violence. Still other jurisdictions require that the evidence of a complainant's prior prostitution provide a basis for proving motive to fabricate and a minority of those jurisdictions limit that admission to circumstances in which the evidence specifically involved former extortionate threats.

IV. PRIOR PROSTITUTION FOR DRUGS TO PROVE CONSENT AND BIAS

Increasingly, courts have been faced with cases in which the rape defendant claims that what occurred on the instance in question was a slightly different kind of prostitution–sex in exchange for drugs. Often the victims in these cases are addicted to narcotics and have a history of exchanging sexual acts for drugs. Given current research on female addicts, this kind of desperate behavior is not surprising. In a survey of Chicago substance abuse treatment programs, for example, 60-100% of women in these programs had regularly exchanged sex for drugs or money (O'Leary & Howard, 2001).

Cases involving women who have previously exchanged sex for drugs may present even more serious credibility problems for the women than cases involving those who have previously exchanged sex for money. Studies indicate that, all other factors being equal, the victim's and defendant's inebriation during a rape tends to increase the blameworthiness people assign to the victim, while it decreases the blameworthiness people assign to the defendant (Norris & Cubbins, 1992; Stormo, Lang, & Stritzke, 1997). Although these studies involved alcohol instead of illegal narcotics, the same may be true if the defendant and the victim were high on drugs.

The Maryland case of *Johnson v. State* (1993) provides an example. The complainant in that case was addicted to crack cocaine and was allegedly raped by three men at "the culmination of an evening and night of drug use, which consumed all, or virtually all, of the victim's previous weeks wages," the court noted (p. 153). Johnson himself testified that the complainant was "freaking" (p. 153)–or exchanging sex for drugs–with the three men but that she became angry when none of them gave her drugs as promised. At trial, Johnson wanted to cross-examine the complainant about her prior prostitution in exchange for drugs. In a private hearing in front of the judge, the complainant acknowledged that she had exchanged sex for drugs in the past, including one week before the rape. The trial judge excluded the evidence, however, concluding that the risk that it would sway the jury unfairly outweighed the evidence's relevance. The highest court in Maryland, the Court of Appeals, disagreed. That court explained:

> As we have seen, the critical issue is whether, on this occasion, the victim was freaking for cocaine or was raped. And, because these are the only two explanations for what occurred, evidence that she had freaked for cocaine in the past and, particularly, the very recent past, has special relevance to the issue; such evidence . . . is relevant to and probative of the victim's motive. From a finding that on this occasion she was freaking for cocaine but did not receive the bargained for cocaine, the jury could infer that the victim had an ulterior motive for making a false accusation of rape against the petitioner. (p. 159)

The court concluded that the evidence was necessary because prostitution was the central issue in the case. This *Johnson* case appears to admit evidence of the complainant's prior prostitution whenever the defendant claims that what happened was an act of prostitution. The only difference between this and other such cases is that the type of prostitution alleged here is the exchange of sex for drugs instead of sex for money.

The Maryland Court of Appeals in *Johnson v. State* (1993) made the same prohibited "yes/yes" inference (*yes* to sex for drugs previously means *yes* to sex for drugs now) that the Supreme Court of New Mexico rejected in *State v. Johnson* (1997) (see the preceding section). The prior instances of sex for drugs here did not involve extortionate threats to lodge false claims or engage in other retributive behavior on the part of the complainant. Nevertheless, the Maryland court mandated that the evidence be admitted.

V. THE REALITY OF PROSTITUTION TO PROVE RAPE

In some cases involving the admission of evidence of an alleged rape victim's prior prostitution, courts seem to misunderstand the realities of street prostitution. In a California case, for example, the complainant testified that, after a friend had dropped her off at 11:30 at night a few blocks away from a bus stop, two men accosted her, took her to a nearby house, and orally and vaginally gang-raped her (*People v. Varona*, 1983). The defense argued that the complainant had solicited the men to engage in acts of prostitution, gone voluntarily to the house, and engaged in the sexual acts consensually. The defense argued that the woman became enraged when she realized that they had no money to pay her, so she falsely accused them of rape. To bolster its position, the defense attempted to introduce evidence that the woman had previously pled guilty to a charge of prostitution and was on probation for that crime at the time of the trial. The trial judge excluded the evidence of her prior conviction for prostitution but the California appellate court reversed. As in similar cases, the court stated, "We do not here hold that, in every rape case where the prosecutrix is a prostitute, evidence of that fact must be admitted to show consent" (p. 46). However, the court said, because of the "peculiar facts here involved," the prior prostitution conviction should have been admitted. The court detailed those "peculiar facts" in the following manner:

> The official records offered here show, not only that the woman was a prostitute, but: (1) that in pursuit of her profession, she walked the night streets in this very area to solicit customers; and (2) that, in the practice of that profession, she not only engaged in normal intercourse, but that she specialized in oral copulation. (p. 46)

What is striking about these "special factors," as the court later called them, is that–far from being unique–they reflect the everyday reality of street prostitution. One would expect that, if a woman prostituting on the street were raped, it is likely that she would be raped in the area where she was prostituting. Research indicates that 68% of street prostitutes are raped while working as prostitutes, which would be in the area where they work (Farley & Barkan, 1998). One would also expect that the vast majority of prostitutes would "specialize" in oral sex, given that it is the most commonly bargained for sexual act in prostitution (Kandel, 1992; Monto, 1999).

The appellate court in *Varona* decided, however, that the fact that the woman was allegedly raped where she had previously prostituted "is here of special significance in that it casts light on the woman's story that she walking to the bus stop because the 'friend' who had driven her from the friend's home had callously refused to drive two blocks further, to the bus stop because the friend had, at 11:30 p.m., an urgent appointment at home" (p. 46). This language suggests that the court believed that the complainant was lying about whether she was prostituting on the evening in question. Prostituting on the evening in question and being raped that same evening are not mutually exclusive.

The court also decided that the fact that the woman previously "specialized" in oral sex was "very significant in that it tends to support the defense claim that the oral copulation, on which count IV was based, was voluntarily engaged in by the woman" (p. 46). The court offered no further analysis on this point. How one's "specialization" in oral sex suggested consent to an act of oral sex alleged to have been rape was assumed to be self-evident. This analysis is exactly the "yes/yes" inference (*yes* to oral sex previously mean *yes* to oral sex now) that a number of courts have rejected. Courts' failure to understand the nature of street prostitution and the violence connected with it may result in a lack of justice for both victims and defendants.

CONCLUSION

The experience of rape for prostitutes is particularly traumatic not only because the rapes prostitutes suffer tend to be more violent than other rapes, but also because of the prejudice many people harbor against prostitutes. Miller and Schwartz's (1995) interviews with women prostituting on the street revealed several distinct prejudices: that prostitutes cannot be raped, that prostitutes are not harmed even if they are raped, and that prostitutes deserve the violence they suffer. Most of the victims in that study did not go to the police when they were raped. As one woman explained, the police "don't have no pity for no prostitutes. They figure if you out there whoring, you supposed to take what's coming to you" (Miller & Schwartz, 1995, p. 13). Of those who did report rapes to the police, law enforcement officers often treated them with contempt. The women reported that police showed a lack of concern and one police officer even laughed about the sexual violence she had reported. Additionally, the women pointed out that it was not uncommon for a man to pick a prostitute up, refuse to pay her, force sexual acts on her against her will, and then give her money once those acts were complete, as if the money legitimized the violence and as if the man was entitled to purchase the experience of rape (Miller & Schwartz, 1995).

Health practitioners who treat physical and psychological trauma would improve their ability to help their clients by understanding the use of prior sexual history in rape law. Psychologists helping women recover from rape and prostitution, social workers counseling those who were sexually abused as children, substance abuse counselors working with women who have bartered sex for drugs, as well as others in public health would appreciate more deeply their clients' experiences by comprehending how the law has constructed both the crimes their clients have suffered and the crimes they may have committed.

Too many courts continue to routinely admit evidence of a rape complainant's prior prostitution. This injustice stems from the historical importance of a woman's sexual chastity in rape law. Unless the evidence of a complainant's prior prostitution involves extortion or extortionate threats, the relevance of such evidence is very low and it should be excluded. If a raped prostitute reports having been assaulted to the police and is lucky enough to have the police and prosecutors take her claim seriously, she will end up on the witness stand in front of a jury. Because of courts' willingness to admit evidence of their prior prostitution, raped prostitutes may suffer humiliation and traumatic stress on the witness stand. The judicial system's bias against prostitutes who are raped mirrors the mistreatment they face elsewhere.

REFERENCES

Anderson, M. J. (2002). From chastity requirement to sexuality license: Sexual consent and a new rape shield law. *George Washington Law Review, 70*(1), 1701-1818.

Bureau of Justice Statistics, U.S. Department of Justice. (1997). *Criminal victimization in the United States, 1994* (Report No. NCJ-162126). Washington, DC: U.S. Government Printing Office.

Commonwealth v. Houston, 722 N.E.2d 942 (Mass. 2000).

Commonwealth v. Joyce, 415 N.E.2d 181 (Mass. 1981).

Farley, M. & Barkan, H. (1998). Prostitution, violence, and posttraumatic stress disorder. *Women & Health, 27*(3), 37-49.

Farley, M., Cotton, A., Lynne, J., Zumbeck, S., Spiwak, F., Reyes, M. E., Alvarez, D., & Sezgin, U. (2003). Prostitution and Trafficking in Nine Countries: An Update on Violence and Posttraumatic Stress Disorder (M. Farley, ed.). *Prostitution, Trafficking, and Traumatic Stress.* Binghamton, NY: The Haworth Press, Inc.

Greenfeld, L. (1997). *Sex offenses and offenders: An analysis of data on rape and sexual assault.* (NCJ Publication No. 163392). Washington, DC: U.S. Department of Justice, Bureau of Justice Statistics.

Johnson v. State, 632 A.2d 152 (C.A. MD 1993).

Kandel, M. (1992). Whores in court: Judicial processing of prostitutes in the Boston Municipal Court in 1990. *Yale Journal of Law & Feminism, 4,* 329-352.

Katz, B., & Burt, M. (1988). Self blame in recovery from rape. In A. W. Burgess (Ed.), *Rape & sexual assault II,* (pp. 51-66). New York: Garland Publishing, Inc.

Kilpatrick, D. G., Edmunds, C. N., & Seymour, A. E. (1992). *Rape in America: A report to the nation.* Arlington, VA: National Crime Victim's Center.

Lee v. State, 179 S.W. 145 (Tenn. 1915).

Lizotte, A. J. (1985). The uniqueness of rape: Reporting assaultive violence to the police. *Crime and Delinquency, 31*(2), 169-190.

Madigan, L., & Gamble, N. C. (1991). *The second rape: Society's continued betrayal of the victim.* New York: Lexington Books.

Miller, J., & Jayasundara, D. (2001). Prostitution, the sex industry, and sex tourism. In C. M. Renzetti, J. L. Edleson, & R. K. Bergen (Eds.), *Sourcebook on violence against women,* (pp. 459-480). Thousand Oaks, CA: Sage Publications, Inc.

Miller, J., & Schwartz, M. D. (1995). Rape myths and violence against street prostitutes. *Deviant Behavior, 16,* 1-23.

Monto, M. A. (1999). *Focusing on the clients of street prostitutes: A creative approach to reducing violence against women* (Grant No. 97-IJ-CX-0033). Final Report for National Institute of Justice.

Norris, J., & Cubbins, L. A. (1992). Dating, drinking, and rape: Effects of victim's and assailant's alcohol consumption on judgments of their behavior and traits. *Psychology of Women Quarterly, 16,* 179-191.

O'Leary, C., & Howard, O. (2001). *The prostitution of women and girls in metropolitan Chicago: A preliminary prevalence report.* Chicago: Center for Impact Research.

People v. Abbot, 19 Wend. 192 (N.Y. 1838).

People v. Varona, 192 Cal. Rptr. 44 (Cal. App. 1983).

Robinson v. State, 575 So.2d 699 (C.A. Fla. 1991).

Rules of evidence; admissibility of evidence of victim's sexual conduct in sex offense cases, NY Crim. Pro. § 60.42. (1992).

Silbert, M. H., & Pines, A. M. (1982). Victimization of street prostitutes. *Victimology, 7,* 122-133.

Silbert, M., Pines, A., & Lynch, T. (1980). *Sexual assault of prostitutes* (Grant No. RO1-MH-32782-01). Delancey Street Foundation, National Institute of Mental Health.

State v. Coella, 28 P. 28 (Wash. 1891).

State v. Johnson, 133 N.W. 115 (Iowa 1911).

State v. Johnson, 944 P.2d 869, (N.M. 1997).

State v. King, 925 P.2d 606 (Wa. 1996).

State v. Slovinski, 420 N.W.2d 145 (C.A. Mich. 1988).

Stormo, K. J., Lang, A. R., & Stritzke, W. G. K. (1997). Attributions about acquaintance rape: The role of alcohol and individual differences. *Journal of Applied Social Psychology, 27*(4), 279-305.

Tjaden, P., & Thoennes, N. (2000). *Full report of the prevalence, incidence, and consequences of violence against women: Findings from the national violence against women survey.* (NCJ Publication No. 183781). Washington, DC: U.S. Department of Justice, Center for Disease Control and Prevention.

United States v. Footman, 66 F. Supp. 83 (D.C. Mass. 1999).

United States v. Harris, 41 M.J. 890 (Army Crim. App. 1995).

Valentiner, D. P., Foa, E. B., Riggs, D. S., & Gershuny, B. S. (1996). Coping strategies and posttraumatic stress disorder in female victims of sexual and nonsexual assault. *Journal of Abnormal Psychology*, *105*(3), 455-458.

Winfield v. Commonwealth, 301 S.E.2d 15 (Va. 1983).

Gay Male Pornography's "Actors":
When "Fantasy" Isn't

Christopher N. Kendall

Rus Ervin Funk

SUMMARY. Gay male pornography harms men. It harms some of the men who are used to perform in it and more broadly, men in general once used and distributed. It is, at its core, harmful to the movement for social, sexual, gender, and racial justice. In this article, we examine gay male pornography under the lens developed by over twenty years of feminist scholarship and activism relative to heterosexual pornography. We find that, like heterosexual pornography, gay male pornography uses real people, many vulnerable and easily exploited, to sexualize racism and promote both homophobia and sexism. Rather than being a tool for liberation, as some gay and bisexual men have argued, we conclude that gay male pornography promotes degradation, violence and harm–and as such, *is* degradation, violence, and harm.

Christopher N. Kendall, LLB, SJD, is Professor of Law and Dean at the School of Law, Murdoch University, Perth, Western Australia 6150. He can be reached at: (C.Kendall@murdoch.edu.au).

Rus Ervin Funk, MSW, is at the Center for Women and Families, PO Box 2048, Louisville, KY 40201. He can be reached at (rfunk@cwfempower.org).

Christopher N. Kendall would like to thank Professor Catharine MacKinnon for her support and guidance throughout the writing of some of the arguments that appear in this work.

Printed with permission.

[Haworth co-indexing entry note]: "Gay Male Pornography's 'Actors': When 'Fantasy' Isn't." Kendall, Christopher N., and Rus Ervin Funk. Co-published simultaneously in *Journal of Trauma Practice* (The Haworth Maltreatment & Trauma Press, an imprint of The Haworth Press, Inc.) Vol. 2, No. 3/4, 2003, pp. 93-114; and: *Prostitution, Trafficking, and Traumatic Stress* (ed: Melissa Farley) The Haworth Maltreatment & Trauma Press, an imprint of The Haworth Press, Inc., 2003, pp. 93-114. Single or multiple copies of this article are available for a fee from The Haworth Document Delivery Service [1-800-HAWORTH, 9:00 a.m. - 5:00 p.m. (EST). E-mail address: docdelivery@haworthpress.com].

http://www.haworthpress.com/store/product.asp?sku=J189
10.1300/J189v02n03_05

No job
No money
No self-esteem
No confidence
All I have is my looks and body,
And that's not working anymore.
I feel washed up.
Drug problem.
Hate life.
HIV-positive

–Joey Iacona Stefano, gay pornography actor who died of a drug overdose
(Isherwood, 1990, p. 162)

INTRODUCTION

Little has been written about the lives of the men used in gay male pornography. More frequently, authors have attempted to distinguish gay male pornography from heterosexual pornography, arguing that it is harm-free, that it is a source of gay male liberation and central to the formation of gay male sexual identity (Stychin, 1995; Burger, 1995).

Those who support the production, use and promotion of gay male pornography argue that the pornographic presentation of gay and bisexual men using or being used sexually by other men is an act of rebellion against the heterosexist norms of our society and a liberating and even necessary act in response to what Adrienne Rich has called the "compulsory heterosexuality" of mainstream US culture (Rich, 1980). According to this argument, gay male pornography is good and is a right that should absolutely be protected and promoted.

Others, including the authors, recognize the individual and systemic harms caused by gay male pornography, and counter that gay male pornography does much more than present sex between men. Rather, like heterosexual pornography, gay male pornography uses real people, many of them prostituted in real life, to eroticize inequality, degradation, and abuse while simultaneously promoting sexist, heterosexist, and racist gender stereotypes (Kendall, 2001; Kendall, 1999; Kendall, 1997; Kendall, 1995; Stoltenberg, 1989; Stoltenberg, 1990a and 1990b; Jensen, 1998). The result is the promotion of the same sex-based harms that result from heterosexual pornography.

A review of the content of the gay male pornography now sold world-wide reveals a sexualized identity politic that relies on the inequality found between those with power and those without it; between those who are top and those who are bottom; between straight men and gay men; between men and women. From these and other materials, we are taught to glorify a sexualized, hyper-masculine, muscular ideal. Gay male pornography, like heterosexual pornography, offers a virulent form of propaganda promoting a masculinity that is associated not only with degradation of women, but also with the degradation of men who are seen and sexualized as "other"–men of colour, poor men, men who are disabled, and gay and bisexual men (Kendall, 2001; Stoltenberg, 1990a; Funk, 1993; Funk, 2003, Connell, 1995; Frosh et al., 2000; Pease, 2000).

The result is that men who are deemed feminine are degraded as "queer" and "faggots" and are subjected to the same dehumanizing epithets usually used against women, such as "bitch," "cunt," and "whore." These effeminate men are in turn presented as enjoying this degradation. Gay male pornography reinforces a system in which "a victim, usually female, always feminized" is actualized (MacKinnon, 1989, p. 141).

Far from the fantasy or mere fictional representation that its promoters would have us believe it is, gay male pornography presents and therefore is a form of male power, using real people to market and normalize through sex the inequality and harms it causes. This sexuality of dominance, in which men sexually violate women, leads to the oppression of gay men as well.

Because gay male pornography glorifies the masculine and denigrates the feminine, it reinforces the male/female social dichotomy and male supremacy seen everywhere else, resulting in those actions and practices that make both homophobia and sexism a threat to physical safety and social equality. Pornography enacts and promotes, and relies for its sexual value upon, a hierarchy that keeps straight on top of gay by keeping men on top of women.

The threat to equality posed by these materials has received some attention in recent years from authors concerned about its use by gay men and its negative impact on gay male identity. In this paper we will discuss one aspect of gay male pornography's harms that has not received critical analysis: the harm and trauma resulting from an industry which exploits and uses men who are economically and socially disadvantaged for the financial gain and sexual gratification of other men (gay and non-gay alike). Specifically, we look at the harm perpetrated against some of the men who have been used to produce gay male pornography and the way that gay male pornography uses already traumatized people–thus denying and minimizing the harm they have experienced, and interfering both with their healing process and our collective ability to respond more appropriately to the harm they have experienced.

While not every person who has been used to produce gay male pornography claims to have been harmed, and while not every producer of gay male pornography sets out to exploit those used to make his product, given the documented links between the production of heterosexual pornography and harm (MacKinnon and Dworkin, 1997; Lovelace, 1980; Dines, Jensen, & Russo, 1998; Factum of the Intervener Women's Legal Education & Action Fund, 1990), and given the experiences of some of the men who have been used to make gay male pornography (Isherwood, 1996; Edmonson, 1998), there is reason to believe that some pornography producers do harm, or at least turn a blind eye to the exploitation of the men they use. These men–the men sold as sex–matter to us, as do the men who take their place once they are no longer wanted or no longer exploitable through sex.

Although little research has examined the extent of childhood trauma in the lives of the gay or bisexual men used in gay male pornography, there is a body of research that shows that many of the women used in heterosexual pornography experienced childhood trauma. From the research available on the gay male pornography industry, which we discuss below, it is evident that at least some of the men used in gay male pornography are also suffering sequelae of traumatic events from childhood or adolescence. The research on heterosexual pornography further suggests that a substantial majority of the women used are abused, victimized and traumatized through their experience of heterosexual pornography. In this paper, we offer some examples illustrating that the same can be said of some of the men used in gay male pornography.

Our analysis begins with a brief overview of psychological trauma. We will then examine what some gay and bisexual men have said about their experiences in gay male pornography and how its impact on them. Far from being a tool for sexual liberation, gay male pornography reinforces the same sexist, heterosexist and racist stereotypes as heterosexual pornography–thereby maintaining those social prejudices and stereotypes that ensure the oppression of gay and bisexual men. We will discuss the ways in which the impact of the traumatization inherent in gay male pornography undermines the ability of gay and bisexual men to build and sustain community, the foundation of which is the basis for any struggle for social justice.

TRAUMA OVERVIEW

Trauma is a physically or emotionally overwhelming, often horrifying, event. It can also be a series of events. Here, we will focus on childhood physical and sexual abuse and its effects on adult gay and bisexual men. We have included the voices of men used in gay male pornography, many of whom have been abused as children. Thus, we provide a brief overview of child abuse trauma and its subsequent effects on adults.

Child abuse is traumatic and has lasting effects (Briere, 1992; Herman, 1992). Physical and sexual assault of children results in pathological adjustment responses that leave adults vulnerable to being manipulated and abused in adult relationships. These include: difficulty creating or sustaining trust, inability in setting and enforcing personal boundaries (including sexual boundaries), lowered self esteem (including self doubt, self-blame, and lowered self image), difficulty in recognizing cues for danger, and relationships characterized by an imbalance of power (Briere, 1992; Herman, 1992; Higgins & McCabe, 2000). The message to children sent by child abusers is that the children themselves are unworthy of love and that they are deserving of the maltreatment they receive because of some inherent flaw. For abused gay and bisexual youth, their sexual orientation is often used as an excuse for the abuse. Sexual abuse has particularly insidious ramifications because of the way that sexual abuse connects bad feelings (being used, exploited, harmed, etc.) with good feelings (being attended to, physical sensation, etc.). This can be especially confusing and damaging for children.

Gay male pornography offers men who have been maltreated as children a way to feel good about themselves through attention and income but in ways that reinforce the messages they received as a result of the abuse inflicted on them as children. Children who were abused often suffer from poor self-image and a lack of confidence (Briere, 1992; Herman, 1992; Higgins & McCabe, 2000). Incorporating the perpetrator's view of himself, the sexually abused child may eventually come to see himself as good for nothing but sex (Farley, 2003, citing Putnam), which is to say, he concludes that he is a prostitute. Acting out sexually may be a way to express himself in a positive light. Gay pornography offers men who have been maltreated as children attention and income in ways that reinforce the contempt and objectification coupled with the positive feelings of attention they experienced from child abuse. For others, being sexualized may be an attempt to reclaim what was taken from them as children. Either way, these behaviors result from attempts to heal the harm they suffered as children. Without appropriate support and care by their community, however, their attempts are unlikely to succeed.

Thus, some men's "participation" in pornography can be better understood as a traumatic re-enactment than as personal choice. Adults who have survived childhood abuse struggle to actively master the trauma in a multitude of ways, including enacting abuse scenarios in pornography and prostitution (Cassese, 2000; Gill & Tutty, 1997; Meston, Heiman, & Trapnell, 1999; Meston & Heiman, 2000; Maltz & Homan, 1987). Sadly, many who use their involvement in gay male pornography as a way to recover from their abusive pasts find more exploitation, more demands that they "perform" to please someone else, and more of the same dynamics experienced as children.

Gay male pornography is based on Eurocentric definitions of male beauty and hyper-masculinity, and, like heterosexual pornography, defines and describes sexuality and sexual relations as being based solely on physical performance and sensation with no regard for emotional connection. The use of beauty and imageries of masculinity are often used in the abuse of male children. Men may be abused because they are either "so beautiful" and/or because they "aren't man enough" (Cassese, 2000; Gill & Tutty, 1997; Ray, 2001). The narratives below of gay men used to produce gay male pornography reveal that some gay and bisexual men who were abused as children have sought out gay male pornography and the industry that produces it as a way to validate their beauty and/or to prove their masculinity. Mirroring the powerlessness of abused children, we see that these men have little voice in their sexual "performances," and have little power or agency vis-à-vis the producers. They don't choose what they will do, they aren't given a choice of how long to "perform" or when to stop if they so desire, have little choice in "partners," and as we will show later, often are given no choice to practice safe sex. They are used for a short time and are then discarded when those who use them choose a new object for sexual use. Within this relationship, we again see a parallel to childhood sexual abuse.

The narratives that follow include histories of drug and alcohol dependence, dynamics that are common amongst traumatized individuals. Self-medication via drug or alcohol abuse is often used in attempting to manage the overwhelming feelings related to trauma (Langel & Hartgers, 1998; Ouimette, Kimerling, Shaw, & Moos, 2000; Hughes, Johnson, & Wilsnack, (2001). All of the narratives offered here include stories of substance use/abuse. Although certainly not representative of all of men who are used in gay male pornography, these narratives do demonstrate how, for these men, the pain of performing required some use or abuse of substances. From these narratives, we see the connection between childhood trauma and substance use/abuse and how ongoing experiences re-trigger their traumatic experiences–thus leading to even more substance abuse. The stories show the ways that their being used by the gay male pornography industry has harmed and further traumatized these men.

WOMEN HARMED IN HETEROSEXUAL PORNOGRAPHY: IMPLICATIONS FOR GAY MALE PORNOGRAPHY

Women are harmed in and by the pornography industry (MacKinnon, 2001; Dworkin, 1989; Dworkin & MacKinnon, 1989; MacKinnon & Dworkin, 1997; Cole, 1989; Dines, Jensen, & Russo, 1998; Lederer & Delgado, 1995;

Russell, 1989; Russell, 1993). In 1991, the Canadian Supreme Court, in its decision in *R v. Butler*, accepted the evidence that physical and psychological harm is inflicted on real people in order to make some pornography, particularly visual pornography. These findings revealed that many women were coerced into pornography and that the massive pornography market provides a profit motive for harming people and treating them as second-class citizens (LEAF, 1990).

In its submissions before the Supreme Court of Canada in *Butler*, the Women's Legal Education and Defence Fund (Factum of the Intervener Women's Legal Eductaion and Action Funds, 1990) outlined the harms suffered by the women used to produce heterosexual pornography. Known for her role in the film *Deep Throat*, the life of Linda Marchiano illustrates the harm suffered by women used to produce pornography. Marchiano exposed an industry which exploited the most psychologically and economically vulnerable and thus most easily abused during the production of pornography (Lovelace, 1980) and described the sadistic, abusive and non-consensual practices common in the pornography industry. From Marchiano and others we have learned that the harms caused by heterosexual pornography include prostitution, that many women enter the sex industry as children, that many women feel trapped once they enter the industry and are unable to leave as a result of the abuse inflicted on them by pimps or as a result of drug addiction or because they feel they have nothing else to offer other than their bodies, and that many women are physically coerced into making pornography (MacKinnon, 2000; Dines, Jensen, & Russo, 1998; Lederer, 1980). As a result of this work, we now understand that heterosexual pornography causes harm both directly to the women used in its production, but also to women generally because of the misogyny that is inherent in its production and consumption (MacKinnon & Dworkin, 1997).

The *Butler* trial did not raise the issue of the harms of same-sex pornography in detail, although subsequent litigation has revealed that same-sex pornography causes the same sex-based harms as heterosexual pornography.[1] Unfortunately, neither this litigation or past writings about heterosexual pornography have inquired as to whether the harms inflicted on those used to produce heterosexual pornography are also inflicted on the men used to make gay male pornography. Given what we know about effects of the gay male pornography sold worldwide (Kendall, 2001); however, it would be naive to assume that gay male pornography is somehow completely different from heterosexual pornography in terms of how it is produced and consumed, and the harm it causes and perpetrates.

Some gay men argue that, because of the homophobic silencing of gay male sexuality, the effects of gay male pornography are qualitatively different than the effects of heterosexual pornography.[2] We disagree. When we examined the content of the gay male pornography now available to gay men (Kendall 2001) we discovered that the gay pornography industry risks placing its "models"[3] in situations, which promote and hence are violence, cruelty, degradation, dehumanization, and exploitation. While described as "representational," "fictional," or "fantasy," gay male pornography uses real people. We should not assume that these men are not harmed because they are gay men, rather than women.

From the documented experiences of Marchiano and other women (MacKinnon & Dworkin, 1997), we know that many of the women involved in the production of pornography are subjected to behind-the-scenes abuse, degradation and violence in addition to the sexualized abuse, degradation, and violence through which they are victimized during the production of pornography. Unfortunately, the abuse, degradation or violence that is presented is frequently denied or minimized under the guise of being protected as "freedom of speech and expression," not real (i.e., "just acting" or "part of the script"), or interpreted as being "chosen" by the "actors." Slapping and kicking thus become foreplay, degradation and rape become consensual, cuts and bruises become signs of pleasure, and tears of pain become tears of sexual ecstasy.

We accept Marchiano's and other women's accounts of their abuse in the production of pornography. Given what we now know about the content of gay male pornography and the extent to which it mimics the individual and systemic harms in heterosexual pornography (Stoltenberg, 1989; Kendall, 2001), we must ask whether the men used to produce gay male pornography are also harmed in ways similar to the ways that women are harmed in heterosexual pornography.

GAY RIGHTS: DON'T THE MEN USED TO PRODUCE GAY MALE PORNOGRAPHY HAVE ANY?

Given the negative response to those exceptional women who have spoken out about the abuse and trauma they were subjected to in the pornography industry, it is not surprising that few gay men have been willing to report their own experiences of harm or address the harms perpetrated against men in the gay pornography industry. The little information that has been made available, however, discussed below, reveals that the industry producing gay male pornography is similar to its heterosexual counterpart.

A 1985 study[4] examined the histories of gay and bisexual men used in and by the gay male pornography industry. This study exposes the financial and emotional vulnerability of some of those men, how they view themselves, and how others see them. These young men begin to see themselves in the same ways that they are viewed and sexualized by the industry. This view eventually results in considerable harm:

> Chris J. is 26 years old and has appeared in over one hundred gay films and numerous magazines. He "enjoys" heavy S&M ("all the queens in the leather bars are a bunch of pansies"), and is known for his "ravenous rectum." At a recent gay filmmakers awards show he was publicly whipped, led around the stage by a chain attached to a dog collar around his neck, and then penetrated by a large dildo; he says he loved it. He was recently arrested and charged with assault with a deadly weapon, after having tied up and beaten black and blue (with a belt) [another pornography actor]. (Los Angeles Study (1985), reported in Kendall, 1993)

Chris J. is not only known for his ravenous rectum, but *as* his ravenous rectum. He, the young man, becomes invisible except as a rectum desperately waiting to be filled/raped/fed by a cock. In the discourse of pornography, this becomes his identity which he appears to internalize. The practice of combining humiliation (such as being publicly whipped or led around the stage by a chain) with sexual expression seems counter to sexual liberation, if sexual liberation includes sexual justice, equality, mutuality, and respect. Where is justice in the whipping of another person? Where is the liberation in watching someone being led around by a chain? Who here is liberated; who is experiencing justice? Where is the equality, the mutuality, the respect?

Some gay or bisexual men leave home because of a homophobic response to their sexual orientation. Because they are young and poorly educated, sex businesses are one of the few economic options open to them. Because gay men and bisexual men are defined by both society and the gay community itself in sexual terms, many of these young men come to view themselves exclusively in sexual terms. Being used in pornography thus becomes a means of validating their sexuality in a society and subculture that defines them as their sexuality while simultaneously degrading them because of it. For many of these men, sex businesses, while initially appealing, become a dead end.

Little is known about the men held forth as the paradigm of gay male attractiveness, the pornographic images from which, we are told, gay male identity is derived. Interviews with the young men from the Los Angeles Study noted above, however, suggest that their actual experiences are very much like the realities of the pornography they are used in. The fictionalized "depictions" of harm, mistreatment, abuse, scorn, ridicule, and humiliation become, upon closer examination, presentations of real people, suffering real abuse:

Jim Y. was raised by abusive, alcoholic parents. When Jim told his parents he was gay, at age 13, his father tried to kill him with a large kitchen knife. Jim left home at 17. At 19 he met Frank H., about ten years his senior, who was to become his lover. Frank was making a pornographic film at the time. He convinced Jim to appear in it. Jim played a new arrival to the big city who engages in S&M, including bootlicking, bondage, beating with a belt, fisting, and implied murder. This film was the first to show fisting and Jim says he is convinced that it created the gay interest in fisting as a sexual behavior. The film also reflected the S&M relationship that Jim and Frank were to share for the next decade . . . Jim has been trying to avoid S&M sex, and believes that his sexual behaviour was a way he sought out contact with his abusive father. He also recognizes that much sexual "fantasy" can be destructive. Jim was diagnosed with AIDS, and now fears that he has lost whatever chance he might have had to turn his life around. (Los Angeles Study, 1985, page 20)[5]

Jim's story articulates the use of extremely vulnerable men for the production of pornography. A severely abused child, Jim describes the impairment that his childhood abuse created in his ability to form a mutual, equitable, and healthy adult relationship. Stating that his sexual behavior was a way that he sought out contact with his abusive father, Jim appears to have "chosen" an adult relationship that mirrors the abusive, degrading childhood relationship he had with his parents. He attempted to find a corrective experience for the abuse he was subjected to as a child, only to find that abuse reinforced through sex. This is commonly seen in adults with histories of childhood abuse (Meston, Heiman, & Trapnell, 1999; Higgins & McCabe, 2000; Dilorio, Hartwell, & Hansen, 2002).

Reynolds (1995) interviewed a number of gay pornography actors and arrived at a conclusion similar to the 1985 Los Angeles Study. With respect to child sexual abuse, for example, Reynolds notes:

One of the less pleasant things I learned in researching this article is that there's another thing which many of the models have in common: sexual molestation as children. Ray is a prime example of that horror. 'I didn't know my father until I was nine years old and I went to live with him. He was a drug addict and when I was ten, he held a knife to my throat and told me he would show me what men and women did. I was raped so brutally that I had to go to the emergency ward of the hospital. The doctors ignored the evidence and sent me home, where he continued to rape me for three years, often trading me out to his friends in exchange for drugs.' (Reynolds, 1995, page 15)

Ronnie Larsen, director of the documentary, *Shooting Porn* and the off-Broadway production of *Making Porn*, has worked with many of today's better-known gay porn "actors." Discussing some of the men he interviewed and worked with, Larsen explains that "to work with them was to see them as they are: immature and deeply disturbed-men who desperately need psychotherapy." Illustrating the link between pornography and prostitution, and the harms of both, he states:

> . . . Ryan Idol has cried on my couch that he didn't ever want to make another porn video or turn another trick. Well, he's still advertising . . . as an 'escort'! Everyone pretends the Industry is such a big happy family–bullshit! They're miserable, unhappy people. So many of the models say they don't like turning tricks, but they continue to do it because they cannot see any other way to make a living–they can't act and most come and go so quickly. Christ, it's such a pathetic industry. . . . so many are sick and need help. (Reynolds, 1988, p. 59)

Nicholas Iacona (whose stage name was Joey Stefano), who acted in more than 35 hard-core gay pornography videos, ran away from home at age 15, shortly after the death of his father (Isherwood, 1996). With little education and "in search of the American dream," Iacona was exploited by an industry quick to market his youth and good looks. The result was tragic. Although Iacona eventually "hustled his way through thousands of dollars paid to him by clients around the globe" (Isherwood, 1996), all of the fame and contacts could not save this young man's life, and evidence suggests that few of his "fans" even tried. From pornography, Iacona entered prostitution, believing that the wealthy men who used him "as their trophy" (Mitchell, 2000, p. 9) would help him land roles in TV commercials and Hollywood blockbusters–none of which happened. Iacona, naïve and vulnerable, was swept up in an industry that only "loved him for his body and sexual prowess, nothing more" (Mitchell, 2000, p. 9).[6]

In time, Iacona's star status faded as fresher, younger men replaced him as gay men's preferred sex object. Having done nothing with his life but "sell sex," and finding that his friends in the industry had less time for him than for the fresher, more popular and now in demand newer boys, and increasingly addicted to a drug habit and eventually HIV-positive, Iacona, like many before him, fell into a state of despair from which he never recovered. On February 20, 1994, he was found dead at the age of 26 in a motel from an apparent drug overdose (Isherwood, 1996).

Like many young prostitutes, Iacona was a traumatized adolescent, searching for a home, swept into a community that exploited his traumatic history. The pornography industry in turn benefited from his vulnerability. Iacona sold the only things he thought he had to an industry willing to exploit his insecurities and lack of self-confidence: his appearance and ability to perform. Once addicted to drugs and marketed as a sex-toy in prostitution, his exploitation and sexual use became easier.

Perpetration of physical harm against men in pornography is also evident in the life of Cal Culver, who appeared in gay pornography in the 1980s as Casey Donovan (Edmonson, 1998). Like Iacona, Culver's life typifies the fall from favour and eventual self-destruction of some of the men used to produce gay pornography. Culver too assumed that he could use pornography as a step toward mainstream success–success that was not forthcoming. However, his transformation from "smiling preppie" to "sexual predator" (Jordan, 1994, p. 47; Edmonson, 1998) was immortalized in his final movie, *Fucked-Up*, described by one of Culver's friends as follows:

> '*Fucked Up* was the saddest thing I had ever seen,' Rob Richards confided. 'It was a horrible film . . . Cal was so far gone, and he was being so used and abused. He was holding . . . a mayonnaise jar full of poppers or ethyl chloride . . . sitting in the corner of a room. These faceless people arrive and push toys and fists up into him. He's drooling, and it is absolutely terrifying . . . It was . . . a haunting study in self-destruction . . .' (Edmonson, 1998, pp. 223-224)

PORNOGRAPHY'S HARMS:
DOCUMENTING INEQUALITY AND EXPLOITATION

Despite the realities of men like Culver, some activists ignore the fact that some gay and bisexual men's actual physical and emotional abuse has been documented on film. Stychin (1995, p. 83), for example, has argued that there is no reason to believe that gay men are harmed during the production of pornography. This assertion risks trivializing abuse and overlooks the fact that gay male pornography uses real people, sexualized in situations that both promote and are violence, cruelty, degradation, dehumanization, and exploitation. Stychin states that statements which attempt to prove harm are unrealistic because, although:

> the Hollywood film industry in general is highly exploitive of workers, it would be trite to suggest that the actors who portrayed Jews in the film

Schindler's List, for example, were degraded in the way the characters they portrayed were within the narrative structure of the movie. (Stychin, 1995, p. 83)

In response, it is not trite to assume that the pornographic presentation of a young man being penetrated by a 12 inch dildo might actually do some real physical damage to him or that the burning of a cigarette on human flesh, presented as a sexual stimulus, might cause tissue damage. Not is it trite to argue that the pornographic presentation of unsafe sex involves two real men engaging in an unsafe sexual practice and that the actual deaths of some of these people could have been avoided if, as Stychin asserts, this presentation had in fact been fictional. Describing the production of heterosexual pornography, Torres explains:

> . . . the nature of adult motion picture production encourages unusual and unsafe working conditions. Producers have been known to force actors to do sexual acts that they would really rather not do. In most of the productions, producers do not test the performers for sexually transmitted diseases and do not require that performers practice safe sex. Additionally, some producers ignore the risks associated with allowing a performer, who may be infected with HIV, to perform in a film. In these situations, the performers are faced with the greatest risk of contracting AIDS. (Torres, 1989, p. 99)

Similar dangers exist in the gay pornography industry. In his work on the life of Joey Stefano, Isherwood describes the industry's reluctance to reveal Stefano's HIV+ status either to the public or to the men paired with Stefano in his films. Nor were precautions taken to ensure that condoms were used to protect Stefano or his fellow actors in his early films (Isherwood, 1990).

The gay pornography industry promoted safer-sex early in the AIDS crisis by introducing condoms into their pornographic videos and incorporating their use into their storylines (Skee, 1997, p. 53). However, unsafe sex is now creeping back into gay porn videos. One director justifies this trend by arguing that:

> . . . being gay is about sex for gay men and it's about dick, and we've been denied that. While I may have some personal problems with it, pornography is only porn if it represents the culture it is a part of. Gay men want unsafe sex. I don't give a damn about responsibility. This is business, and someone is going to do a video without condoms and get rich doing it, so it may as well be me. (R. Douglas quoted in Skee, 1997, p. 53-54)

Surely, there is more to being gay or bisexual than sex and dick. Perhaps more eloquently than he realizes, Douglas exposes the abusiveness, degradation and harm inherent to and caused by gay pornography, as well as the callous disregard for the well being of the men used to produce it. His definition of being a gay male includes the notion of a dick that proves itself (and thus the manliness and gay identity of the human being to which it is attached) by being stuck into someone else, often through force sexualized as normal. This is similar to the definition of masculinity found in and promoted through heterosexual pornography, which reinforces the rigid gender hierarchies that are at the core of both sexism and homophobia.

RACISM IN GAY PORNOGRAPHY/PROSTITUTION

The production and use of sexually explicit materials that sexualize racist stereotypes and degrade members of racial minorities for the purpose of sexual arousal is common in both heterosexual and gay male pornography. The message conveyed in some gay male publications, for example, is one in which gay Asian men are presented as wanting to be sexually subordinated and violated by a more dominant, stereotypical white male.

An example of this type of publication is the magazine *Oriental Guys (OG)* which, although about Asian men, is directed at the Caucasian gay male market. Although the magazine does not present violence or physical pain, it sexualizes youth and Asian ethnicity while connecting the use of these young men with stories of, among other things, older white men cruising Asian boys and male prostitutes. Young Asian men are described as "pearls of the orient," "easy to find," "sushi," "accessible," and "available." The photo spreads of young Asian men face down with buttocks elevated, are often accompanied by "news" articles that tell the reader how, for example, to recruit young Balinese men.[7] *Oriental Guys'* "letters to the editor" detail the success of the magazine's Caucasian readers' overseas sexual conquests.

OG sexualizes racism and sexual exploitation. This is its intended result and it is marketed as such. The publication justifies through sex the attitudes and inequalities that powerfully interconnect racism and sexism: the white male is described as one who seeks out an inferior Asian other; The young Asian is presented as ready and willing to serve the white man's sexual fantasies. The white male is superior; the Asian male inferior. The resulting harm to racial justice is an affront to all persons seeking equality.

In a similar vein, the gay male pornography user is offered materials in which African-American men are presented as violent sexual predators with large sexual organs who want to emasculate white men through rape or in which the same men are presented as sexually desiring to be the slaves of white men who need to reaffirm a masculinity threatened by the Black male.

Many of the stories in the magazine, *Sex Stop*,[8] for example, sexualize racial difference, and sex ·with or between young boys and incest. In the story, "Boy Buys Bicycle by Riding Man's Face," for example, the author describes how he and his friend were paid by an older Black male for sex when they were boys. Similarly, in the drawings of *Tom of Finland*,[9] African American men are portrayed as predators (for example, one white man is shown being assaulted by four Black men) or being exploited by groups of white men (for example, in one drawing a Black man is whipped with a belt by two white men). In the same collection, a Black man is restrained by two white police officers who are holding their penises and are preparing to rape him. Racial inequality appears to be the norm throughout these publications and much of what is sexualized relies heavily on racial stereotype.

With respect to the pornography now available via the Internet, in the recent documentary, *The Fall of Communism as Seen Through Gay Porn* (Horton, 1999), we see first hand the use of young Russian boys and men who, trying to survive in a devastated economy, find themselves trapped in prostitution and, exploited by pornographers, photographed or filmed for little if any money. The film powerfully documents what some gay men will buy and what others will do to ensure that the product they want is available via the Internet or other media. While horrifying in its own right, the documentary reveals only the tip of the iceberg in so far as the abuse of these young men is concerned. The film does not, for example, discuss the 1996 "discovery that boys from Bratislava were being abducted and transported to Holland to make films in which they were tortured" (Horton, 1999).

Reviewing the content of the Internet pornography now being distributed by some pornographers, it is also clear that unsafe sexual practices are being performed by and on young men with few life choices. Men wanting food and shelter or who are addicted to drugs are not empowered enough to demand safe sex practices when filmed or photographed. Add to this the growing number of websites that now sell "homemade" pornography (sometimes of men who are unaware that they are being filmed, and of others who are unaware that the pictures taken will be sold or seen by others), and one questions how "safety" of any sort can be guaranteed.

Given what we know about the pornography industry as a whole, about the lives of some of those who work in it, and about the content of gay male pornography specifically, it seems unreasonable to argue that all of the materials that are now being sold to gay men worldwide present only "fictional" scenarios of abuse. It is easier and cheaper to simply show the real thing–practices which will likely continue as long as vulnerable young men are sexually available and unable to demand safety and so long as gay and bisexual men continue to demand materials which market and sexualize harm and inequality.

CONCLUSION

If anything can violate a person's freedom and integrity more than direct sexual and physical abuse, it is the mass marketing of that abuse as sexual entertainment (LEAF Factum, 1990). Scenarios of sexual violence and pain presented as pleasurable in pornography may document real degradation that is neither pleasurable nor fiction. The implication for gay male equality is this: the use and abuse of young men in scenarios of degradation, dehumanization and violence must not be viewed as integral to gay liberation. Those who are marginalized as a result of abuse history, class, and race (or a combination of these) are also the men who are most in need of community support. At best, it is insensitive to use them for the sake of someone else's sexual expression and "enjoyment." At worst, it amounts to participation in their abuse.

The argument has been made that the harms inflicted on these young men will be reduced once more gay men themselves are provided a greater role in the production of gay male pornography (Stychin, 1992). We are not convinced. Even if efforts can be made to use less vulnerable "actors," the fact remains that the presentation of what is presently justified as the source of gay male identity (that is, abuse and inequality) is precisely what makes gay male pornography lucrative. Such a foundation makes suspect the industry's commitment to equality, justice, and freedom.

Eroticized racism, for example, is remarkably profitable. Discussing the racial objectification of Asian men in gay male films produced by Asian men, Fung explains that "the race of the producer is no automatic guarantee of 'consciousness' about these issues" (Fung, 1991, p. 160). Similarly, the pornographer's sexual orientation does not guarantee that his product will be less harmful for those used to produce the inequality which makes gay pornography financially rewarding in the first place. Gay male pornography is profitable precisely because it presents what those who purchase it find pleasurable: sexual hierarchy. The use of young men in scenarios of degradation and objectification is required for this model of gay male identity. The pornography market provides a profit motive for exploiting the most vulnerable in our community and the availability of expendable youth provides little incentive to protect them when the alternative is reduced profit. As one young man prostituted on the street explained

The established gay community will never really do anything for young, poor gays because poverty will force young gays to provide economical sex services. Let's face it. Who wants to have sex with an old troll? (Seto, 1993, p. 18)

Gay male pornography justifies, through sex, the subordination and object-ification of real people. While we support the political advocacy of sexuality rights, we do not favor ignoring pain, suffering, and sexual inequality in the guise of sexual freedom. From the evidence reviewed in this paper and else-where, it is clear that, within the context of a racist, misogynist, and homopho-bic culture, when gay and bisexual men defend the production and distribution of gay male pornography in the name of liberation, they inhibit liberation by sexualizing and trivializing trauma. Working for our own healing and social liberation requires that we address this inequality directly rather than deny it, minimize it, and re-enact it within and through pornography.

NOTES

1. On December 20, 2000, the Supreme Court of Canada ruled unanimously in the case of *Little Sisters Book and Art Emporium*, a case concerning the right of Canada customs to detain lesbian and gay male pornography, that gay male pornography vio-lates the sex equality test for pornographic harm first set down by the Court in its 1992 decision in *R v. Butler*. In *Butler*, the Court ruled that legal efforts aimed at prohibiting the distribution of pornography were constitutionally sound because pornography un-dermines the rights of all Canadians to be treated equally on the basis of sex. In *Little Sisters*, the Court ruled that lesbian and gay male pornography should not be excluded from the same sex equality-based approach.

2. In *Little Sisters*, a number of gay rights groups argued that the entire framework of production for gay male pornography is different from the framework for the pro-duction and consumption of heterosexual pornography, primarily because it is pro-duced by gay men for a gay male audience. Because of this, these groups suggested that gay pornography avoids the harms that result from the production of heterosexual por-nography (Little Sisters Factum, 1999, page 24). The arguments raised in the *Little Sis-ters* case are examined in more detail in Kendall (2001).

3. The use of the words "model" or "actor" risks glamorizing the very real experi-ences of many of the people presented as "actors" and the reality that they, as real people, do experience. The seriousness of this point should not be underestimated. Those who support gay male pornography tend to overlook the fact that the "images/models" in gay male pornography are real people, upon many of whom direct physical contact, often in the form of violence presented through sex, is inflicted in order to produce that which is defended as fantasy–a political euphemism or cover for abuse. It should not be assumed that these young men are always willing participants, particularly when free will is largely defined by one's ability to exercise some social and economic independence. The young men who appear in gay male pornography do so for a number of reasons, but

"choice" is not always a factor. This corresponds to the findings of those who have documented the lives of the women used in heterosexual pornography.

4. The study was unpublished because the author wanted to ensure confidentiality to his sources. In 1993, Christopher Kendall was granted permission to publish some of the author's findings on the condition that he did not identify him or the men he interviewed. He agreed to this request and we continue to protect the author's identity and sources in this paper. See Kendall (1993).

5. Jim's description of fisting, as first promoted in his films and then copied by gay men, is reminiscent of the forced oral penetration inflicted on Linda Marchiano in the film "Deep Throat"–a sexual practice later copied by men and directed at their female partners, many of whom suffered considerable physical harm as a result (MacKinnon & Dworkin, 1988, p. 215).

6. Stefano's use of hustling for drugs is documented by Isherwood (1990). Initially, Stefano's status as "the" gay porn star, commanded huge prostitution fees. The higher fees did not, however, command any more self-respect: The decision to escort wasn't exactly an agonizing one for Stefano. He had hustled for drug money in Philadelphia from an early age. . . . One of LA's biggest music moguls used to pay him $1,000 to go have sex with him. . . . It was on a call to the same music mogul that it was brought home to Stefano that if he had moved up the scale in his own eyes, an expensive prostitute, in the eyes of others, he was hardly different from a cheap one. "He came home really hurt and upset. He felt like now he was a big porn star, but people still treated him the same way: 'Here's the money–do your thing.'" Stefano's already fragile self-esteem would suffer even more when, after his status as one of the best had vanished, he was left having to hustle for far less money in order to pay for a drug habit which had peaked during his heyday as a performer. Although Stefano had sworn he would not return to the industry, he soon felt and found that sex was all had and all he was wanted for. Desperate, he again found himself turning to an industry quick to exploit his vulnerability (Isherwood, 1996, p. 178).

7. From *Oriental Guys*, Issue 4, Spring 1989, p.10. The specific examples provided in this paper are pornographic materials that were defended by gay activists in the *Little Sisters* trial. A more in-depth overview of the exhibits, how they were summarized and their effects is provided in Kendall (2001).

8. Little Sisters Trial Exhibits, Exhibit number 200, *Sex Stop: True Revelations and Strange Happenings From Wheeler, Volume 3*.

9. Little Sisters Trial Exhibits, Exhibits 29 and 30, *Tom of Finland Retrospective I and II*.

REFERENCES

Alien, D.M., "Young Male Prostitutes: A Psychological Study," (1980). 9 *Archives of Sexual Behavior 9: 399.*

Altman, D. (1980). What Changed in the Seventies? in Gay Left Collective (eds.) *Homosexuality, Power, and Politics*. London: Alyson and Busby. 52-63.

Anonymous (1985). Gay Pornography: Sometimes Men Possess Men. Unpublished paper. Los Angeles, California.

Briere, J. (1992). *Child abuse trauma: Theory and treatment of the lasting effects*. Newbury Park, CA. Sage Publications.

Browne, A., and Finklehor, D. (1986). Impact of child sexual abuse: A review of the research. *Psychological Bulletin 99: 66-77.*

Burger, J. (1995). One Handed Histories: The Eroto-Politics of Gay Male Video Pornography. NY: Harrington Park Press.

Cassese, J. (2000). Introduction: Integrating the experience of childhood sexual trauma in gay men. *Journal of Gay and Lesbian Social Services* 12(1/2): 1-17.

Cole, S. (1989). *Pornography and the Sex Crisis. Toronto,* CA: Amanita Press.

Coleman, E. (1989). The Development of Male Prostitution Activity Among Gay and Bisexual Adolescents. *Journal of Homosexuality* 17(1): 131-140.

Connell, R.W. (1995). *Masculinities.* University of California Press. Los Angeles, CA.

Dilorio, C., Hartwell, T., and Hansen, N. (2002). Childhood sexual abuse and risk behaviors among men at high risk for HIV infection. In *American Journal of Public Health.* 92(2): 214-221.

Dines, G., Jensen, R., & Russo, A. (1998). *Pornography: The Production and Consumption of Inequality.* New York: Routledge Press.

Dworkin, A. (1989). *Pornography: Men Possessing Women.* New York: Putnam's.

Dworkin, A. & MacKinnon, C. (1988). Pornography and Civil Rights: A New Day for Women's Equality Organizing Against Pornography. Minneapolis, MN.

Edmonson, R. (1998). *Boy in the Sand: Casey Donovan–All American Sex Star.* Los Angeles: Alyson Books.

Factum of the Intervener. (1990) Women's Legal Education and Action Fund (LEAF) in R v. Butler, File No. 22191, 1990. Available from the Supreme Court of Canada.

Factum of the Appellant Little Sisters Book and Art Emporium 1999. In the case of Little Sisters Book and Art Emporium v AG Canada. Court File No. 26858, July 30, 1999.

Fajer, M.A. (1992). Can Real Men Eat Quiche Together? Storytelling, Gender-Role Stereotypes and Legal Protections for Lesbians and Gay Men. 46 *U. Miami L. Rev* 511.

Farley, M. (2003). Prostitution and the Invisibility of Harm. *Women & Therapy* 26(3/4): 247-280.

Fischer, B. (1980). Young Male Prostitutes: A Psychological Study. *Archives of Sexual Behavior* 9: 399.

Frosh, S. (2001). *Young Masculinities.* London: Palgrave Publishing.

Fung, R. (1991). Looking for My Penis: The Eroticized Asian in Gay Video Porn. In *Bad Object Choices* (eds.) *How Do I Look: Queer Film and Video.* Seattle: Bay Press. P 145-160.

Funk, R.E. (1993). *Stopping Rape: A challenge for men.* Philadelphia: New Society Publishers.

Funk, R.E. (2003). Creating a collaborative community response to teen dating abuse. In A. Grieg (ed.) *Partners in Change: Working with Men to End Gender-based Violence.* Geneva: INSTRAW Publishing. p. 104-126.

Furnold, R. (1998). Male Juvenile Prostitution. Unpublished Masters Thesis University of Southern California, Los Angeles, CA.

Gill, M., & Tutty, L.M. (1997). Sexual identity issues for male survivors of childhood sexual abuse: A qualitative study. *Journal of Child Sexual Abuse* 6(3): 121-135.

Herman, J. (1992). *Trauma and Recovery.* Thousand Oaks, CA: Sage Publications.

Higgins, D.J., & McCabe, M.P. (2000). Relationships between different types of maltreatment during childhood and adjustment in adulthood. *Child Maltreatment* 5(3): 261-272.

Horton, A. J. (1999). Building a New Europe: William E Jones's The Fall of Communism As Seen in Gay Pornography. *Central European Review*: 35. *http://www.ce-review.org*. Accessed May 24, 1999.

Hughes, T.L, Johnson, T., & Wilsnack, S.C. (2001). Sexual assault and alcohol abuse: A comparison of lesbians and heterosexual women. *Journal of Substance Abuse* 13: 515-532.

Isherwood, C. (1996). *Wonder Bread and Ecstasy: The Life and Death of Joey Stefano*. Los Angeles: Alyson Publications.

Itzin, C. (1992). *Pornography: Women, Violence, and Civil Liberties*. Oxford: Oxford University Press.

Jeffreys, S. (1996). Heterosexuality and the Desire for Gender. D. Richardson (ed.) *Theorizing Heterosexuality*. Buckingham, England: Open University Press. p. 75-90.

Jensen, R. (1998). Getting it up for Politics: Gay Male Sexuality and Radical Lesbian Feminism. In S. Miles & E. Rofes (eds.) *Opposite Sex*. New York: New York University Press. p. 147-170.

Jordan, P. (1994). The Naked VCR *Outrage* 131: 45-48.

Kendall, C. (2001). The harms of gay male pornography: A sex equality perspective post Little Sisters Book and Art Emporium. *Gay and Lesbian Law Journal 10:* 42-80.

Kendall, C. (1999). Gay Male Pornography/Gay Male Community: Power Without Consent, Mimicry Without Subversion. In J. Kuypers (ed.) *Men and Power*. Halifax, Nova Scotia: Fernwood Press. p. 157-172.

Kendall, C. (1997). Gay Male Pornography After Little Sisters Book and Art Emporium: A Call for Gay Male Cooperation in the Struggle for Sex Equality. *Wisconsin Women's Law Journal* 1 (1): 21-82.

Kendall, C. (1995). Gay Male Pornography and the Sexualization of Masculine Identity. In Lederer, L. and Delgado, R. (eds.), *The Price We Pay: The Case Against Racist Speech, Hate Propaganda and Pornography*. New York: Farrar, Strauss, & Giroux. 141-150.

Kendall, C. (1993). Gay Male Pornography and the Pursuit of Masculinity. *Saskatchewan Law Review* 57(1): 21-58.

Koppelman, A. (1994). "Why Discrimination Against Lesbians and Gay Men is Sex Discrimination." *New York University Law Review* 69: 197.

Koppelman, A. (1988). "The Miscegenation Analogy: Sodomy Law as Sex Discrimination." *Yale Law Journal* 98: 145.

Langeland, W., & Hartgers, C. (1998). "Child sexual and physical abuse and alcoholism: A review." *J of Studies on Alcohol* 59(3): 336-348.

Law, S. (1988). "Homosexuality and the Social Meaning of Gender." *Wisconsin Law Review 187* at 218.

Lederer, L. (1980). Then and Now: An Interview with a Former Pornography Model. In L. Lederer (ed.) *Take Back the Night*. New York: William Morrow. p. 57-70.

Lederer, L., & Delgado, R. (1995). *The Price We Pay: The Case Against Racist Speech, Hate Propaganda and Pornography*. New York, NY. Hill and Wang Press.

Lovelace, L. (1980). *Ordeal* New Jersey. Citadel Press.

MacKinnon, C. (2001). *Sex Equality*. New York: Foundation Press.

MacKinnon, C., & Dworkin, A. (1997). *In Harm's Way: The Pornography Civil Rights Hearings*. Boston: Harvard University Press.

MacKinnon, C. (1989). *Toward a Feminist Theory of the State*. Boston: Harvard University Press.

Maltz, W., & Homan, B. (1987). *Incest and Sexuality: A guide to understanding and healing*. Lexington: Lexington Books.

Meston, C.M., & Heiman, J.R. (2000). Sexual abuse and sexual function: An examination of sexually relevant cognitive processes. *Journal of Consulting and Clinical Psychology* 68(3): 399-406.

Meston, C.M., Heiman, J.R., & Trapnell, P.D. (1999). The relationship between early abuse and adult sexuality. *Journal of Sex Research* 36(4): 385-395.

Mitchell, S.P. (2000). Ifs and Butts: The Life and Death of a Porn Star on the Stage. *West Side Observer*, February 4, 2000.

Ouimette, P.C., Kimerling, R., Shaw, J., & Moos, R.H. (2000). Physical and sexual abuse among women and men with substance use disorders. *Alcoholism Treatment Quarterly*, 18(3): 7-17.

Pearlman, L. (1994). Theorizing Lesbian Oppression and the Politics of Outness in the Case of Waterman v National Life Assurance: A Beginning in Lesbian Human Rights/Equality Jurisprudence. *Canadian Journal of Women and the Law* 7(2): 454.

Pease, B. (2000). *Recreating men: Postmodern masculinity politics*. Thousand Oaks: Sage Publications.

Pharr, S. (1988). *Homophobia: A Weapon of Sexism*. Little Rock: Clarendon Press.

Ray, S.L. (2001). Male survivors' perspectives of incest/sexual abuse. *Perspectives in Psychiatric Care* 37(2): 49-59.

Reynolds, D. (1995). I'm Ready for My Cum Shot Mr. De Mille. *Outrage* 147: 12-15.

Reynolds, D. (1998). Documenting America's Schizoid Sexuality. *Outrage* 178: 58-62.

Rich, A. (1980). Compulsory Heterosexuality and Lesbian Existence. 5(4) *Signs: Journal of Women in Culture and Society* 5(4) 63.

Russell, D. (1989). Pornography and Rape: A Causal Model. *Political Psychology* 9, 41.

Russell, D. (1993). *Pornography: The Evidence of Harm*. Berkeley: Russell Publications.

Seto, D. (1993). Caste and Castaways: Welcome to Polk St. *Bay Area Reporter*. July 29.

Skee, M. (1997). Laid Bare. *Frontiers Magazine* 16(8): 53.

Stoltenberg, J. (1989). *Refusing to Be a Man*. New York: Meridian Books.

Stoltenberg, J. (1990a). You Can't Fight Homophobia and Protect the Pornographers at the Same Time: An Analysis of What Went Wrong With Hardwick. In D. Leidholt and J. Raymond (eds.) *The Sexual Liberals and the Attack on Feminism*. New York: Athene, Press. p 184-190.

Stoltenberg, J. (1990b). Gays and the Pro-Pornography Movement: Having the Hots for Sex Discrimination. In M. Kimmel (ed.) *Men Confront Pornography*. New York: Crown Publishers. p 248-262.

Stychin, C. (1992). Exploring the Limits: Feminism and the Legal Regulation of Gay Male Pornography. *Vermont Law Review* 16: 857-910.

Stychin, C. (1995). *Law's Desire: Sexuality and the Limits of Justice*. London: Routledge Press.

Sunstein, C. (1994). Homosexuality and the Constitution. *Indiana Law Journal* 70:1.

Torres, F.G. (1989). Lights, Camera, Actionable Negligence: Transmission of the AIDS Virus During Adult Motion Picture Production. *Hastings Communication and Entertainment Law Journal* 13: 89.

Valdes, F. (1995). Queers, Sissies, Dykes, and Tomboys: Deconstructing The Conflation of "Sex," "Gender," and "Sexual Orientation" in Euro-American Law and Society. *California Law Review* 83: 3-376.

CASES

R v. Butler, [1992] 1 SCR 452 (SCC).

Little Sisters Book and Art Emporium v. Canada (Minister of Justice), 2000 SCC 69, File No. 26858, unreported. The case can be found at *http://www.lexum.umontreal. ca/csc-scc/en/rec/html/sisters.en.html.*

Prostitution Online

Donna M. Hughes

SUMMARY. The technological innovations and unregulated use of the Internet have created a global medium for men's sexual exploitation and abuse of women and children. The sex industry has aggressively adopted every new information technology to increase men's sexual access to women and children. A mutually beneficial relationship exists between the Internet and sex industries. New technologies enable pimps to market women and children in prostitution or related activities, such as online strip shows, sex shows, and commercial voyeurism. The global communications forums have increased the visibility and exposure of women and children being exploited and abused, while conversely, increasing the privacy and communication of the men who exploit and abuse them. These forums normalize men's exploitative and abuse behaviors. Violence and humiliation are eroticized. The combined experience of using new information technologies, finding a supportive community on the Internet, and having a sexual experience is positively reinforcing and empowering to perpetrators. Viewing and interacting with women in online sex sites causes a loss of empathy for them as human beings. Women used in online sex shows are exploited and abused in ways that are both similar to the regular sex industry and unique to being online. In some instances, the abuse and exploitation is worse. More research is needed on

Donna M. Hughes, PhD, is Professor and Carlson Endowed Chair at University of Rhode Island, 316 Eleanor Roosevelt Hall, Kingston, RI (Email: dhughes@uri.edu). Printed with permission.

[Haworth co-indexing entry note]: "Prostitution Online." Hughes, Donna M. Co-published simultaneously in *Journal of Trauma Practice* (The Haworth Maltreatment & Trauma Press, an imprint of The Haworth Press, Inc.) Vol. 2, No. 3/4, 2003, pp. 115-131; and: *Prostitution, Trafficking, and Traumatic Stress* (ed: Melissa Farley) The Haworth Maltreatment & Trauma Press, an imprint of The Haworth Press, Inc., 2003, pp. 115-131. Single or multiple copies of this article are available for a fee from The Haworth Document Delivery Service [1-800-HAWORTH, 9:00 a.m. - 5:00 p.m. (EST). E-mail address: docdelivery@haworthpress.com].

http://www.haworthpress.com/store/product.asp?sku=J189
10.1300/J189v02n03_06

the use of new information technologies for the sexual exploitation and abuse of women and children.

> . . . it's pretty bad working at [an] adult [Web] site. . . . the abuse is way beyond what goes on at strip clubs . . ." (Email from Renee, May 19, 2000)

INTRODUCTION

The technological innovations and unregulated use of the Internet have created a global medium for men's sexual exploitation and abuse of women and children. Internet forums are used to advertise prostitution and compile men's experiences buying women and children in prostitution. Technological advances, such as live video chat, have enabled pimps to sell a range of sexually exploitative and abusive entertainment.

The global communications forums have increased the privacy and decreased the isolation of the men who exploit and abuse women and children. The Internet provides an anonymous network of support for perpetrators to share their experiences, legitimize their behavior, and advise and mentor less experienced men. Little pimps can advertise the availability of a few women; big pimps can offer live sex shows and online prostitution with women from anywhere in the world.

The Internet has enabled pimps and pornographers to distribute unlimited amounts of pornography, including extremely violent pornography and child pornography. At the end of 2001, there were 300,000 pornography sites on the Web. This is a 350% increase in the number of pornography sites from January to December 2001. From 1996 to 2001, the FBI documented a 1,280% increase in child pornography (Kellog, 2002).

The first section of this paper describes new Internet Web technologies and how they are used to promote prostitution and deliver online prostitution. These new Web technologies have increased sexual exploitation and abuse by making women and girls more visible and exposed, while enabling men to exploit and abuse women and children with more privacy and anonymity. The paper then describes men's increased capacity to harm women and children through new information technologies. Men's use of online communities as information networks is discussed and women's experiences in online stripping, sex shows, and voyeurism are described.

NEW WEB TECHNOLOGIES AND THEIR USE FOR PROSTITUTION

The sex industry has aggressively adopted, and in a few cases invented, Internet technologies to increase men's sexual access to women and children.

There are many modes of communication and forums online: email, ftp (file transfer protocol), newsgroups, the Web, chat, newsgroups, and peer-to-peer servers. Although a variety of forums are used, most of the activities related to prostitution are found on the World Wide Web (also called the Web). In a few cases, the content of newsgroups are archived on Web sites.

The Web started growing rapidly in 1994, after Netscape introduced the Netscape Web browser, which enabled transmission and viewing of Web pages with text, images, sound, and video.[1] From the beginning, sites on the Web became meeting places for sex offenders and exploiters of women and girls. The first Web-based prostitution business, A Personal Touch Services, from Seattle, Washington appeared in 1994 (Bosley, 1995). *The Internet Business Journal* described this site as the most significant Internet marketing innovation of 1994 (Strangelove, 1995). This endorsement of the sex industry's marketing on the Internet was an early indication of the mutually beneficial relationship between the Internet and sex industries (Hughes, 2000).

Advertisements for prostitution tourism followed in 1995. Alan J. Munn, from New York City, advertised group prostitution tours to the Dominican Republic and Nevada, USA on the Web in 1995. Calling himself PIMPS 'R' US, he offered four days and three night trips to a "wonderful setting" which includes "many female prostitutes." A tour guide on the trip provided "practical information about how to find and deal with prostitutes and how to arrange group orgies." On one night, Munn boasted, "oral sex (fellatio) is provided by an attractive female whore chosen by the tour guide" (Munn, 1995).

Advertisements for prostitution tours to Asia, Europe, and South America soon followed. Pimps offered "Tropical Paradise Vacations" to Central America and the Caribbean for "single men." An advertisement for Erotic Vacations to Costa Rica quoted a price, which included double occupancy rooms and intra-country flights, booked for two. Men were told: "Your companion [a euphemism for prostituted woman] will meet you at your hotel . . ." (The Travel Connection, 1995).

Before the Web came into popular usage, newsgroups on Usenet offered information regarding prostitution. The newsgroup alt.sex.services (later renamed alt.sex.prostitution) was formed for men to write about their experiences buying women and girls in prostitution, and to give advice to other men (Atta and M., 1997). When the Web became available, postings from this newsgroup were archived into a Web site called The World Sex Guide, which provides "comprehensive, sex-related information about every country in the world." The slogan of The World Sex Guide in 1996 was "Fuckers of the world unite!" In 1997, it changed to "Where do you want to fuck today?" and in 1998, changed to the more pretentious sounding "A research project about prostitution worldwide" (Atta and M., 1996, 1997, 1998).

Other Web sites dedicated to information about finding women in prostitution in one region appeared online, such as PunterNet, which specializes in locating and reviewing women in prostitution in the United Kingdom (http://www.punternet.com). In these forums, men use misogynistic and pornographic language to rate their experiences with prostituted women. The women are rated more favorably if the men are able to coerce them into sex acts that are painful, risky, or humiliating. Men specify street addresses on where to find special kinds of sex or victims. The following posts from the World Sex Guide offer tips on obtaining children in Europe:

> (1). Street girls, Some of the girls are young, really young, but don't imagine them "clean." They live more or less on the street. They will join your car. They have places which you can reach in about 10 minutes by car. Mostly empty parking lots. (Frankfurt, Germany, 2000)

> (2). [. . . . .], the street where very young girls hang out. You might find 12-15-year-old girls here . . . (Copenhagen, Denmark)

> (3). On down the street . . . some younger scared looking girls in doorways. They didn't come out to talk. (Berlin, Germany, 1996)

In 1995, a new information technology called live videoconferencing enabled live video and audio connection between users (White Pine & Cornell University, 1995). Pimps immediately adopted this new technology for online prostitution through live person-to-person video and audio transmission. By late 1995, live videoconferencing was delivering live strip shows and sex shows to buyers over the Internet (Rose, 1997). By either keyboard or telephone, the buyers could communicate with the women in the sex show and make requests for what they wanted the women to do. The viewer could be in another state, or even another continent from the actual show. One of the first live videoconferencing sex industry sites was Virtual Dreams. The site advertised itself as follows:

> Virtual Dreams uses cutting-edge technology to bring you the most beautiful girls in the world. Using our software and your computer, you can interact real time and one-on-one with the girl of your dreams. Ask her anything you wish–she is waiting to please you! (Virtual Connections, 1995)

In 2002, all large sex industry subscription sites on the Web included live strip and sex shows, referred to as live video chat. Viewers can watch passively, interact by voice or keyboard, or direct the sex acts performed. Multiple viewers can be linked at one time, or viewers can pay extra for a private show.

Specialized companies produce "streaming video content" for sex industry sites on the Web. For example, women act out pornographic scenarios in 8-by-8 foot cubicles setup in a warehouse in Seattle, at one company (Wired for Sex, 1998). Stage sets included a health club, bedroom, shower, and dungeon, each with a microphone and speakers so the strippers and the buyers can communicate. The men often ask the women to give special signals to indicate that the performance is live, and that they are in direct contact with the women (Rose, 1997).

In 1999, the scope of live video chat for online prostitution came to world attention when a man from the U.S. announced that he was opening a live "rape camp" online (http://www.rapecamp.com). Men were given the opportunity to pay for and watch acts of rape and torture perpetrated against Asian women in Phnom Penh. Viewers made requests for acts that they wanted to see committed against the women (Hughes, 2000b).

Sex offenders or exploiters may use video capture technology to record the transmissions of the live video chat sessions. Thus, live sex shows can be recorded and repeatedly watched. The videos may be considered "trophies" if the women or children responded to the men's requests.

Web sites facilitate the marketing of women by pimps. Many escort services and brothels advertise on the Web. Photographs of women in the brothels are increasingly available on Web sites.

Men communicate with the pimps and book "appointments" through the Web or by email. Message boards on brothels' Web sites encourage men to inquire about what sex acts they can buy with different women. The following is from the Web message board of a brothel in Prague.

> I understand . . . you have, 6 girls our more, ATT [sic] the time, girls are from Ukraine. I will be in Praha, late August 2000, . . . me [sic] flights is from Iceland to Copenhagen and from Copenhagen to Praha. . . . I wold like to stay in your house the first 2 nights when I am testing your girls after that I will know which of your girls I like. . . . I will have one of your girls, one hour at the time in your house . . . I wold prefer to have sex with all of them, and then chosen one of the to stay in me hotel four 2 night after thatch, is thatch [sic] ok with you? Are your girls shaved? [full name] Iceland [Email address] 01.07.00. (Milas Holiday and Escort Service, 2001)

Pimps use computer technologies to maintain surveillance of women in prostitution. Cameras linked to computers (Web cams) transmit live images.

With these cameras, pimps monitor women from remote locations, which could be either another room in a brothel or any location with an Internet connection. In Yorkshire, England, one pimp planned to maintain control of an 18-year-old girl from his prison cell. After his arrest, he transported her to a studio for live sex shows on the Internet. He planned to continue to pimp and monitor her online performances from prison (personal communication with anonymous source in UK, May 2001).

Live video broadcasting on the Internet enabled pimps to sell online voyeurism. By setting up houses with live video cameras (video cams) in each room, they created commercial voyeurism. Members pay a subscription fee to watch the women eating, sleeping, taking a shower, dressing, and going to the toilet (VoyeurDorm.com, 1999).

As new technologies become available, pimps, exploiters, and abusers of women quickly adopt them.

INTERNET TECHNOLOGIES: INCREASING THE IMBALANCE OF POWER

In some cases, prostitution Web sites are little more than electronic versions of telephone yellow pages or free advertising tabloids from the sex industry. However, the Web is a unique communications system. The ways that men access and interact with prostitution-related images and texts on the Web creates new experiences and influences offline attitudes toward women. In an online environment of exploitation and abuse, new Internet technologies shift the balance of power toward the perpetrators.

WOMEN'S VISIBILITY AND MEN'S ANONYMITY

In prostitution, women are exposed and vulnerable. They stand on street corners; they strip in clubs and bars; they are used in making pornography; and their photographs are used to advertise escort services, massage parlors and other venues for prostitution. The purpose of sex businesses is to increase women and children's sexual accessibility to men. While women have never been able to control the pornographic photographs and videos made of them in the sex industry, the global network of the Internet makes the distribution of these images both vaster and more unknown.

Increasingly, Web sites for escort services and brothels publish photographs of the women. Men's texts in the online guides to prostitution graphically describe specific sex acts the women were paid to perform, and often include cruel comments. In some cases, individual women are named, described, and their addresses and locations posted for other men to find them. For example, for several years, men maintained a special Web site on specific women in brothels in Nevada (Hughes, 1999).

Having their photographs on the Web exposes women to the public as prostitutes. Some of the women may not realize that their photographs are on Web sites (personal communication with NGO representatives). This public exposure as prostitutes adds to women's humiliation and trauma.

Men post evaluations of women's appearances and "performances" on Web message boards on brothel's Web sites. In the following message, a man asks a pimp about a woman's weight:

> Dear Milla: What happened to Alina? Alina's new photos indicate that she has gained some extra weight!! She must not be 52Kg as written on her page Please advise what is her weight currently. (Milas Holiday and Escort Service)

Men and pimps frequently photograph or videotape women in prostitution, sometimes without their knowledge or permission. Women have no control over these pictures once they are taken. Men take the photographs and videos home as trophies or souvenirs. The following is a man's description of his trophy video:

> They have full video equipment at their premises. Prices for video services start from 1000 Danish Kronor for 30 minutes with one girl, including a strip, vibrator action and to finish, a hand job with a condom. For 3000 Kronor you get 30 minutes with one girl with a bit of everything–oral, straight sex and anal. I chose _____a perfect young body with a hint of puppy fat, and an amazingly tight pussy. The only fault was that she was so cool and unresponsive throughout. That apart, great value and the video of our fuck is still a prized possession. (Anonymous, 2000)

A woman who lived in a house equipped for commercial voyeurism (VoyeurDorm.com) described feeling very upset that men distributed nude pictures of her on the Web (*Tech TV, 2002*).

Some Web sites consist of "amateur" images and videos, where men post pornographic pictures of their girl friends, wives, or women they bought in prostitution. Bill Bensen of Memphis, Tennessee, for example, displayed and sold images and videos of "streetwalkers," bragging that: "All the whores on my site I personally picked up and paid to pose nude" (http://www.StreetwalkerPics.com, March 4, 2001). Bill measures his success by the number of photographs he gets of the woman. The following are comments that accompany women's photos on the Web site:

> This cute little white trash natural redhead says she hasn't been working the streets to long but she sure acts like a pro. Maybe that is just cause she has been fucking for so long. She got her cherry popped at the age of 12 by a 10-year-old that lived down the street. <Lucky Little Fucker> And since then she was hooked. . . . I picked her up on the warm sunny morning of Sept 1st 98. I took 88 pics of her.

> Meet Sharron of Knoxville, TN, a 33-year-old with a fetish for pain. She likes to get burned with cigarettes and beaten by her girlfriend during sex. You can see some of her 'love scars' (as she calls them) in her pics. . . . I picked her up on the street beside the hotel in which they live. (http://www.streetwalkerPics.com, August 21, 1999)

New technologies are used for the invasion of women's bodies to make her sexual anatomy visible for inspection. On sex industry Web sites there are advertisements for "dildo cams," tiny cameras inside dildoes.

In contrast, men who use women and children in prostitution prefer to remain invisible and anonymous. Men are rarely scrutinized as they go into sex industry businesses (personal communication with Nikki Craft, 29 July 2001). One man wrote:

> I don't like . . . the waiting room where you are seemingly expected to sit down together with other customers . . . the chance of having other males enter this room while I am there makes me cringe on the inside. (Aarhus, Denmark, 1999, http://www.worldsexguide.org)

The Internet is popular because it gives men greater access to pornography, live strip and sex shows, and information about prostitution, while giving them more privacy. Previously, they had to visit pornography stores and theaters to view pornography. Video cassettes and VCRs made it possible for men to view pornographic videos in their homes and not have to go to poor sections of town where peep shows were zoned and risk being seen by others. Computers and the Internet have further privatized men's viewing and access to pornography, strip and sex shows, prostitution, and voyeurism. The increased privacy and anonymity give men more protection from social stigmatization and law enforcement interference with their exploitation and abuse of women.

ONLINE COMMUNITIES FOR PERPETRATORS

On the Web, there is unfettered operation of the sex industry (Hughes, 1999, 2000a). Perpetrators who buy women and children in prostitution can find like-minded men for support. For boys and men who have not yet exploited or abused a woman or child, these images and text legitimize the exploitation and abuse and provide how-to-guides.

Their online writings and images reveal that men who buy women and girls in prostitution are not all alike or looking to use women and children in the same way. They range from apparently lonely men who think it is acceptable to use a woman for a short period as long as they pay to serial rapists.

Men online describe "the hunt" for women offline. They describe, often at length, looking for the right woman they want to buy. Men circle the block in cars, or go from bar to bar, looking for a woman who meets their requirements. Some men write that the anticipation and excitement they feel during "the hunt" is more enjoyable than the actual sexual act that follows. A man who photographs "street walkers" for his Web site describes his search for women:

> I have always had a thing for hookers whores prostitutes no mater what you call them they are all women of the street. I guess I am one sick fuck ... Around the time I got my drivers license I would drive around town and look for hookers. . . . I didn't need to do anything with them though cause I could feel it in the pit of my stomach that scared excited feeling when I would see them. . . . To this day I still get that scared sick feeling in the pit of my stomach when I pick up a prostitute even though it's just for some pics and videos. (http://www.streetwalkerpics.com)

> He also writes: "If you want to consider me a predator fine. You might even be right" (Email from Bill Bensen www.streetwalkerpics.com, April 24, 2000).

Men write about their experiences as a way of reliving the experience. One man wrote, "I'm getting a hard-on as I remember this night to write about it" (Anonymous, 2000). Some men include graphic descriptions indicating they are getting enjoyment out of reliving the experience through writing about it.

Men write about "good" and "bad" experiences buying women in prostitution. They have "good" experiences when women comply with everything the men want them to do, focus all their attention on the men, and pretend they like the men and enjoy the sex acts. Men express great satisfaction in being able to ejaculate on a woman's face or in her mouth (Raymond, Hughes, & Gomez,

2001, p. 77). They consider it a stroke of luck when they find a woman who does not insist on a condom, and are happy to find a woman who permits anal intercourse. Men have "bad" experiences when women will not do everything they want, or are disinterested, perfunctory, and try to minimize the physical contact with them.

Sometimes, the men write that they coerce or force the women to do what they want. The men often claim they like or even love women, but write about them using misogynistic, pornographic language. Violence, degradation, and humiliation are eroticized. Because women and children smile in pornography, perpetrators are convinced that women and children enjoy abuse and exploitation. Researchers who interviewed sex offenders who used the Internet to collect child pornography found that they lacked the ability to perceive harm being done to the children.

> Offenders talk of a lack of any objective measure as to whether the child in the picture was actually being abused . . . A frequent comment refers to the smiling faces of the children in the pictures, as proof of their enjoyment . . . (Taylor, Quayle, & Holland, 2001)

Over time, watching women and sex shows online causes people to lose empathy for the women and children or even see them as real. A woman who lived in Voyeur Dorm with 24 live video cameras broadcasting all her activities—eating, undressing, showering, and eating—to paying subscribers said:

> One member wrote a letter, he said he couldn't accept that we were real people. We were just little people who lived in the computer. Sometimes, I look at them that way. I have a hard time thinking of them as real people. (Tech TV, 2002)

When Tampa, Florida officials shut down the commercial voyeurism site for violation of zoning laws, the operator claimed that no activity was occurring at the house, it was all in cyberspace: "People don't show up at the house and pay money to get in. Everything's happening in virtual space and not at that location" (Roos, 2002).

Men who write about buying women usually try to present themselves positively. The most frequent fantasy is that the woman had an orgasm. These self-aggrandizing writings normalize the activity and reinforce the offender's perception of the activity.

These publicly accessible writings, which number in the thousands, legitimize the perpetrator's activities to others who read them. The accessibility of this material produced by the sex industry and individual perpetrators often leads men (and boys) to search for increasingly violent and extreme pornography, and travel to locations throughout the world where they exploit and abuse women and children without likelihood of arrest.

"DOING IT" ON THE INTERNET:
COMPUTER SKILLS
AND THE EMPOWERMENT OF PERPETRATORS

The extent to which men's experiences and behaviors are affected by using Internet technologies is not known. Early research in this area indicates that the impact is high and contributes to an escalation of exploitation and abuse of women and children. Using the Internet to access prostitution related information and engage in virtual prostitution empowers men to sexually exploit women and children. The combined experience of using high tech computer hardware and software, finding a supportive community on the Internet, and having a sexual experience (masturbating to pornography, live sex shows, and writings about prostitution) is reinforcing and empowering.

Max Taylor, head of the Combating Pedophile Information Networks in Europe (COPINE) Project, investigated use of the Internet by child pornography collectors and found that sex offenders are empowered by using the computer to locate child pornography (Taylor, Quayle, & Holland, 2001). Pedophile behaviors are reinforced in that the perpetrator acts in an environment with no social rules, and with minimal chance of being held accountable.

> . . . through Net experience people come to reinterpret society, relationships, and self. Through the Internet we see a potential change in the offender's beliefs, values and cognitive styles. The fact that through the Internet users can in the main go anywhere and say anything without any official governing body restricting those actions means that for some people this will be their first experience of acting outside the confines of a conventional hierarchy . . . Such experiences may empower some people such as sex offenders who have otherwise felt marginalized in conventional society. Those who have never been able to function at an optimal level in the real world may feel that they have the chance to do so now that conventional structures are broken down. (Taylor et al., 2001)

Collecting child pornography is a psychological process and is directly connected to acquiring new computer and Internet skills. The offender is reinforced by the combination of a physical collection, sexual satisfaction, computer skills, and a supportive online community.

The rapid acquisition of images largely goes hand-in-hand with the acquisition of technical skills. Collecting also leads to an increase in fantasy and sexual activity, particularly masturbation in relation to images or through engaging in mutual fantasies with others while online. With increasing mastery of the Internet comes a sense of power and control. (Taylor et al., 2001)

The technology is part of the excitement. The newest, fastest technology becomes the sexiest, and enables the best sexual experience online. Possessing the latest computer equipment is compared to masturbating to a live strip show:

Here's something that will make your modem sizzle! I was sitting at home . . . when I stumbled across "Video Fantasy" on the net. With Windows, my 486, and their software, I called a pretty girl's studio with my modem and watched her undress. All of this was live and in color on my computer monitor. What will they think of next. Sitting at home being entertained by a beautiful girl. Talk about "safe sex"! I love it! Check out their website at http://www.videofantasy.com. This is lot's of fun. (Hamilton, 1995)

Using the Internet to access pornography leads to an escalation in accessing, collecting, and using pornography. Among child pornography collectors, offenders usually start out downloading adult pornography, but move on to child pornography as they acquired more computer skills and find an online support community (Taylor et al., 2001). Accessing sexual material on the Internet lowered sexual inhibitions and increased online sexual activity of some men convicted of downloading child pornography. Some men tried to maintain an erection the entire time they were online. One man said:

I was with the masturbation . . . almost avoiding coming . . . because if I was online for an hour or so I would actually be masturbating on and off for an hour . . . and wanting to maintain the state of arousal. (Taylor et al., 2001)

WOMEN'S EXPERIENCES ONLINE

In prostitution and pornography, women and children's experiences are distorted and fabricated; yet, little is known about women's experiences in online sex shows. The newsgroups and web sites only include the men's voices and experiences, and the sex industry promotional claims.

Prostitution is not a victimless crime. Each sex act, whether online or not, is a violation of women's dignity and bodily integrity. Each sex act adds to the accumulation of trauma in prostitution (Farley, Baral, Kiremire, Sezgin, 1998; Iliina & Kalugin, 2002). Only glimpses of women's experiences online are available. During the live strip shows and commercial voyeurism, multiple men can be connected simultaneously, watching the same show. Men who pay for the shows often expect the women to respond directly to them and do what they request. That's how the shows are advertised. In these situations, the men compete for the woman's time and attention. One woman reported that it is overwhelming to have a number of men expecting her attention at one time.

> It's really disconcerting. Suddenly, the phone will pop on and a man will say hello, and when another one pops on it's like two kids tugging on your arm. A lot of them are very clear about what they want to see and what they want you to say. (Rose, 1997)

Women in the live strip and sex shows are usually in the same constrained economic circumstances with limited opportunities as women who strip in clubs. In 1998, the women stripping at one of the largest online sex sites were paid US $20/hour when they were online (Wired for sex, 1998). One woman said that she stripped online because her other job did not pay enough for her to support her family. She concealed the stripping from most of her friends and family. She described the same depersonalization as other women undergo in pornography and prostitution. She took on another personality to act out the scenarios required. "Out there, I'm a completely different person than I am in [the online studio]. This is my shadow side." (Wired for sex, 1998)

A woman from Voyeur Dorm said:

> We use stage names. That way if you're ever out, your walking down the street and someone calls you by the name you use here at the dorm, then you know not to turn around. Just keep walking. Get out of there. (Tech TV, 2002)

In online stripping, women do not have to physically interact with men as they do in clubs and bars. Madeleine Altmann, who was formerly in pornography, runs her own online strip site, Babes4U. She records herself dancing and stripping, and then transmits it to buyers on the Internet. She says, "I would never be a stripper or a prostitute. I don't want to be near the clients or see them." Although Altmann herself does not want to have any contact with the men, she pays other women to engage in sexually explicit "chat" with the men while they are logged on to the site (X-rating sites pace online, June 24, 1997).

A woman who does live shows on the Internet wrote about the exploitative conditions, poor pay, and degrading treatment she experienced.

> I used to be a dancer . . . Now cyber sex sites like www._____.net is very much like dancing at a club, we are "independent contractors" yet they charge a membership and we lose an additional percentage of our "50% cut" of what rate we charge per min to transmit live video. . . . I quit dancing to work at an adult site. . . . but it's pretty bad working at adult site . . . the abuse is way beyond what goes on at strip clubs, men requesting the women and men to penetrate with toys, vaginally and anally . . . Phone sex for less than 1.00 per minute . . . (Email from Renee, May 19, 2000)

Women can be identified by men unknown to them when they are offline. One woman on an online voyeurism site described being afraid of being recognized when she went out in public.

> Like I can't go out in public. I'm always looking around. Especially when you go out to a club . . . then you look in the corner and see this old guy in the corner like staring you down. Oh, my god, it's a member. . . . I always feel like I'm being watched. (Tech TV, 2002)

FUTURE RESEARCH

Little is known about men's use of Internet technologies for the purpose of sexual exploitation. The criminal activities of downloading and distributing child pornography, and contacting and meeting children for sex have received the most law enforcement attention (Taylor, 1999; Quayle, Holland, Linehan & Taylor, 2000; Taylor, Holland, & Quayle, 2001; McLaughlin, 2001). These first studies contribute to an understanding of child sex offenders and their use of the Internet. There are a few descriptive reports on the use of the Internet for sexual exploitation globally (Hughes, 1999, 2000a, 2001).

According to James McLaughlin, Keene Police Department, New Hampshire, USA, who has been involved in the arrest of numerous offenders using the Internet:

> Presently there is no profile for people who go on to the Internet and seek out child pornography, sexual contacts with children or who want to engage in cybersex with children. At this time there is not enough

data collected to determine if there is any difference between those who engage in the sexual abuse/exploitation of children in traditional ways as compared to those who employ computer technology to do so. (McLaughlin, 2001)

Conducting research within the present legal standards can make it difficult to understand who the victims are and how they have been hurt, and who the perpetrators are and how they harm the victims.

Stating that that it is not possible to understand the scope of collecting and the motivation of men with a sexual interest in children by looking only at what is illegal by present standards, which varies widely, COPINE Project's research on sex offenders' collections of child pornography is not based on legal standards. Taylor et al. (2001) emphasize the importance of examining and analyzing all the images and videos collected by men with a sexual interest in children.

Although the focus of the researchers at the COPINE Project is on child pornography and sex offenders who target children, they note the lack of information about consumers of adult pornography.

The Internet is a collection of innovative communication applications, with new ways of transferring information becoming available each year. To date, each new application has been adopted for the transmission of sexually exploitative and abusive material, or networking among perpetrators.

The sexual exploitation of women has been normalized by the sex industry. There appears to be no limit to what can be done to women if men pay for it and it is transmitted online (Hughes, 2000b). The current trend is for continued and expanded use of Internet technologies for promotion of prostitution, sex shows, and voyeurism. Glimpses of the impact that Internet technologies are having on men's increased exploitation and abuse of women and children indicates greater harm to women and children in the future.

NOTE

1. The Web browser Mosaic preceded the Netscape browser, but lacked the functionality of Netscape.

REFERENCES

Anonymous (2000). Copenhagen, Denmark. World Sex Guide, http://www.world sexguide.com.

Atta and M. (1997). World Sex Guide, [Web site] Retrieved June 1997 from: http://www.paranoia.com/faq/prostitution.

Atta and M. (1998). World Sex Guide, [Web site] Retrieved 1998 from: http://www.worldsexguide.org

Bosley, A. (1995). Escort agency: A Personal Touch Services, Selling sex in Cyberspace. *The Internet Business Journal*, Jan. 1995, p. 4.

Craft, N. (1991). Unmasking male privilege. ICONoclast, 3 (2). Retrieved July 29, 2001 from: http://www.nostatusquo.com/ACLU/Porn/ Unmask.html.

Farley, M., Baral, I., Kiremire, M., & Sezgin, U. (1998). Prostitution in five countries: Violence and post-traumatic stress disorder. *Feminism and Psychology*: 8 (4): 405-426.

Hamilton, D. (1995). Retrieved Nov, 21, 1995 from: alt.sex.prostitution. [Newsgroup].

Hughes, D.M. (1999). Pimps and Predators on the Internet: Globalizing the Sexual Exploitation of Women and Children. Kingston, Rhode Island: Coalition Against Trafficking in Women.

Hughes, D.M. (2000a). The Internet and sex industries: Partners in global sexual exploitation. *IEEE Technology and Society Magazine*, p. 35-42. Spring 2000.

Hughes, D.M. (2000b). "Welcome to the Rape Camp": Sexual exploitation and the Internet in Cambodia. *Journal of Sexual Aggression* 6 (1/2): 29-51.

Hughes, D.M. (2003). The Impact of the Use of New Communications and Information Technologies on Trafficking in Human Beings for Sexual Exploitation: A Study of the Users. Strasbourg, France: The Council of Europe. February 2003.

Iliina, S., & Kalugin, I. (2002). The Russian customer of sex service's attitudes towards prostitution and violence. Unpublished paper.

Kellog, B. (28 February 2002). Number of Internet porn sites, victims rising. *Focus on the Family*.

McLaughlin, J.F. (2001). Cyber child sex offender typology. Retrieved March 2001 from: http://www.ci.keene.nh.us/police/Typology.html.

Milas Holiday and Escort Service (2001). [Web site] Retrieved April 21, 2001 from: http://www.prag-girls.de/frame_hallo_e.htm.

Munn, A.J. (1995). PIMPS 'R' US goes to the Dominican Republic. The World Sex Guide [Web site] Retrieved Fall 1995 from: http:// www.panix.com/~zz/ exDR.html.

Quayle, E., Holland, G., Linehan, C., & Taylor, M. (2000). The Internet and offending behavior. A case study. *Journal of Sexual Aggression*, 6, 78-96.

Raymond, J. G., Hughes, D.M., & Gomez, C.G. (2001). Sex Trafficking of Women in the United States: International and Domestic Trends. Amherst MA: The Coalition Against Trafficking Women.

Roos, D. (2002). Talkback: Voyeur Dorm next door? Tech TV. Accessed Feb 26, 2002 at http://www.techtv.com.

Rose, F. (1997). Sex Sells: Young, ambitious Seth Warshavsky is the Bob Guccione of the 1990s. *Wired*, December 17, 1995, p.5.

Strangelove, M.E. (1995, January). Internet advertising review: The Internet has hormones, Selling sex in Cyberspace. *The Internet Business Journal*, p. 10.

Taylor, M. (1999). The nature and dimensions of child pornography on the Internet. US/EU International conference, Combating Child Pornography on the Internet, Vienna, Austria. Retrieved September 1999 from: http://www.stopchild pornog.at/.

Taylor, M., Holland, G., & Quayle, E. (2001). Typology of pedophile picture collections. *The Police Journal*, 74: 97-107.

Taylor, M., Quayle, E., & Holland, G. (2001). Child pornography, the Internet and offending. ISUMA. *The Canadian Journal of Policy Research.* 2(2): 94-100.

Tech TV. (2002). Meet the women of Voyeur Dorm (Video interviews). Accessed March, 26, 2002 at http://www.techtv.com.

The Travel Connection. (1995). A tropical paradise vacation is waiting for you! [Web site] Retrieved November 18, 1995 from: http://www. travelxn.com/fer/fer2.htm.

Virtual Connections. (1995). Live nude video teleconferencing. [Web Site] Retrieved on October 29, 1995 from: http://www.cts.com/~talon.

White Pine & Cornell University. (1995). News Release: White Pine and Cornell team up to bring real-time desktop videoconferencing to Internet users worldwide. [Web site]. Retrieved May 3, 1995 from: http://www.wpine.com/press.htm.

Wired for sex (1998): A growing cyberporn empire in Seattle takes a new twist on an old trade. Seattle Post-Intelligencer. (April 27, 1998).

X-rated sites pace online. (1997) June 24, 1997. *Chicago Sun Times.*

From Duty to Despair:
Brothel Prostitution in Cambodia

Wendy Freed

SUMMARY. This article summarizes findings from interviews with prostituted women and adolescent girls in Cambodian brothels. In this article we review the psychosocial and cultural context for brothel prostitution in Cambodia. The social attitudes towards women and the cultural role of being a good daughter are discussed with respect to entry into prostitution. The findings summarize the respondents' histories of being sold into prostitution and their subsequent sexual trauma and victimization. We discuss the stages of adaptation to captivity with a focus on understanding the public behavior of the women and adolescent girls in prostitution. We discuss the ways in which prostitution interrupts normal adolescent development. We discuss the psychological sequelae of self-blame, shame, grief and depression, fear and disruption of trust. We also look at resilience and coping in a cultural context.

INTRODUCTION

There are about two million women in prostitution in Asia and half of them are children (Bunch, 1997). Poverty and widespread psychosocial disruption,

Wendy Freed, MD, is at Harborview Center for Sexual Assault and Traumatic Stress, 325 Ninth Avenue, Box 359947, Seattle, WA 98104 (Email: freed@ u.washing ton.edu).
Printed with permission.

[Haworth co-indexing entry note]: "From Duty to Despair: Brothel Prostitution in Cambodia." Freed, Wendy. Co-published simultaneously in *Journal of Trauma Practice* (The Haworth Maltreatment & Trauma Press, an imprint of The Haworth Press, Inc.) Vol. 2, No. 3/4, 2003, pp. 133-146; and: *Prostitution, Trafficking, and Traumatic Stress* (ed: Melissa Farley) The Haworth Maltreatment & Trauma Press, an imprint of The Haworth Press, Inc., 2003, pp. 133-146. Single or multiple copies of this article are available for a fee from The Haworth Document Delivery Service [1-800-HAWORTH, 9:00 a.m. - 5:00 p.m. (EST). E-mail address: docdelivery@haworthpress.com].

http://www.haworthpress.com/store/product.asp?sku=J189
10.1300/J189v02n03_07

along with the subjugation of women, and cultural attitudes that normalize violence against women, all influence the context in which women and children are prostituted in the developing world. The violence, threat of violence, and degradation inherent in prostitution are universal (Farley & Barkan, 1998; Farley, Baral, Kiremire, & Sezgin, 1998). This study documents the psychological harm to women and adolescent girls in brothel prostitution in Cambodia (Freed, 1997).

Cambodia has experienced more than thirty years of civil war, trauma and severe psychosocial disruption. The number of women and adolescent girls being prostituted in Cambodia has increased dramatically since the early 1990s. Two trends in Cambodia and throughout Asia that account for this increase are that younger adolescent girls are being recruited into the sex industry and an increasing number of them are trafficked for prostitution.

When women and adolescent girls are trafficked into the sex industry they often are paying off a loan given to their parents or relatives. Traffickers have offered parents money, promises of education, a new skill or a good job for their daughters. These women and adolescent girls are taken from their home villages or towns, brought to a distant part of Cambodia or occasionally to other countries, then sold to pimps in brothels, bars, restaurants, massage parlors and other sex businesses (Human Rights Vigilance of Cambodia, 1995).

It is difficult to obtain accurate information about the age of adolescent girls and women in prostitution. With increased public scrutiny and government crackdowns of juveniles, the adolescent girls are under pressure from the brothel owners to say that they are at least 18 years old. But in three separate surveys conducted by the Cambodian Women's Development Association (CWDA) from 1992 to 1995 the youngest reported age of adolescent girls in prostitution dropped from 18 to twelve (CWDA, 1995).

Surveys conducted in Cambodia in 1993 indicated that about 50% of prostituted women and adolescent girls had been sold into brothels (UNICEF, 1995). Two years later another survey showed increasing numbers of women and adolescent girls sold into prostitution (UNICEF, 1995). Of those individuals sold into prostitution, 45% reported they were deceived by pimps and 55% reported they were sold by people they knew and trusted: parents and relatives (40%), boyfriends (10%), and friends (5%). These statistics reflect the profound economic and psychosocial disruption affecting families and communities. Since the mid-1990s, the sex industry in Cambodia has expanded with increased sex tourism by Western men and more trafficking of young girls from Viet Nam (Hughes, 2000; Hall, 2003).

The typical scenario that prostituted women and adolescent girls report is as follows: a recruiter comes to an economically destitute village and tells parents that there are jobs available in the city for their daughters as restaurant workers, maids, or factory workers. The recruiters tend to be women since they engender more trust from the families. The recruiter offers a sum of money as a salary advance for the family. This becomes the first layer of debt. The recruiter transports the woman or adolescent girl to the city where she is then sold to a brothel owner. The money paid by the brothel owner becomes the second layer of debt that she is supposed to pay off. Her living expenses and medical costs are added to that debt. This situation quickly becomes economic enslavement. The women and adolescent girls are deliberately taken far from their homes and communities. This adds to their dependence on the traffickers and brothel owners. Alternatively, some women and adolescent girls leave home on their own to escape an abusive situation or to help their impoverished families. Other women give histories of being abandoned by husbands or boyfriends and being unable to provide for their children. Pimps and brothel owners use the same deceptive practices with adolescent girls and with divorced, widowed, or abandoned women (UNICEF, 1995; Freed, 1997).

In Cambodia it is common for adolescent girls to be kept locked up until the first customer buys her. Her virginity is purchased for approximately $500 US and the customer keeps her captive for up to a week, usually imprisoned in his hotel room. Following the rapes and loss of virginity, her commercial value rapidly declines. She is resold to a lower level brothel where she is bought by 6-7 customers a day each paying an average cost of $2 US. Half of that sum is applied against her debt and the brothel owner keeps the rest (Human Right Vigilance, 1995; UNICEF, 1995).

Examining the social and cultural attitudes towards women, sexuality and marriage is essential for understanding the exploitation of women. In Cambodia a woman's identity is based upon getting married, serving her husband and caring for her children. The honor and reputation of a woman and her family are represented by first her virginity and later her marital fidelity (Surtees, 2003). She is expected to remain a virgin until she marries. If she loses her virginity, she is considered "damaged goods" (Phan, 1994). Once in prostitution, women remain in brothels in part because of social contempt and an internal sense of being dirty (Putheavy, 1997). Men are believed to have limitless sexual urges and it is acceptable for them to seek sexual experiences outside of marriage (Phan, 1994). It is threatening for a man to form an emotional attachment outside of marriage; thus, visiting brothels becomes a socially sanctioned activity for men.

METHOD

The author collected data on two trips to Cambodia in April and July 1996. Twelve in depth interviews were conducted: 6 were women and adolescent girls living in brothels in Phnom Penh and six were adolescent girls rescued from brothels one year earlier and living at the International Catholic Migration Commission's (ICMC) New Life for Young Women project in Battambang. Several subjects were interviewed multiple times. Only one subject living in the brothel area was found on the second visit and she was interviewed several times. The adolescent girls living at the ICMC center were available for second interviews. The qualitative methodology of this project documented how these women and adolescent girls viewed their own experiences.

The interviewees ranged in age from 14-23 years with a mean age of 17.5 years. Interviewees were referred to as women if they were 18 years of age or older, and as adolescents if they were 14 to 18 years. The length of time in the brothels ranged from three weeks to one year. The mean length of time in brothels was 5.5 months. Ten of the 12 women and adolescent girls interviewed were sold to brothel owners. Four were sold by relatives, two were sold by boyfriends and four were sold by people who offered them false jobs. One woman entered prostitution after being widowed and one adolescent girl had been sold to a brothel, escaped and then had no option but to enter another brothel. We inquired about the following: demographics (province of origin, age, socioeconomic status, education and family constellation); childhood history and quality of family relationships, account of entry into prostitution, description in her own words of living conditions in the brothels. We also asked about the psychological impact of prostitution, inquiring about: depression, trauma, fear and anxiety, shame, somatic concerns, and how these were related to age and developmental status. We explored their concerns about health, including HIV and condom use. Finally, we asked about the meaning of the experience to her, her family and within the larger social context. We assessed for areas of strength, coping skills, and hopes for the future.

The interviews lasted from forty-five to ninety minutes and were audiotaped with each informant's permission. The interviews were conducted in Khmer (Cambodian) with the help of two female interpreters. The author prepared case notes then reviewed each tape several times to identify common psychological issues and themes related to the experiences in brothel prostitution.

RESULTS

Multiple Stories, Layers of Truth

What is the meaning of "the story" and of telling one's story? The stories reflect what the women and adolescent girls are able to communicate about their experiences. The ambiguities, uncertainties, denials, omissions, distortions, and historical inaccuracies must be understood as an important communication in the telling. It is the challenge to the listener to sort out the many layers of truths.

Many of the women and adolescent girls appeared to have been coerced into making up stories about themselves in the brothels. The brothel owners often demanded that they use false names and forced them to say they were from a different province in order to keep them from being located by families or friends. The brothel owners distanced the women and adolescent girls from their prior identity and constructed a new identity in order to more effectively use and control them. Some women and adolescent girls may make up a name in order to protect a private part of themselves. They may also make up stories to engender sympathy in the hopes that a customer gives them extra money, treats them less violently, does not rape them, or even helps them escape the brothel. They learned to deceive with words and affects in the interest of their survival.

The accounts of the women's and adolescent girls' experiences in the brothels were remarkably consistent. In contrast, the stories of how they entered the brothels were vague and inconsistent, especially when trickery or betrayal was involved. What seemed to be missing were clear narratives of how the deception occurred. When she blamed herself for how she was tricked, the story became very confusing to follow. They omit parts of the story for which they feel the most shame, either the role of family members in betraying or selling them, or their own misplaced trust in an individual or a situation. The distortions in the stories serve to protect self-esteem and psychological integrity. An example of this was a 19-year-old woman who reported that a man she knew for only five days had sold her to a brothel. It was later learned that they lived together five months before he sold her. It was likely less painful for her to say that the deception occurred earlier in their relationship. Another example was a 16 year old adolescent girl who was so saddened by her stepmother selling her to a brothel that initially she said she left home on her own then met a woman on a train who promised to help her, but later sold her to a brothel. It was less painful for her to say she was betrayed and sold by a woman whom she barely knew, than by the stepmother who "fed her all her life."

The women and adolescent girls may become so disconnected from their own feelings and sense of self that when the brothel life is over they feel fragmented psychologically. They have used dissociation in the service of their psychological survival and that persists. Ultimately, reconstructing one's story and addressing the trauma can become a means of regaining internal cohesion. It is a slow process that occurs over time, and a process that can only begin once the women and adolescent girls leave the brothel and are in a place of safety.

Sexual Trauma and Victimization

Sexual trauma is a violation of the most intimate and personal aspect of the self. One's own body becomes the setting in which the atrocities are perpetrated. For the women and adolescent girls living in a brothel, the sexual violations take place inside the tiny cubicle (smaller than most prison cells) that is their only private living space. There is no safe haven for them.

Rape occurs not only when overpowering force is used and the rape victim fights back; rape implies lack of consent between individuals and lack of other options for survival. When an individual has been beaten into submission, and has become passive and accepting of what is done to her because she is captive, then any sexual encounter she has is a rape. Even if she has worked hard to attract the customer, because she has no right to refuse consent, she is being raped.

The women and adolescent girls held captive in prostitution experience the psychological reactions that accompany victimization. They feel helpless, damaged and degraded, and often betrayed by people close to them. They are impacted by social prejudice that dictates that when a young girl is no longer a virgin she has lost her value. One adolescent girl believed that she had no choice but to allow herself to be sold to a brothel after her stepfather raped her. She felt tremendous shame and believed her future had been taken away from her. She feared that if she stayed at home she would be raped again and because she had been raped, no one would want to marry her.

Disruption of Normal Development

Most of the women and adolescent girls interviewed were between the ages of fifteen and twenty. In traditional Cambodian society, they would be caring for younger siblings or helping families with work, either in the rice fields or at the market. They would be learning about a woman's role in the family and they would be preparing to marry. In stark contrast, they are removed from their homes, confined in brothels, and forced to perform sex acts with strangers.

Separation from family is a difficult part of the experience for the women and adolescent girls, whether she is escaping an abusive home situation, was deceived and sold, or left home on her own looking for work. There are important relationships she will miss. She may have been taking care of younger siblings and she is also separated from extended family, friends, and her community. This separation adds to the disorientation and vulnerability she experiences when confined to a brothel. In the brothel, she is forced to rely on new relationships with other prostituted women and adolescent girls and with the brothel owner.

Shame

The women and adolescent girls felt shame for having been sexually violated and for having been prostituted. Even when they saw themselves as victims and did not blame themselves, they still suffered shame. The shame is generated from internalized social attitudes. They were very concerned with how other people would view them now and they were aware of negative social stigma. Even those who were doing well in the recovery process had not yet told their families about what had happened to them because of their sense of shame.

Trust and Betrayal

More than half of the women and adolescent girls were sold to brothels by someone they knew, either family members or acquaintances. The closer the relationship, the deeper and more painful the betrayal of trust. They have been exploited and their basic trust in people has been damaged. They are vigilant regarding the possibility of additional betrayal. One earns their trust slowly; they do not give it freely. The social workers at the ICMC program report that it may take four or five conversations before the adolescent girls reveal accurate details of their stories. Sometimes they do not disclose their true village of origin in an attempt to minimize feelings of shame and protect against exposure.

Self-Blame

Many of the young women blamed themselves for ending up in a brothel. They believed it was their fault for trusting someone who betrayed them. They did not make the connection between their vulnerability at the time that led them to trust people they hardly knew, or make poor judgements. They had an exaggerated sense of their own complicity in the interactions that led to disastrous consequences. One example of this is the story of a 23-year-old widowed woman with two children who came to the capital city. She stayed with relatives and was trying to find work in a garment factory. She met a motorbike driver whom she hired to take her to the factory. Instead he took her to the nearby brothel area and sold her to a brothel owner. She blamed herself for trusting the motorbike driver.

Grief and Depression

Many of the women and adolescent girls reported depression, hopelessness, inability to sleep, nightmares, poor appetite, and a sense of resignation and despair. They appeared sad, subdued, withdrawn and ashamed. They suffered grief for many losses: the loss of freedom, safety, family, childhood, innocence, and virginity. They have lost a sense of safety and trust in the people most important to them. Depressive affect was not always immediately evident as they restricted what they talked about in order to modulate the level of depression they could tolerate. When they spoke about family situations that put them at risk, the reasons they left home and their betrayal by close family members, much more emotional pain and depression became apparent. One adolescent girl confined in a brothel told the author that she was always sad and wished she could go back to her old life. She was orphaned young and used to work in construction, building roads until she was tricked and sold to a brothel. She hated being prostituted, had bad dreams at night, ate very little, was scared and cried every day. She said she now had no choice, no freedom. If her parents were alive, she would never have had to live like this.

Fear

Many women and adolescent girls reported high levels of fear and anxiety. They described panic attacks and frequent nightmares. Their greatest fear was of beatings and physical punishment by the brothel owners. They were beaten if they refused to accept a customer, even if they had an infection. They reported fear of violent, drunken customers. The fear of HIV/AIDS was ever present. All of the individuals interviewed knew about HIV and AIDS and expressed fear about acquiring the infection. They knew that using condoms every time they had sex was the best means of preventing the infection. The women and adolescent girls in captivity said that they could not insist that their customers always use condoms. If the customer was unhappy he might get violent or the brothel owner might beat them. They felt that the knowledge about AIDS prevention without having the means to insist on their own protection left them feeling more terrified and powerless.

Captivity

These women and adolescent girls had been in captivity for a period of weeks to months or years. At first, when they realized that they were sold, they protested the brothel owner's demand that they accept customers. Refusal led to beatings, being locked up in a room and even starvation. They were threatened with electric shocks and other forms of torture. This persisted until their resistance was broken and they realized they were trapped with no other options. At some point in this process, they submitted in order to avoid further beatings and torture. Their spirits were broken. They surrendered, became resigned and accommodated to the circumstances of captivity. Autonomy, self-agency, and control over one's fate were no longer possible.

One 19-year-old woman described the details of being sold into a brothel by her boyfriend. He told her he was taking her to meet a family member because he planned to marry her. When they got to the brothel, he told her he had no intention of marrying her and was going to sell her. He and the brothel owner beat her when she refused to accept customers. She was about to be tortured with electric shocks but could not bear that possibility so she capitulated to their demands. One adolescent girl told of being locked up inside a room for a week until she agreed to have sex with a customer. Another adolescent girl said the brothel owner threatened to throw acid on her face and threatened to kill her if she did not agree to his demands.

Relationships with the other women and adolescent girls were conflicted. While there was some camaraderie and support, this was not always the case. There was rivalry to earn money or compete for customers and there were reports of some brothel owners using the women and adolescent girls to torture and beat each other.

As people find the best way to survive, some of their behaviors may raise questions if viewed out of context. For example, the women's and adolescent girl's flirtatiousness, seeking out clients, and getting clients to feel pity or love for them may represent strategies aimed at enhancing their survival. If they accept customers they may not be beaten. If they bring in more income they may pay off their debt more quickly in order to escape prostitution. If they elicit pity or love from their customers, they may be treated less violently.

Meaning to the Young Woman: The Value of Being a Good Daughter

Being a respectful and dutiful daughter was important to most of the interviewees. They felt compassion for their families' hardships and poverty. In particular, they spoke of wanting to alleviate their mothers' suffering. They saw themselves as being in a position to help their families survive. This was crucial to the overall meaning they attributed to being prostituted. For example, helping to finance the purchase of a small plot of land, or providing the means for younger siblings to attend school, gave value and some meaning to their personal sacrifice. If the family valued and respected her sacrifice, this decreased the negative impact of being prostituted. If the family did not appreciate her sacrifice, this led to more unhappiness and feeling worthless, damaged, and without a future.

One 16-year-old prostituted adolescent had agreed to let her stepmother bring her to a brothel in exchange for money that the family needed because her younger brother was sick. She expected to work hard for three months in exchange for the money and then return home. When she asked to leave, after three months, the brothel owner told her that her stepmother had unbeknownst to her come and taken an additional sum of money. She felt betrayed and became suicidal once she realized how she had been used.

Often, however, even the knowledge that being prostituted kept the family from starving could not make the experience tolerable. A 22-year-old woman who was tricked by a woman who came to her village, promised her a job and gave money to her mother, said, "My mother was given a small sum of money as an advance. She bought a small plot of land to grow rice. She is able to send my younger brothers to school. This has made a difference for my mother. She is able to survive . . . this gives me some comfort but I would rather be with them and starve than be here, forced to work in the brothel."

Resilience and Coping

The ICMC project was a residential center for adolescent girls rescued from brothel prostitution run by Cambodian social workers. The adolescent girls participated in a variety of activities designed to help them address their trauma as well as help them prepare for their future: supportive group meetings several times a week, literacy classes, and instruction in hairdressing and sewing. They wrote and produced a play called "My Life," which was a compilation of their stories about how they ended up in brothels. This play, which was performed around the country, was a creative way for them to address their traumatic experiences.

Social workers evaluated each individual's family situation to determine whether or not reunion with their families was possible. Even in the face of extremely traumatic experiences these adolescent girls showed strength and ways of coping, both in captivity and afterwards. While they still struggled with depression, shame, fear, and other sequelae of victimization, they acquired skills and developed their capacity to care for one another. The ability to concentrate, learn, be creative, form new attachments and have hope for the future were indicative of their capacity for healing, once they were safe.

DISCUSSION

The devastating impact of brothel prostitution involves psychological, physical, and social damage to survivors. These include depression, persistent terror, post traumatic symptoms, and disconnection from self and others. They also experience multiple losses: of innocence, trust in others, value to herself and to the social order. They also suffer long-term damage to their health caused by physical violence experienced at the hands of pimps and customers. The Cambodian Women's Development Association (CWDA) survey in Phnom Penh documented high rates of harassment, extortion, and rape by police against women in prostitution and also high rates of violence against prostituted women by brothel owners and customers (CWDA, 2002).

The impact of being involved in brothel prostitution in Cambodia is similar to that described in other studies of brothel prostitution. A 1993 report by Asia Watch studied the situation of Burmese women fleeing civil war who were trafficked to Thailand. The report found that these women were subjected to brutal violence and imprisonment, and suffered traumatic stress reactions, depression, fear, and anxiety. Because of their illegal status the women were terrified to seek help from the authorities. Studies of Nepali adolescent girls trafficked to the brothels of India described similar scenarios: adolescent girls from impoverished families being lured with promises of jobs, being betrayed by family and friends, and being victimized by traffickers (Human Rights Watch Asia 1995). In her discussion of prostitution in Asia, Brown (2000) describes similar patterns of recruitment, exploitation of the porest communities, adaptation to captivity, debts that can rarely be repaid, profound social stigma and psychological devastation.

It is critically important to understand the cultural context in which prostitution occurs. In Cambodia, the role of duty and obligation to the family is crucial to an individual's sense of belonging. Thus, prostitution becomes a mean of helping one's family. In Cambodian culture, there is also a Buddhist belief in accepting Karma or predestined fate. If people find themselves in a situation of great suffering, they assume it is probably because they have committed some transgression in a past life. If a woman or adolescent girl provides financial assistance to her family (through prostitution), she may believe that her next life will be better. This attitude towards accepting prostitution as the workings of Karma is thus consistent with a Buddhist worldview. Acceptance is often misinterpreted by people outside the culture as passivity.

Similarly, Bates described how force, violence, and psychological coercion in slavery convince people that they must inevitably accept their fate. The Thai women and adolescent girls he interviewed had been told that their families would suffer if they did not cooperate with their own enslavement. They were encouraged to believe that they had committed horrible sins in a past life and that slavery was payment for past sins. For their psychological survival the young Thai women redefined slavery or debt bondage as penance (Bates, 2002).

Consistent with the findings of this study, Muecke (1994) writes that in Thailand, women and adolescent girls who are prostituted and send money home to support their families are fulfilling cultural obligations to their parents. However, if the family squanders the money she will feel that she has lost everything. Not only will she have lost her earnings; she will have also lost the moral justification for suffering the degradation of prostitution. She is then rendered worthless.

There are limitations inherent in data obtained in this type of study. In the brothels, the women and adolescent girls are in captivity and can neither move about nor speak freely. No matter how "good" the brothel owner may be the women and adolescent girls were totally dependent on the good will of the brothel owner. The "worst" of the brothel owners were unlikely to let the women and adolescent girls they control be interviewed. Efforts to interview younger adolescent girls were met with resistance and one interview had to be stopped early on in the process because the environment was too controlled and became menacing even though the brothel owner ostensibly had given permission for the interview. The individuals at risk for the worst victimization were the least accessible to this study. The unavailability of those who are the most harmed and most vulnerable has also been noted by Vanweesenbeeck (1994) and Farley et al. (1998). The brothel owners approached for interviews were the ones with the best working relationships with the NGOs. Thus the sample is skewed towards the women and adolescent girls in brothels who were in a slightly better situation.

Although no attempts were made to directly corroborate what the informants said, the validity of the findings is suggested by several factors. First, what the interviewees said is consistent with what people who have been working with prostituted women in Cambodia have said about their lives. Second, these case studies were clinical and anecdotal reports, and there was a consistency in what was heard from interview to interview. Third, the author verified tentative findings with informants, both interview subjects and local service providers.

When adolescent girls or women in prostitution escape, they are assisted by projects that offer physical and emotional safety, housing, violence prevention programs, information about gender inequality, training in job skills that allow for realistic sustainable economic development, and access to healthcare and counseling to address the traumatic impact of prostitution. Psychosocial interventions aim to address the trauma in culturally appropriate ways, to rebuild self-esteem, trust, and a cohesive sense of identity. In order to reduce self-blame, the adolescent girls and women need to appreciate their own victimization and realistically understand the power dynamics operating within their families, their social networks and the larger society.

The need to belong, to be a part of a family or a group in Khmer society is very strong. Some women and adolescent girls wish to return to their families yet for others that may not be safe. In situations where family members were involved in trafficking, there is a higher risk that the individual will be trafficked again (Dersks, 1999). The stigma and shame of having been prostituted or of having AIDS makes return to their villages extremely difficult. In Cambodia, up to 50% of those escaping prostitution have contracted HIV. New families or extended families of those in similar circumstance can provide alternatives to the traditional family. Material survival is crucial and without profitable sustainable employment there is a strong likelihood that the women and adolescent girls will have no choice but to return to prostitution.

Ultimately, these therapeutic, public health, and vocational efforts are meaningless unless the social and political supports for prostitution are ended. The demand for young adolescent girls, the abuses perpetrated by traffickers and brothel owners, and the social attitudes toward the women who become their victims are all issues that need to be addressed on a global level. The institutions that support prostitution and the individuals who perpetuate and maintain such abuses for personal and financial gain need to be stopped.

REFERENCES

Asia Watch and the Women's Rights Project. (1993). *A Modern Form of Slavery: Trafficking of Burmese Women and Girls into Brothels in Thailand.* New York: Human Rights Watch.

Bates, K. (2002). The Social Psychology of Modern Slavery. *Scientific American.* April 2002. 286 (4): 80-88.

Brown, L. (2000). *Sex Slaves: The Trafficking of Women in Asia.* London: Virago Press.

Bunch, C. (1997). The Intolerable Status Quo: Violence Against Women and Girls. *http://www.unicef.org/pon97/women1.htm.* Accessed April 10, 2002.

Cambodian Women's Development Association (CWDA). (1994). Prostitution Survey Results from CWDA February 1994. In The Trafficking and Prostitution of Children in Cambodia: A Situation Report, Appendix 2, p. 30-33. Phnom Penh: UNICEF CAMBODIA. December 1995.

Cambodian Women's Development Association (CWDA). Aug/Sept 2002 posted on http://archives.healthnev.net/sex-work.

Dersks, A. (1999). Results of the research on the reintegration of victims of trafficking in Cambodia. Presented at National Workshop on Reintegration Strategies February 4 and 5, 1999. Published in Proceedings of the National Workshop on Reintegration Strategies. 11-18. Phnom Penh: International Organization for Migration.

Farley, M., & Barkan, H. (1998). Prostitution, Violence, and Posttraumatic Stress Disorder. *Women & Health* 27(3), 37-49.

Farley, M., Baral, I., Kiremire, M., & Sezgin, U. (1998). Prostitution in Five Countries: Violence and Post-Traumatic Stress Disorder. *Feminism & Psychology* 8(4): 405-426.

Freed, W. (1997). *Commercial Sexual Exploitation of Women and Children in Cambodia. Personal Narratives: A Psychological Perspective. Report prepared for Physicians for Human Rights.* Report published by Physicians for Human Rights, Boston.

Hall, M. (2003). The darker side of travel. The Telegraph Group Limited. Accessed September 13, 2003. at http://www.telegraph.co.uk/travel/main.jhtml?xml=/travel/2003/ 091/13/etsextr.xm.& sShee t=/travel/2003/091/13/ixtrvhome.html.

Hughes, D. (2000). Welcome to the Rape Camp: Sexual Exploitation and the Internet in Cambodia, *Journal of Sexual Aggression* 6(1/2): 29-51.

Human Rights Vigilance of Cambodia. (1995). Rapid Appraisal on Child Prostitution and Trafficking. In *The Trafficking and Prostitution of Children in Cambodia: A Situation Report*, Appendix 2, p. 9-22. Phnom Penh: UNICEF Cambodia, December 1995.

Human Rights Watch Asia. (1995). *Rape For Profit. Trafficking of Nepali Girls and Women to India's Brothels*. New York: Human Rights Watch.

Muecke, M. (1994). Mother Sold Food, Daughter Sells Her Body: Prostitution and Cultural Continuity. *Social Science & Medicine* 35:7: 891-901.

Phan, H., & Patterson, L. (1994). "Men Are Gold, Women Are Cloth." A Report on the potential for HIV/AIDS spread in Cambodia and implications for HIV/AIDS education. Phnom Penh: CARE International.

Putheavy, P. (1997). 'Strategies and services to address gender violence' Paper presented at the Global NGOs Initiative International Workship, Manila. Quoted from Surtees, R. (2003) Rape and Sexual Transgression in Cambodian Society. In L. Manderson and L.R. Bennett (eds) *Violence against Women in Asian Societies*. London: Routledge.

Surtees, R. (2003). Rape and Sexual Transgression in Cambodian Society. In L. Manderson and L.R. Bennett (eds.) *Violence against Women in Asian Societies*. London: Routledge.

UNICEF, Cambodia (1995). *The Trafficking and Prostitution of Children in Cambodia. A Situation Report*. Prepared by UNICEF Cambodia for the Regional Workshop on Trafficking of Children for Sexual Purposes. Phnom Penh, December 1995.

Vanweesenbeeck, I. (1994). *Prostitutes Well-Being and Risk*. Amsterdam: VU University Press.

Prostitution and Trafficking of Women and Children from Mexico to the United States

Marisa B. Ugarte
Laura Zarate
Melissa Farley

SUMMARY. The historical background of sex trafficking from the United States to Mexico is briefly described. We also summarize two case examples that illustrate the complexity of providing physical and emotional safety, as well as immigration protection to victims of trafficking. We emphasize the importance of understanding the varied cultural contexts in which sexual exploitation, rape, prostitution and trafficking occur. Two agencies: Arte Sana in Dripping Springs, Texas and the Bilateral Safety Corridor Coalition in San Diego, California, of-

Marisa B. Ugarte is affiliated with the Bilateral Safety Corridor Coalition, 5348 University Avenue, Suite 119, San Diego, CA 92105 (Email: sdbscc@yahoo.com).

Laura Zarate is affiliated with Arte Sana, Austin, Texas (Email: lazarate@yahoo.com).

Melissa Farley is at Prostitution Research & Education, San Francisco (Email: mfarley@prostitutionresearch.com).

The authors thank Wendy Freed, MD, Gloria Gonzales-Lopez, PhD, and Frank Lostaunau, LCSW, for their thoughtful reviews of this paper and their helpful comments. They also thank Chuck Goolsby for his assistance in providing references for the paper.

[Haworth co-indexing entry note]: "Prostitution and Trafficking of Women and Children from Mexico to the United States." Ugarte, Marisa B., Laura Zarate, and Melissa Farley. Co-published simultaneously in *Journal of Trauma Practice* (The Haworth Maltreatment & Trauma Press, an imprint of The Haworth Press, Inc.) Vol. 2, No. 3/4, 2003, pp. 147-165; and: *Prostitution, Trafficking, and Traumatic Stress* (ed: Melissa Farley) The Haworth Maltreatment & Trauma Press, an imprint of The Haworth Press, Inc., 2003, pp. 147-165. Single or multiple copies of this article are available for a fee from The Haworth Document Delivery Service [1-800-HAWORTH, 9:00 a.m. - 5:00 p.m. (EST). E-mail address: docdelivery@haworthpress.com].

http://www.haworthpress.com/store/product.asp?sku=J189
10.1300/J189v02n03_08

fer a range of culturally appropriate services to Latina survivors of sexual assault, sexual exploitation, prostitution, and trafficking.

INTRODUCTION

Prostitution and trafficking are sexual violence that result in economic profit for perpetrators. Other types of gender violence such as incest, rape and wife-beating are hidden and frequently denied but they are not sources of mass revenue. Described by survivors as "paid rape," prostitution provides buyers (johns, tricks, dates) constant sexual access to women and children. Prostitution and trafficking can take place in massage parlors, strip clubs, escort agencies, lap dance clubs, on the street, in a car or motel, or in a tent set up at the edge of a field being cultivated by migrant workers.

Women are trafficked (moved) by pimps to wherever there is a demand for prostitution, for example military bases, tourist destinations, conventions or migrant communities. The current US trafficking law places the burden of proof on the victim to show evidence of force, fraud or coercion.[1] Since pimps/traffickers move people to wherever they are sold for sex, we think a better definition of trafficking would include movement of people within a country as well as across international borders for the purpose of sexual exploitation. Trafficking is a direct result of cultural and economic forces which sweep a woman or child into prostitution including not only coercion, manipulation, deception, initial consent, family pressure–but also past or present family and community violence, economic deprivation, racism, and conditions of inequality between the sexes. This broader definition of trafficking is appropriate if governments seek to decrease sex businesses, taking into account the range of forces that channel people into prostitution.

SEX TRAFFICKING FROM MEXICO TO THE UNITED STATES

Mexico-to-United States immigration has been described as the longest-running labor migration in the world (Ehrenreich & Hochschild, 2002). The 7.9 million Mexicans living in the United States comprise 27% of all foreign born persons (Chiquiar & Hanson, 2002). However, restrictions against illegal immigrants, combined with anti-immigrant hostility in the United States, have created an economy that consists of generally undesirable jobs. In addition to exploited labor, this illegal economy includes both prostitution and trafficking.

Non-Latino US men, as well as men from immigrant communities, are customers of prostitutes supplied by Mexican traffickers (Heinzl, 2003). Every day, thousands of male tourists enter Mexico from the United States to purchase women and girls in prostitution.

Of the 50,000 people annually trafficked to the United States, a third are Latin Americans (Richard, 2000). Women and youth seeking work in the USA must rely on labor traffickers (coyotes) to help them cross the border in search of work. Sex traffickers lure poor women and youth with false promises of jobs, sometimes kidnapping those they transport and selling them.

Mexico is both an origination and destination point for trafficking women and children, as well as being a stopover for transportation of people along several trafficking routes (for example, from Brazil or Guatemala to the United States) (Lederer, 2001). Although accurate numbers are impossible to obtain, one report noted that 16,000 girls in Mexico were sexually exploited through networks involving immigrants, military personnel, police, governmental officials, and businessmen (Azaola, 2001). There is great danger of sex trafficking occurs along the Mexican-U.S. border, where unemployment is high and thousands of US citizens cross into Mexico daily for the purpose of buying Mexican youth in prostitution (British Broadcasting Report, 2002; Taino, 1998). Castillo, Gomez & Delgado (1999) estimate that there are 15,000 women in street prostitution in Tijuana with many more working in the city's more than 200 club/brothels.

THE SAN DIEGO TRAFFICKING CORRIDOR

According to health workers interviewed by the first author, trafficking of women and children for prostitution in San Diego is common but is rarely reported to US or Mexican police. Although prostitution/trafficking are in fact human rights violations based on sex, race, and class, they have been prejudicially dismissed as "the problems of illegal immigrants." As a result, trafficking of people across the Mexico/US border has become a lucrative business.

When women and children migrate illegally, they are at the mercy of traffickers. Many are raped or murdered in transit. If their families are known to have money, migrants may be held for ransom. Coyotes who transport people across the Mexico/USA border are aware that neither victims nor their families will report these crimes, since the victims themselves would risk felony charges for illegal entry into the United States.

Pimps often work in concert with coyotes. In a scenario of brutal exploitation, coyotes transport victims from Mexico to the United States for a reduced fee, sexually assaulting and prostituting the women as payment for passage. Instead of being reunited with families across the border, children may be considered saleable by coyotes and may never arrive at their intended destination. Children may be sold to gangs who prostitute them. Their families are then told that they died during the border crossing. Children who are unaccompanied or who have run away from abusive homes are at especially high risk for prostitution/trafficking.

Women and girls are often moved from the Mexico/California border to northern San Diego County, where they are placed in apartments controlled by women pimps hired by the traffickers. Brothels have been identified in communities from San Diego to as far north as Canada. Prostitutes are transported in a sex trafficking corridor that supplies them to the shifting locations of migrant labor communities (sometimes called camps) near Fresno, Barstow, Sacramento, and Seattle. In San Diego, a wide range of commercial sexual exploitation exists, including adult prostitution, child and youth sex tourism, mail order brides, pornography, peonage, and bondage.

Hernandez (2003) investigated the trafficking of Mexican girls to brothels near San Diego. Over a ten-year period, hundreds of girls aged 12 to 18 from rural Mexico were either kidnapped or tricked into US border crossings by traffickers/pimps. Criminal networks in San Diego county control more than 50 brothels and outdoor farm labor sexual exploitation camps. Trafficked girls are sold to migrant farm workers, US tourists, and US military personnel. In one typical case, caves made of reeds served as brothels at the edge of the fields. Many of the girls had even younger children of their own, who were then held as hostages so their mothers would not try to escape. Hundreds of farm workers were transported each day to these sexual slavery camps, where they sexually assaulted girls in prostitution.

A US physician who worked for a clinic that provided health care to migrant workers said, "The first time I went to the camps I didn't vomit only because I had nothing in my stomach. It was truly grotesque and unimaginable." Many of the girls were 9 to 10 years old. On one occasion the physician counted 35 men raping a girl for money during a single hour. When police raided the brothels, they found dozens of empty boxes of condoms, each box having held a thousand condoms (Hernandez, 2003).

Under instruction from her supervisor, the physician worked with the pimps for five years. After she reported the girls' sexual assaults in prostitution the physician was instructed by US officials that prostitution was "not a migrant health concern." Advised by her superiors to work with the pimps, she limited her practice to "prevent[ing] HIV/AIDS and other venereal diseases in the exploited minor girls" (Hernandez, 2003). This tunnel vision regarding the health of those in prostitution is commonly seen in clinics and in AIDS organizations. Although at first glance the public health attention to HIV and STD includes the prostituted woman herself, on closer inspection it becomes apparent that the overarching concern is to decrease the customer's exposure to disease (Farley & Kelly, 2000). The overwhelming health consequences *to the victim* of captivity, terrorization, traumatic psychological stress and violence are officially ignored, as in this case.

CASE EXAMPLE: SOFIA, AGE 15

A child protective officer brought Sofia, a victim of prostitution and trafficking, to the Bilateral Safety Corridor Coalition (BSCC). Her sexual abuse did not fit the guidelines for receiving assistance from California Child Protective Services because the abuse had not been perpetrated by a family member, relative or family friend. Furthermore, Child Protective Services declared that they did not have the resources to assist Sofia.

Sofia attended an initial interview with a representative of the BSCC, a representative of the sheriff's department and a child protective service worker. Sofia stated that her pimp had kidnapped her one-year-old son in Mexico. The pimp then forced her to work in the field brothels under threat that her son would be killed if she refused to prostitute. She described seven prostitution camps where women and girls were rotated weekly. Although she was paid, she did not actually keep any of the money. She was prostituted to migrant laborers without condoms, used by 20-30 men in four hour shifts. The sheriff's department intervened when her pimp beat her after Sofia refused to go to one of the field camps.

The first goal was to provide Sofia with safe housing and crisis services. Since there was no emergency housing for minors in San Diego, Sofia was admitted to a battered women's shelter where she remained for six months.

Coordinated case management was crucial in order to assist Sofia, as it often is with members of marginalized populations who do not have comfortable access to social, medical and legal services. With the battered women's shelter and the BSCC functioning as advocates, Sofia's needs were addressed by more than twenty agencies, including:

- Bilateral Safety Corridor Coalition (victim advocacy and coordination of services)
- Battered Women's Shelter (housing, group counseling, case management)
- San Diego Sheriff's Department (investigation of the crime)
- Planned Parenthood (gynecological care)

- Community Health Clinic (other medical treatment and lab tests)
- Catholic Charities (certified victim's needs, vaccinations, management of funds through Office of Refugee Resettlement, Health and Human Services)
- Mexican Judicial Federal Police (legal charges in Mexico, assistance in rescue of the baby)
- DIF (Desarrollo Integral de la Familia: Mexican Social Services) (investigation of victim's family, rescue and shelter for Sofia's child)
- Federal Bureau of Investigation (investigation, administration of Office of Victim Services funding)
- Immigration and Naturalization Service (investigation, legal documentation provided to victim)
- Mexican Consulate Minor Protection (supervision of victim's rights, investigation and retrieval of Sofia's child)
- Pre-trial Services (legal advice, case monitoring, payment for psychological evaluation, supervision of court appearances)
- Criminal attorney
- Immigration attorney (functioned as legal guardian, coordinated T-Visa application and humanitarian visa application)
- US Attorney (prosecution of traffickers)
- Services for Youth (shelter and case management)
- Psychologist (evaluation)
- Children's Hospital (trauma counseling)
- Human Rights Mexico (public denunciation of the crime)
- Group home in Georgia (placement of Sofia's rescued child)
- Juvenile Justice system in Georgia (victim became ward of the court).

Because it was physically unsafe to remain in San Diego, Sofia was moved out of California, and services for her were managed by another state's social service agency, along with continued coordination of services by BSCC. Her child was rescued, and Sofia was given a US visa for victims of trafficking.

CASE EXAMPLE: GUADALUPE, AGE 12

In an Immigration and Naturalization Service (INS) exit interview during the process of deportation to Mexico, this transgender youth stated that she had been trafficked into the United States for the purpose of prostitution by a criminal gang that operated in her home town in Mexico. They had transported her to a number of cities on both US coasts, selling her on the gay/transgender prostitution circuit. In the INS interview where she was identified as a boy, she reported extensive family violence and abandonment at a young age by her father, at which time her mother permitted (and probably took in money from) the child's prostitution. Although it was not known whether she had been sexually assaulted by family and neighbors, her prostitution was child sexual abuse. The US Justice Department and DIF (Mexican Social Services) determined that Guadalupe should remain in the United States pending further investigation of her home environment. As with Sofia, many agencies in both the United States and Mexico were involved and the BSCC functioned as an advocate and coordinator of services for the child.

Guadalupe was traumatized as a preadolescent by a homophobic social environment in which she was surrounded with contempt and physical violence, including rape. Gender roles are narrowly defined in Mexico, and when a boy is perceived as feminine (derisively called *joto* or *maricon*), he is loathed, socially shunned and often banned from family events such as weddings, funerals, and holiday gatherings.

There is confusion regarding the difference between sexual orientation and gender identity in both Mexico and the United States. Because those who identify as transgender often do not hide their birth gender, they are stigmatized not only by homophobia, but also by prejudice within gay communities against those who do not "pass" as sufficiently masculine.[2] In addition to being gay, Guadalupe openly expressed her identity as female, which resulted not only in social stigma but escalated to contempt and physical violence. This violence is sometimes extended even to the family of the transgender person (Lostaunau, 2003).

Homelessness may be a consequence of family violence including homophobia. Transgender adolescents prostitute for food and shelter and also as a way to send money home to families. At an emergency shelter Guadalupe was retraumatized by other children's prejudice toward gay and transgendered youth. The humiliation and social isolation were intolerable and she ran away from the shelter.

Shortly afterward the US border patrol arrested Guadalupe as an undocumented minor, identifying her this time as a girl, unaware that she had been previously trafficked and prostituted. Guadalupe was placed in custody of Child Protective Services and deported to Mexico. At that point her history of trauma, neglect, abuse, and trafficking was discovered. Out of concern for the child's safety Guadalupe was returned to the United States. There she was taken to a specialized facility where she received support for both her sexual orientation and gender identity.

Angry that her child was out of her control, Guadalupe's mother filed a complaint against DIF (Mexican Social Services) with the Mexican Human

Rights Commission demanding the return of her son. Guadalupe was emotion-ally blackmailed into silence by her mother and she denied her history of ne-glect, violence, and prostitution. Bowing to political and legal pressure, US and Mexican law enforcement agencies permitted Guadalupe to be returned to her mother in Mexico. Subsequent reports from DIF noted that Guadalupe did not attend school. Instead, she worked in a restaurant at her mother's request, supporting the family.

DIF again filed a complaint against the mother. In the meantime, Guadalupe ran away from her mother's home to a large city in Mexico. At age 12, she ob-tained identification that listed her age as 18. She is currently working in a strip club as a female table dancer, which almost always involves prostitution (Farley, Cotton, Lynne, Zumbeck, Spiwak, Reyes, Alvarez, & Sezgin, 2003). The fetishized sexuality in strip club prostitution may have provided a social niche that Guadalupe failed to find elsewhere. BSCC monitored Guadalupe's status via messages from other street children. BSCC staff felt that it would further harm the child to offer her services that would not adequately address her complex needs. Treatment for Guadalupe should necessarily include: long term housing, medical care, safety planning to protect her from violence by pimps, addiction treatment, and voca-tional training. Psychotherapy would address childhood trauma, prostitution/traf-ficking trauma, and at the same time address race and cultural prejudice, traumatic homophobia, prejudice against transgender persons, and repeated betrayals by so-cial and legal systems, as well as betrayals by friends and family. Peer support should be an integral part of the healing process (Hotaling, Burris, Johnson, Bird, & Melbye, 2003; Rabinovitch, 2003).

HISTORICAL BACKGROUND
OF THE SEXUAL EXPLOITATION
OF MEXICAN AND LATIN AMERICAN
WOMEN AND CHILDREN IN PROSTITUTION

Most women in prostitution in Mexico come from rural areas, having sur-vived extreme poverty, family violence, and often leaving abusive homes to migrate to cities (Castillo, Gomez, & Delgado, 1999). A conservative estimate of the prevalence of trafficking is that 100,000 women are moved across Latin American states' borders annually for the purpose of prostitution (Kovaleski, 2000; Maki & Park, 2000).

For centuries, religious and legal institutions in Mexico and across Latin America have reinforced male supremacy. Fueled by belief in the subordina-tion of women, the Spanish conquest of the peoples of Latin America included the colonization of indigenous women. These attitudes toward women persist as for example in Mexico's granting women the right to vote only as recently as 1953 (Jordan, 2002). Across Latin America, 20% to 40% of women are raped each year (Casteneda, 2000), yet rape is often treated as a lesser crime than stealing a cow, with only 1% of rapes resulting in criminal charges (Jordan, 2002).[3] In some Mexican states, a girl who brings charges of rape against an adult is required to first prove her chastity. Kidnapping and rape are accepted methods of obtaining marital partners in some regions (Jordan, 2002).

Prostitution occurs throughout Latin America (as elsewhere) in contexts of brutal poverty and family violence. A girl's first "sexual" experience is often sexual abuse by an adult family member, co-worker or acquaintance (UNICEF, 1999). Sexual and physical abuse in their homes often lead children to run away, with homelessness documented as a risk factor for prostitution of both children and adults (Tyler, Hoyt, & Whitbeck, 2000). According to one estimate, 16,000 children are prostituted in Mexico (Azaola, 2001). Approximately 135,000 Mexican children have been kidnapped and were presumed to have been trafficked into illegal adoption, prostitution, and pornography from 2000-2002 (Hadden, 2002).

Mexican federal law prohibits procuring, thus making prostitution technically illegal. However, most states have legalized and regulated prostitution in *zonas de tolerancia* (red light districts) (Gonzalez de la Vega, 1968).

The sexual exploitation faced by women and girls worsens considerably during national and regional conflict. For example, the conflict between the Mayan people and the Mexican state (also called the Zapatista uprising) involved widespread rape and prostitution of indigenous women and girls by the Mexican Army (SIPAZ, 1999).[4] Throughout the 1980s thousands of indigenous and other poor, mostly rural women were raped and many were murdered in Central American civil wars (Harbury, 1997). During the civil wars in El Salvador and Nicaragua, women were sexually assaulted by army personnel and civil police. Following these assaults, the women themselves as well as their families viewed them as *mujeres marcadas* (dirty, tainted, or ruined). As a result, women migrated not only to escape conditions of war, but also to escape family shame.

MUJERES DECENTES: THE INTERNALIZATION OF MALE SUPREMACY IN LATIN AMERICA

While Olmec gender roles are considered to have been nonhierarchical and even "fluid" two thousand years ago (Joyce, 2000), sexist beliefs in female inferiority have affected all people in Mexico today, including indigenous people. In many Latino cultures, the influence of the Catholic Church controls women's and girls' lives through dogma that controls sexuality and reproduction. Just as Franciscan Catholics urged Nahua parents to instruct daughters not to go out in public, not to laugh, not to enjoy themselves, not to look or smile at men–Latina girls today are warned about the disastrous consequences of being a 'bad' girl (Overmyer-Velazquez, 1998).

Mexican and other Latin American men generally assume the right to sexually exploit any female. A consequence of this attitude has been a deliberate lack of educational opportunity for women that has increased their dependence on men. If domestic violence precipitates escape from a marriage or if they are abandoned by men, women and girls become vulnerable to further sexual exploitation, including prostitution.

According to Latina participants of Arte Sana workshops (see below) *dichos* (popular sayings) are passed down through generations, delivering the message that girls are worth less than boys. When daughters are born it is still common to hear them referred to as *carne para los gallotes* (meat for the roosters). For the girl, being labeled as meat will affect everything in her life; her mother's duty will be to protect her daughter from the inevitable dangers that her gender poses until she leaves home, hopefully 'in tact.' The Mexican saying *tengo suerte que me ha durado* (I am lucky that she has lasted) reflects a mother's intention to both preserve her daughter's virginity and to prevent pregnancy before marriage. The sexist assumptions are that a sexually active woman is invariably promiscuous and thus damaged. Once damaged, the concept of rape does not apply to her (Domecq, 1992, Zarate, 2002a).

A sexually active woman may be referred to as a "eaten bread," *piruja* (whore) or *cancha reglamentaria* (regulation soccer field) upon which many have "played" or "scored." So extreme is the pressure to remain a virgin that there have even been attempts to medically restore virginity. In Northern Mexico for the past 30 years, a physician conducted plastic surgery to restore Latinas' ruptured hymens. Advertising her services *para reparar la virginidad* with hymenoplasty, women were guaranteed to bleed after the hymen was ruptured (Gonzalez-Lopez, in press).

Shame is a common reaction to sexual assault, including the sexual violence of prostitution and trafficking. Survivors may see themselves as damaged, unworthy of marriage, and as bringing shame to their families. Shame limits the victim's capacity to acknowledge the responsibility of the perpetrator/s. Sexual assault survivors often feel that they failed to sufficiently resist. They may feel especially responsible for sexual violence if they were pressured by poverty or previous abuse to "consent" to a work agreement which included illegal border crossing or smuggling even if they were deceived about what the 'work' really was.

It has been estimated that 80% of Mexican women in prostitution are mothers (Ojeda, 1994). In spite of their exhaustion and in spite of the physical and verbal violence in prostitution, they maintain a separate life which includes family and children, and in which the prostitution, for the most part, remains secret (Castillo, Gomez, & Delgado, 1999). A lengthy history of patriarchal domination, cultural influences and the resulting internalization of oppressive moral codes may hinder immigrant women (and all women) from reporting sexual assault and prevent them from seeking protection from pimps and traffickers. This silence results from shame about having been sexually harmed. The emphasis on virginity before marriage may compound the emotional pain suffered by a Latina victim of sexual exploitation, rape, or prostitution. Family and community may collude with the victim's self-blame if they view her as damaged or responsible for her own victimization.

THE NEED FOR COMPETENT BILINGUAL AND MULTICULTURAL SERVICES FOR PROSTITUTED/TRAFFICKED WOMEN AND CHILDREN

As the diversity of the United States grows, so do the needs of sexual assault survivors for culturally appropriate treatment, including services for those who are victims of sex trafficking (Rodriguez & O'Donnell, 1995). Undocumented immigrant women tend to avoid seeking social services for fear of being reported to the Immigration and Naturalization Service (INS). Once involved in the sex trade, immigrant victims may not attempt to escape for fear of violence or even torture by pimps/traffickers, as well as for fear that traffickers will harm relatives.

Culturally appropriate services are especially important for Latina survivors of prostitution, trafficking and other sexual violence. Not only language, but country and regional nuances need to be addressed in order to meet the needs of Latin American victims of all forms of sexual exploitation. Limited English language skills restricts access to information about rights, services and options, thus increasing a feeling of dependency.

A lack of translators, lack of bicultural/bilingual professionals, and lack of reading materials in the client's native language all pose barriers for victims of sexual exploitation. At some battered women's shelters, for example, other Latina survivors or residents have been inappropriately asked to interpret, just because they happened to be in the agency at the time. The use of resident interpreters may cause embarrassment and silence when sexual violence is addressed. Rather than sharing personal or shameful information with shelter roommates or worse yet–bilingual child residents–a survivor may simply choose not to discuss her sexual exploitation (Zarate, 2002b).

While some Spanish language materials are better than none, the message is lost or distorted when dialect, differences in attitude/awareness of sexual exploitation and class differences are ignored. Materials offered to survivors must take into account race discrimination, socioeconomic segregation, Spanish language limitations, and immigrant women's lack of knowledge about US laws. If a victim does not define her experience as abusive, no matter how adverse her experience, she will not seek help from violence prevention programs. Furthermore, the very label 'victim' may exacerbate her feelings of shame and self-blame. Culturally sensitive screening that incorporates a range of references to sexual abuse can be helpful in reframing the abuse and shifting the responsibility to the perpetrator/s. The phrases *me abusaron* (they abused me), *me falto el respeto* (he disrespected me), *me obligaron a salir con otros* (they made me go out with others) are some of the many ways that Latinas may refer to sexual assault and sexual exploitation.

We briefly describe two agencies which offer very different services to Latin American victims of sexual violence.

Arte Sana (Art Heals)

Arte Sana, based in Dripping Springs and Austin, Texas, offers programs that empower survivors of sex and race-based violence including prostitution and trafficking, through the arts, popular culture, community education, and professional training. Founded by the second author, Arte Sana utilizes the arts and *educacion popular* to address issues that are culturally taboo for Latinas such as sexual assault. Arte Sana addresses the lack of specific information for Latinas via Spanish language materials (such as a bilingual website www.arte-sana.com) and professional training regarding cultural competence and prevention of violence against women to other agencies in the United States and Mexico. The agency promotes collaborations for cyber resource sharing and the development of ongoing theme-based art exhibits in galleries, such as the *Corazón Lastimado* (Healing the Wounded Heart) sexual assault survivor art exhibit.

Survivors of rape, sexual exploitation, prostitution, or trafficking may find themselves in an abusive intimate partner relationship. At her first contact with a battered women's shelter or other women's services, she may not reveal the extent of her experience of sexual exploitation. Maria exemplifies the critical importance of culturally relevant education for Latina survivors of intimate partner violence, including prostitution and trafficking.

Maria graduated from a program that addressed issues ranging from finances to assertiveness. Only after attending an additional psycho-
educational presentation on sexual assault and the needs of survivors
was she able to define her experience as sexual assault. At the program's
graduation Maria expressed her appreciation for the session on sexual
assault and wanted to know if she could address that issue in her life.
Two years previously she had been raped as "additional payment" by the
man who smuggled her across the Mexico/US border. Maria's question
hay ayuda para este tipo de problema? (Is there help for this type of
problem?) arose only after she was offered a culturally relevant vehicle
to address her shame, self-blame, and lack of sexual autonomy.

Arte Sana utilizes popular songs to promote gender equality, positive relationships, and sexual autonomy. By deconstructing popular songs, *platicas*
(heart-to-heart talks) expose the narrowly defined subordinate roles for women
that exist in many Latino cultures. For example, the song *Taco Placero* describes sexual relationships as food, one being a full course, while the other is
cheap and quick. In contrast, the song *Invitame a Pecar* (Invite Me to Sin),
questions the notion of sex as sinful and promotes female sexual autonomy as
in the song's line: *invitame o te invito* (invite me or I will invite you). The Arte
Sana support groups expose the sexism in songs that promote the notion of
mala mujer (woman as intrinsically evil).

The Bilateral Safety Corridor Coalition–A Collaborative Service Agency for Provision of All Forms of Assistance to Trafficking Victims

At a homeless shelter in San Diego county, the first author observed that
90% of the clients seeking services were Mexican or Mexican-American
women and girls who had been raped or coerced into survival sex with gangs
after becoming homeless. Some were legal and some were undocumented immigrants, but many of these young women were involved in prostitution.

Although local medical clinics and specialized services for adolescents
were aware of their clients' prostitution and trafficking, abuse reports were not
filed. This may have resulted from a differentiation between "good" child
abuse victims (stranger abductions) and "bad" child abuse victims (those prostituted or trafficked). In 2001, the local sheriff and other county agencies did
not have resources to work with trafficking victims. UNICEF, the first author,
and Mexican Social Services together arrived at a strategic plan for service
provision and prevention of prostitution/trafficking in a southern California
trafficking corridor.

The Bilateral Safety Corridor Coalition (BSCC) was initially composed of a legal task force led by the local US Attorney's office, an education task force comprising University of San Diego and United Nations/San Diego, a communications task force composed of media, and a health task force with public health agencies. Goals of BSCC are to identify prostituted/trafficked children and adolescents, to establish liaisons between border regions, and to analyze the regional extent of trafficking in order to establish a network of services aimed at stopping trafficking. The BSCC encourages the involvement of human rights advocates, consulates, criminal justice and social services agencies on both sides of the border. Bilateral approaches to prostitution and trafficking have been implemented in other regions, such as Sweden and Finland.

NEEDS ASSESSMENT IS CRITICAL

Assessment of the mental and physical health status of transnationally trafficked women and girls is similar to evaluation of the needs of domestically trafficked (prostituted) women. The following must be evaluated: immediate physical safety, housing, legal or immigration status, physical injury, chronic illness or disability, malnutrition, acuity of psychological distress, access to social services, access to nonexploitive social support, literacy, education, job skills, and level of awareness of human rights.

Once the survivor of prostitution/trafficking is removed from immediate danger, crisis intervention is necessary. Effective intervention depends on establishing rapport and on acknowledging the victim's strengths. A supportive relationship with the provider of crisis services will help the victim cope with the stress of meeting with INS and law enforcement. Service providers must become educated about the systematic methods of brainwashing, indoctrination and control that are used against trafficked/prostituted women. In order to assist in prosecuting pimps and traffickers, women must be protected from physical danger. However, they are rarely offered sufficient protection. Pimps often threaten them with death and have told women that they can be arrested at any moment because they lack legal documents. As in the case of Sofia, pimps threaten to kill her family at home if she discloses criminal activity. In order to survive, the victim has had to comply with all of the trafficker's demands.

It is difficult to establish trust with victims of trafficking. Because of repeated betrayals by pimps, family, police, and government officials, many victims do not trust institutions such as the INS, other law enforcement and social service agencies. Informational errors during initial contacts with victims or in basic language interpretation have confused the police and resulted in failures to prosecute pimps and traffickers.

Because young women are without resources, and because they are paid more for not using condoms, STDs are the rule rather than the exception. In addition to hepatitis C and HIV, poverty-related diseases such as tuberculosis are common but rarely assessed in medical examinations of prostituted/trafficked girls. Sensitively delivered sex education should be standard practice when working with survivors of prostitution and trafficking. It should not be assumed that because women or adolescents are performing sex acts, they therefore understand STD and pregnancy prevention (Freed, 2003). Those who have received education about sex and STDs may later become sources of information, referral and support for others.

Trafficking and prostitution survivors experience multiple layers of trauma. The healing process is lengthy since survivors suffer psychological damage from captivity, terrorization, physical violence, and brainwashing and in many cases a long history of family and community violence (Stark & Hodgson, 2003; Farley et al., 2003). Survivors often feel indebted to pimps/traffickers for not killing them, in a psychological dynamic which has been described as the Stockholm Syndrome (Graham, 1994). Drug/alcohol detoxification and mood stabilization require medical management. Dissociative disorders are common, since hiding or forgetting one's real self makes it possible to survive atrocities (Ross, Farley, & Schwartz, 2003).

Trafficked women and girls have lived in a world of verbal abuse, lies, and physical danger, making adversarial law enforcement efforts an additional threat to their survival. Additional fear and mistrust is generated when women are sent to detention centers or locked medical facilities. Above all, the survivor's dignity must be preserved, and her legal rights must not be violated, especially if she is held as a material witness. An advocate should always be present to support her. Most victims will need to consult with both criminal and immigration attorneys. They may be vulnerable to a number of criminal charges such as illegally entering a country (a felony), prostitution (a misdemeanor), possession of false identification (a felony), or pandering (a misdemeanor). Ideally the local consulate of the victim's country of origin will assist in protecting the victim's rights. Collaboration with the criminal justice system of the victim's country of origin may be needed to investigate a trafficking case.

CONCLUSION

Women and children in Mexico and Latin America are profoundly harmed by the convergence of traditional and modern forms of sexual exploitation. Sex inequality, poverty, lack of educational opportunity, racism, rural-to-urban migration, state governments which protect the rich, tourism, and other structural social factors contribute to the harms of prostitution and trafficking. The expectation across cultures that women must always be sexually available to men leaves women vulnerable to the organized sexual exploitation of prostitution and trafficking. In order to gain control, traffickers and pimps exploit existing views of women as subordinate to men. Traffickers calculatedly reinforce the vulnerabilities of victims who have been neglected, abandoned or previously sexually abused. Traffickers lie to victims about their immigration status.

Exploitive working conditions in border factories place women and girls in extremely vulnerable positions, away from their home communities and vulnerable to sexual exploitation, including prostitution and trafficking. Sex businesses are the largest sector of employment for women who have lost jobs as a result of globalization.[5] Pimps and traffickers take advantage of the subordinate status of women and girls in both the United States and Mexico by exploiting sexist and racist stereotypes of women as property, commodities, servants, and sexual objects (Hernandez, 2001). Traffickers also take advantage of institutional inexperience regarding trafficking by criminal justice, health care, and social services within Latin America and the United States.

Trafficked women experience vulnerability, lack of resources, fears, and lack of control of their own lives that follow patterns similar to those of battered women (Stark & Hodgson, 2003). Additionally, trafficked/prostituted women have been uprooted from their home communities and are often in legal jeopardy due to their immigration status. Until special shelters for trafficking/prostitution survivors are available, battered women's shelters should be used for housing and safety.

Resources to assist victims of domestic and international trafficking must be tailored to meet the needs of people who are culturally and ethnically diverse and whose experiences of harm may differ. Although we are here addressing trafficking between Mexico and the United States, much of what is discussed is relevant to trafficking for prostitution between any sending and receiving country and also between sending and receiving communities within the same country. Meeting the challenge of serving survivors of prostitution and trafficking will require multicultural education regarding the complex issues involved, development of specialized treatment protocols for victims and collaboration across agencies, disciplines and borders.

NOTES

1. The United States defined trafficking in 2000 as occurring when "a commercial sex act is induced by force, fraud, or coercion, or in which the person induced to perform such act has not attained 18 years of age; or (b) the recruitment, harboring, transportation, provision, or obtaining of a person for labor or services, through the use of

force, fraud or coercion for the purpose of subjection to involuntary servitude, peonage, debt bondage, or slavery." US Dept of State, July 2001 Trafficking in Persons Report <*http://www.state.gov/g/inl/rls/tiprpt/2001/index.cfm*>.

2. Many Mexican gay men are married, even if they are not bisexual, to hide their sexual orientation and to protect themselves from intense homophobia.

3. See also Anderson, this volume, regarding similar attitudes toward rape of prostitutes under US law.

4. One Guatemalan official commented that given the mass rapes of Mayan girls by military personnel, it would be difficult to find a girl of 11 to 15 who had not been raped (Rich, 1996). See also Farley et al. (2003) (in this volume) for a description of the effect of Colombia's civil war on women generally, and women and girls in prostitution.

5. The international trafficking of human beings, especially prostituted women, is the world's third largest area of organized crime, and a business that produces $7 billion annually. Greater illegal profits are found only in the drugs and arms trades, according to data from the United Nations Office for Drug Control and Crime Prevention (ODCCP), released during the International Seminar on Trafficking in Human Beings, in the Brazilian capital. (Osava, 2000).

REFERENCES

Azaola, E. (2001). *Infancia robada. Niñas y niños víctimas de explotación sexual en México.* UNICEF-DIF-CIESAS, México.

British Broadcasting Company (2002). Human Trafficking Report from Johns Hopkins University. *BBC Monitoring International Reports.* May 24, 2002.

Burkhart, L. (1989). *The Slippery Earth: Nahua-Christian Moral Dialogue in Sixteenth-Century Mexico.* Tucson: University of Arizona Press.

Castillo, D.A., Gomez, M.G.R., & Delgado, B. (1999). Border Lives: Prostitute Women in Tijuana. *Signs: Journal of Women in Culture and Society* 24: 387-422.

Casteneda, M. (2000). Silence is Also Violence, *Granma International.* Havana: Granma International Digital.

Chiquiar, D., & Hanson, G. (October, 2002). National Bureau of Economic Research–International Migration, Self-Selection and the Distribution of Wages: Evidence from Mexico and the United States. Accessed at: *http://www.nber.org/papers/w9242* on January 16, 2003.

Domecq, B. (1992). Acechando el unicornio: la virginidad en la literatura mexicana. Mexico: Fondo de Cultura Economica.

Ehrenreich, B., & Hochschild, A. (2002). *Global Woman.* York: Holt & Co.

Farley, M., & Kelly, V. (2000). Prostitution: A critical review of the medical and social sciences literature. *Women & Criminal Justice* 11 (4): 29-64.

Farley, M., Cotton, A., Lynne, J., Zumbeck, S., Spiwak, S., Reyes, M.E., Alvarez, D., & Sezgin, U. (2003). Prostitution & Trafficking in Nine Countries: An Update on Violence and Posttraumatic Stress Disorder. In M. Farley (ed.) *Prostitution, Trafficking, and Traumatic Stress* (2003) Binghamton: The Haworth Press, Inc.

Freed, W. (2003). From Duty to Despair: Brothel Prostitution in Cambodia. In M. Farley (ed.) *In Prostitution, Trafficking, and Traumatic Stress* (2003) Binghamton: The Haworth Press, Inc.

Gonzalez de la Vega, F. (1968). *Derecho penal en Mexico: Los delitos.* Mexico: Porrua.

Gonzalez-Lopez, G. (in press). "De madres a hijas: Gendered Lessons on Virginity Across Generations of Mexican Immigrant Women," in Pierrette Hondagneu-Sotel (ed.) *Gender and U.S. Migration: Contemporary Trends.* Berkeley: University of California Press.

Graham, D.L.R., with Rawlings, E., & Rigsby, R. (1994). *Loving to Survive: Sexual Terror, Men's Violence and Women's Lives.* New York: New York University Press.

Hadden, G. National Public Radio News, Reporting from Mexico City: Mexico-Child Kidnappings. Accessed January 15, 2003 at: http://search.npr. org/cf/cmn/segment_dis play.cfm?segID=146969. July 19, 2002.

Harbury, J. CERIGUA Weekly Briefs, No. 48. Dec. 11, 1997.

Heinzl, T. (January 4, 2003). Star-Telegram Immigrant smugglers sentenced Accessed February 27, 2003 at http://www.dfw.com/mld/startelegram/news/local/4873549.htm.

Hernandez, A. (2003). The Sex Trafficking of Children in San Diego: Minors are prostituted in farm labor camps in San Diego. *El Universal.* Mexico City. Jan 11, 2003.

Hernandez, T. K. (2001). Sexual Harassment and Racial Disparity: The Mutual Construction of Gender and Race. *U. Iowa Journal of Gender, Race & Justice* 4: 183-224.

Hotaling, N., Burris, A. B., Johnson, B.J., Bird, Y.M., & Melbye, K.A. (2003). Been There Done That: SAGE A Peer Leadership Model among Prostitution Survivors. In M. Farley (ed.) *Prostitution, Trafficking, & Traumatic Stress.* Binghamton: The Haworth Press, Inc.

Jordan, M. (2002). In Mexico, rape often goes unpunished *Washington Post.* Accessed January 21, 2003 at *http://www.arizonarepublic.com/special03/articles/0701mexico-rape-ON.html.*

Joyce, R. A. (2000). *Gender and Power in Prehispanic Mesoamerica.* Austin: University of Texas Press.

Kovaleski, S F. (2000). Child Sex Trade Rises in Central America: Prostitution is Dark Side of Tourism. Cited by L. Lederer (2001) in Human Rights Report of Trafficking of Women and Children. Washington, D.C.: Protection Project, p. 137.

Larrain, S. (1997). Inter-American Development Bank: Curbing Domestic Violence: Two Decades of Action Accessed online at: *http://www.iadb.org/sds/doc/1077eng.pdf.*

Lederer, L.J. (2001). *Human Rights Report on Trafficking of Women and Children Map: Trafficking routes for Latin America.* Washington, DC: The Protection Project.

Lederer, L J. (2001). *Human Rights Report on Trafficking of Women.* Washington, DC: The Protection Project. p. 62.

Lostaunau, Frank (2003). Personal communication. San Francisco California. February 13, 2003.

Maki, F. T., & Park, G. (2000). Trafficking in Women and Children: The U.S. and International Response. Congressional Research Service Report 98-649C, May 10, 2000. Cited in Trafficking in Persons: USAID's Response Selected USAID Antitrafficking efforts in Latin America and the Caribbean. USAID-Office of Women in Development 2001. Accessed February 27, 2003 at *http://www.usaid.gov/wid/pubs/trw01f.htm.*

Ojeda, N. L. (1994). Postitucion en los noventa. *Nexos* 17 (203): 76-80.

Osava, M. (2000). Trafficking in Humans: A $7 Billion Business. Montevideo Uruguay: InterPress Third World News Agency (IPS). November 29, 2000. Accessed October 1, 2002 at: *http://headlines.igc.apc.org:8080/wnheadlines/975944748/in dex_html.*

Overmyer-Velázquez, R. (1998). Christian Morality Revealed in New Spain: The Inimical Woman in Book Ten of the Florentine Codex. *Journal of Women's History* 10(2), Spring, 1998.

Rabinovitch, R. (2003). PEERS: The Prostitutes' Empowerment, Education and Resource Society. In M. Farley (ed.) *Prostitution, Trafficking, and Traumatic Stress.* Binghamton: Haworth.

Richard, A. O. (2000). International Trafficking in Women to the United States: A Contemporary Manifestation of Slavery and Organized Crime. DCI Report, United States Department of State. Also available online at *http://www.cia.gov/csi/monograph/women/trafficking.pdf.*

Rodriguez, O., & O'Donnell, M. (1995). *Help-seeking and use of mental health services by the Hispanic elderly.* Westport, CT: Greenwood Press.

Ross, C.A., Farley, M., & Schwartz, H.L. (2003). Dissociation among Women in Prostitution. In M. Farley (ed.) *Prostitution, Trafficking, and Traumatic Stress.* Binghamton: The Haworth Press, Inc.

SIPAZ (1998). Women and Low Intensity Warfare. Cited in: The Factbook on Global Sexual Exploitation Mexico The Coalition Against Trafficking in Women. SIPAZ Report 3 (1). Accessed Jan. 20, 2003 at *http://www.catwinternational.org/fb/Mex ico.html.*

Stark, C. & Hodgson, C. (2003). Sister Oppressions: A Comparison of Wife Battering and Prostitution. In M Farley (ed.) *Prostitution, Trafficking, and Traumatic Stress.* Binghamton, NY: The Haworth Press, Inc.

Taino, S. (1998). Women's Work and Unemployment in Northern Mexico, Women on the U.S.-Mexico Border. Cited in: From: "Human Rights Watch Report: Maquiladoras" Accessed February 10, 2003 at *http://www.transnationale.org/anglais/sources/tiersmonde/zonesfranchesMaqui98d-02.htm.*

Tyler, K.A., Hoyt, D.R., & Whitbeck, L.B. (2000). The effects of early sexual abuse on later sexual victimization among female homeless and runaway youth. *Journal of Interpersonal Violence* 15: 235-250.

Zarate, L. (2002a). Victim Blaming. Available at Arte Sana online: *http://www.arte-sana.com/virtual_gallery/exhibits/day_dead_02/gallery_exhibit_ni_una_mas.htm.* Accessed April 7, 2003.

Zarate, L. (2002b). The Challenges Identified by Sexual Assault Programs. Presentation at the Centers for Disease Control-Illinois Coalition Against Sexual Assault National Sexual Violence Prevention Conference. Chicago. May 29, 2002.

Prostitution and Trafficking in Women: An Intimate Relationship

Dorchen A. Leidholdt

SUMMARY. This article, written by the Co-Executive Director of the Coalition Against Trafficking in Women, analyzes the relationship of sex trafficking and prostitution. The author begins by examining prostitution as a system of gender-based domination and as a practice of violence against women that often encompasses specific forms of gender based violence, including child sexual abuse, rape, and domestic violence. She explores legal instruments that address and define trafficking, pointing out that distinctions between prostitution and trafficking in women are relatively recent and have been promoted by organizations and governments working to legitimize and/or legalize prostitution as work. She argues that prostitution and trafficking are fundamentally interrelated, to the extent that sex trafficking can accurately be viewed as "globalized prostitution" while generic prostitution often is a practice of "domestic trafficking." The author concludes by calling for definitions, laws, and strategies that include and challenge all manifestations of local and global sex industries.

Dorchen A. Leidholdt, JD, MA, is Director of the Center for Battered Women's Legal Services at Sanctuary for Families, New York, and Co-Executive Director, Coalition Against Trafficking in Women (CATW). She can be contacted at Center for Battered Women's Legal Services, 67 Wall Street, Suite 2211, New York, NY 10005.
Printed with permission.

[Haworth co-indexing entry note]: "Prostitution and Trafficking in Women: An Intimate Relationship." Leidholdt, Dorchen A. Co-published simultaneously in *Journal of Trauma Practice* (The Haworth Maltreatment & Trauma Press, an imprint of The Haworth Press, Inc.) Vol. 2, No. 3/4, 2003, pp. 167-183; and: *Prostitution, Trafficking, and Traumatic Stress* (ed: Melissa Farley) The Haworth Maltreatment & Trauma Press, an imprint of The Haworth Press, Inc., 2003, pp. 167-183. Single or multiple copies of this article are available for a fee from The Haworth Document Delivery Service [1-800-HAWORTH, 9:00 a.m. - 5:00 p.m. (EST). E-mail address: docdelivery@haworthpress.com].

In 1991 I flew to Strasbourg, France to participate in an international conference on trafficking in women. It was less than two years after I had helped found the international nongovernmental organization, the Coalition Against Trafficking in Women, and I felt confident that I understood what sex trafficking is: the merchandising of women's bodies for the sexual gratification of men in a sex industry that mirrored other industries in its growing globalization. Like drug and arms trafficking, sex trafficking, I believe, is under the control of local and international criminal elements, is fueled by customer demand, and exploits and reinforces inequalities between regions in the global North/West and the South/East. Sex trafficking, I was convinced, is uniquely horrific because the commodity for sale is not inanimate objects but living human beings–almost exclusively women and children–and the conclusion of the trafficking process is a paradigmatically gendered transaction, which the male buyers calls sex or prostitution while the women and children bought liken it to sexual harassment or rape. Sex tourism, military prostitution, brothel prostitution, street prostitution, strip clubs, lap dancing, international trafficking: all these I considered interrelated manifestations of local and global sex industries and components of the human rights disaster known as trafficking in women.

A stop I made on my journey to the conference strengthened not only my belief that I understood what trafficking in women was but also my determination to stop it. I flew into Frankfurt, Germany on my way to Strasbourg, and there I was able to study, up close, the contemporary sex industry in all of its complexity. The Frankfurt city fathers had created a system of legal, regulated brothels, apparently in an effort to stamp out an array of evils, including street prostitution, control of the sex industry by organized crime, and the spread of sexually transmitted diseases. From what I could see, their strategy was a colossal failure. Street prostitution was flourishing; organized crime groups were running underground brothels filled with Asian, Latin American, and Eastern European women and girls; and only the few legal brothels (which were grossly outnumbered by their underground counterparts) made an effort to ensure that customers used condoms.

What had emerged in Frankfurt was a two-tiered system of prostitution. Women and girls who had been trafficked primarily from poor countries were propelled into a competition with white, German-born women for local prostitution customers and a growing number of sex tourists. It was apparent that the quotient of suffering was the most acute for the undocumented women and girls in the illegal brothels: They were forced to endure unwanted sex with half-a-dozen customers each night, unable to protect themselves from HIV and other sexually transmitted diseases (indeed the ability of the customer to refuse condoms was one of the chief attractions of the underground brothels), deprived of travel documents, threatened with violence and deportation, and required to work off exorbitant debt that locked them into conditions of slavery. While not as dire as that of their internationally trafficked sisters, the lot of the legally prostituted women was also dismal. Posing as an American newspaper reporter working on a story on "new developments in the sex industry," I was welcomed by the madam into the brothel, which resembled a four-star hotel in the United States. I was soon surrounded by a group of women eager for a distraction from their late afternoon wait for their "clients." Several of the women's husbands were also their pimps, most of the women were from poor, rural areas of Germany, and all faced bleak futures with few employment skills. The sex of prostitution was an unwanted invasion they had developed a series of strategies to avoid–their favorite was to get the men so drunk that they didn't know what they were penetrating. The women seemed bored and depressed. Their depression deepened when I asked them what they hoped to be doing in five years. Aside from one woman who said that she hoped to help manage the brothel, they were at a loss for words.

When I boarded the train to Strasbourg, it seemed indisputable that prostitution and sex trafficking were closely related phenomena. Once I arrived at my destination, however, the conference organizers–the Dutch government-funded Foundation Against Trafficking in Women–announced in no uncertain terms that they believed otherwise. All of the participants were instructed that the topic at hand was trafficking in women; prostitution was not to be discussed. As the conference proceeded, it became clear that the organizers had developed an exceedingly narrow definition of trafficking. The organizers insisted that sex trafficking was the transport of women across national or regional boundaries and always involved the use of force or deceit. The fact that women were trafficked for the purpose of prostitution was, to the organizers, irrelevant. Indeed, it seemed to make little difference to them whether the women were trafficked for purposes of prostitution or cookie baking. It was irrelevant to them that the women were trafficked into local sex industries; their focus was strictly confined to international criminal networks forcibly moving women across borders.

It became evident that the conference organizers' definition of trafficking and their censorship of the topic of prostitution was a deliberate strategy used to further a specific agenda. The Dutch government, which had funded the conference, was convinced that the sex industry can be a benign and lucrative source of income for countries and women alike if prostitution is legalized and regulated. All of the abuses apparent in local and international sex industries, according to the Dutch government, derives from their illegal status, which drives them underground and under the control of organized crime. Prostitution, if made legal and cleansed of its stigma, can be a job like any other job. A decade after the conference, the Dutch government fully implemented its agenda by legalizing and licensing 2,000 brothels and registering as prostitutes the women and girls in them (Louis, 1999; LifeSiteNews.com, 1999). Once prostitution was legal in the Netherlands, brothel owners began to recruit women into prostitution through government-sponsored job centers for unemployed workers (Ananova.com, 2002).

The conference organizers' efforts to censor discussion about prostitution backfired. Several of the participants insisted on addressing it. One of the dissenting voices was that of Swedish social work professor Sven Axel Månsson, who had conducted studies of male prostitution customers and was convinced that trafficking could not be curtailed without strong measures to confront and eliminate the demand for prostituted women and girls.

Since that conference in Strasbourg, the question of the relationship of prostitution to sex trafficking has taken on greater significance. Over the decade that followed, other nongovernmental organizations (NGOs) joined the Dutch Foundation Against Trafficking in insisting that trafficking and prostitution are separate and unrelated phenomena. These NGOs argued aggressively that trafficking is a human rights violation while prostitution is work–"sex work." Following the Netherlands, some jurisdictions have adopted legislation that legalizes domestic sex industries while directing criminal penalties against international sex traffickers (The Protection Project, 2001). Reports have documented a dramatic increase in trafficking following the legalization of prostitution industries (Sullivan & Jeffries, 2001). Never has it been more critical to address the issue of the relationship between prostitution and sex trafficking. What is prostitution? How if at all is it related to sex trafficking? To other practices of violence against women? Why is there a debate over definitions of trafficking? Is there an agenda behind efforts to restrict the definition of trafficking? In this article, I will grapple with these questions.

PROSTITUTION: A SYSTEM OF DOMINATION

Prostitution is often addressed in the abstract, as a transaction unconstrained by social forces, in which one gender-neutral individual purchases an act of sex from another, exchanging sexual pleasure for compensation. Both parties to the exchange, in this way of thinking, benefit from it. It is conceivable that in a radically different social order–one of complete gender equity and equality–the exchange of sex for money might be just such a gender-free, benign transaction. However, prostitution exists squarely within cultures of gender-based inequality. Indeed, some have persuasively argued, it is the paradigmatic expression of male domination of women (Giobbe, 1990; Dworkin, 1993, 1994).

Far from being gender-neutral, prostitution is gendered to the hilt. The buyers are men whose goal is their sexual pleasure. The bought are largely women and girls whose purpose–if they are enough in control of their destinies to have a purpose–is often economic survival. The businesses are controlled by men, often assisted by women in their employ. Their goal is profit–and the profits figure in the billions (Pateman, 1988; Leidholdt, 1993; Arizona Coalition Against Domestic Violence, April 2002). In Germany alone, prostitution reaps an estimated $6 billion annually (Schelzig, 2002).

The reasons that women and girls enter prostitution are profoundly gendered. Research demonstrates that in the global North and West a large majority of women and girls entering prostitution have histories of sexual abuse by a male relative or family friend–some studies estimate as many as 70 percent (Silbert & Pines, 1982; Silbert, 1983; The Council for Prostitution Alternatives, 1991; Giobbe, 1990; Hotaling, 1999). Whether fleeing abuse, and the homelessness and economic destitution that often ensues, drives girls into prostitution or whether the psychological consequences of abuse render them vulnerable to the wiles of pimps, it is clear that incest and sexual molestation are significant risk factors for prostitution. In the global East and South the low social status of girls often induces poor families to sacrifice their daughters to prostitution (Cambodian Women's Crisis Center, 1999; Diakite, 1999; Huda, 1999; Vasconcelos, 1999; Minnesota Advocates for Human Rights, 2000). Around the world, women escaping abuse by their husbands and members of their husbands' extended families are rendered homeless and, with no means of support, find themselves in prostitution (Minnesota Advocates for Human Rights, 2000).

While male customers of prostitution are rewarded by sexual gratification, and male profiteers of prostitution are rewarded by the enormous sums of money they earn, the financial benefits to prostituted women and girls are usually meager and are almost always outweighed by the profound physical and emotional harms of prostitution: sexually transmitted diseases, internal injuries, depression, traumatic stress, somatic and psychological dissociation, to name a few (Raymond, 1999; Raymond, D'Cunha, Dzuhayatin, Hynes, Rodriguez, & Santos, 2002). Not surprisingly, however, they got into prostitution, the women and children in it usually want to get out–as quickly as possible (Farley, Baral, Kiremire & Sezgin, 1998; Farley, 2003).

The exit of women and children from prostitution does not square with the agendas of the men profiting from it or the men who derive pleasure from it. Thus, pimps and sex industry profiteers have made prostitution into a system of domination that is remarkably consistent across cultures–one that mirrors the dynamics of power and control exerted by domestic violence perpetrators over the women they abuse (Stark & Hodgson, 2003).

Like prisons or concentration camps, prostitution often does not require overt physical coercion or verbal threat since the system of domination perpetuated and enforced by sex industry businessmen and buyers is intrinsically coercive. Women and girls who enter prostitution are seasoned into it; they are in the parlance of pimps, "turned out." The sex industry entrepreneur "turns out" a woman or girl by eradicating her identity, erasing her sense of self, especially any belief that she is entitled to dignity and bodily integrity. "Turning out" often takes place through rape and acts of sexual humiliation. It is facilitated by changing her name, giving her a "makeover" to ensure that she will be viewed as a sex object, alienating her from her family and friends, instilling in her the belief that she is an "outlaw," rejected by yet superior to "straight" society, and teaching her to accept her place in a rigid hierarchy, where she is obedient to the man who profits from the sale of her body and any women he designates as his surrogate (Giobbe, 1990; D'Cunha, 2000). The final step is to instill in her absolute obedience to the entrepreneur's regime, a system of rules designed to ensure that she stays in the place he has designated for her and generates the income he wants (Giobbe, 1990; Minnesota Advocates for Human Rights, 2000). While obedience may lead to rewards, most often to a position of control over other prostituted women or girls, violations of the rules are punished severely, usually by rape and beatings (Giobbe, 1998; Giobbe, 1993; Giobbe, 1992; Giobbe, 1991). Thus, prostitution is not only a system of gender-based domination; it is a system of gender-based totalitarianism.

PROSTITUTION AND VIOLENCE AGAINST WOMEN

While prostitution may be characterized as an expression of sexual freedom or as a form of labor, the reality is that it bears a much closer relationship to–indeed it incorporates–practices of gender-based violence, especially the sexual abuse of girls, rape, and intimate partner violence. It is well established that sexual abuse in childhood is a precondition for prostitution: studies reveal that between 55 and 90 percent of prostituted women have histories of childhood sexual abuse (Parriott, 1994, Silbert & Pines, 1982, Farley, Baral, Kiremire & Sezgin, 1998). It has also been established that the prime targets for prostitution and the most valuable commodities in the sex industry are children and young women barely out of childhood (Cardwell, 2002; O'Leary & Howard, 2001). As women mature they rapidly lose their marketability as sex objects and, marginalized within the sex industry, become valuable only if they are available for sadomasochism or other especially degrading practices (Carter, 2002).

The relation between prostitution and child sexual abuse is even closer. Prostitution does not just chronologically follow childhood sexual exploitation: For most prostituted adults, it perpetuates its dynamics and effects (Giobbe, 1992). Prostitution customers are often significantly older than the women and girls whose bodies they purchase–frequently old enough to be their fathers or grandfathers. The inequality of social, sexual, and economic power between prostitution customers and those they prostitute is usually as extreme as the power differential between adult and child. Most important, prostitution, like child sexual abuse, is a transaction whose goal is the sexual satisfaction of the male; it is for this end that the bodily integrity of the female is violated (Farley, 2003). Prostituted girls and women describe having flashbacks to incidents of incest or molestation as they turn tricks and frequently experience the same psychological damage as incest survivors–depression, suicidal ideations or attempts, self-mutilation, and post-traumatic stress disorder (Farley et al., 1998). Prostitution keeps alive the experience and damage of child sexual abuse for the prostituted girl or woman. One prostitution survivor vividly described to me her revulsion at the gray pubic hair of a "trick" the age of her grandfather. During sexual encounters with "tricks," she told me, she re-experienced the sexual abuse she had been subjected to by her stepfather.

While an extraordinarily high number of prostituted women are subjected to rape throughout the period they are prostituted, they also describe the act of being prostituted as rape-like sex acts that are unwanted, violating, and assaultive. One prostitution survivor memorably described prostitution as "bought and sold rape" (Giobbe, 1999). The dissociative state experienced by prostituted girls and women during the act of prostitution is the same dissociation that rape victims employ to shield themselves psychologically from sexual assault. But whereas for date rape or stranger rape victims, rape is almost always a one time assault, women and girls in prostitution are subjected to "bought and sold rape" over and over, often multiple times in the course of a single evening. Thus, for prostituted women and girls, the rape-like experience they must endure is not a single assault but a prolonged, numbing series of sexual violations, carried out by multiple violators, that resembles nothing so much as gang rape, and not just a single gang rape, but gang rape carried out day after day, often over the course of years (Giobbe, 1991).

The relationship between prostitution and domestic violence is profound but rarely understood. In societies where wives are considered the property of their husbands and their husbands' families, women fleeing domestic violence find themselves in circumstances similar to that of girls fleeing incest in industrial and post-industrial societies: homeless and vulnerable to pimps and other sex industry profiteers. Prostituted women I interviewed in Bangladesh and Mali described the factors that drove them into prostitution as battering by their husbands and the homelessness that ensued when their own families refused to harbor them after they escaped their husbands' homes.

Much prostitution is domestic violence, and many prostitutes are battered women. Across cultures, procurers and pimps are frequently abusive husbands and boyfriends. It is not simply a coincidence that one of the most common slurs that batterers direct against their victims is "whore," "puta," or its linguistic equivalent. Batterers often regard and treat their victims as "whores"–as communal sexual property–pressuring or forcing their victims to engage in unwanted sex with other partners. Batterers also frequently turn their victims into their personal prostitutes, requiring their wives and girlfriends to perform sexual favors in exchange for money for food and other necessities (author's unpublished interviews with battered women, 1994-2002).

Pimps are themselves batterers. They typically start out as the boyfriends of young, vulnerable girls, often runaways, and then persuade the girls to prove their devotion by turning tricks and handing over the proceeds (Giobbe, 1996). The pimp's "stable" resembles a polygamous family, with the wives ordered into a hierarchy of submission. The pimp's "main woman" is the equivalent of the polygamous husband's first wife and, like her, is charged with the responsibility of keeping the other, younger women in line. In both "families," when the wives or "whores" step out of line, the consequence is a beating by the paterfamilias/pimp (Giobbe, 1990, 1991, 1993).

While the pimp with his stable of "whores" is the prototype, prostitution in contemporary societies is often less stereotypical. Over the last decade, in Germany, Mexico, the Philippines, and the United States, I have interviewed women who are pimped solo by abusive husbands and boyfriends to whom they turn over their earnings, hoping that the money will enable them to buy a dream home, financial security, and an end to the prostitution.

Domestic violence has come to be understood not as a discrete series of violent acts but as a system of power and control the batterer institutes and maintains over his victim through the use of an array of interconnected strategies: isolation, intimidation, emotional abuse, economic abuse, sexual abuse, and threats (Power and Control Wheel, Domestic Abuse Intervention Project, Duluth, Minnesota). The criminal justice system's focus on the batterer's violent acts rather than on his tactics of "coercive control" has hidden the fundamental harm of domestic violence–not physical injury but gender-based subjugation (Stark, 2000).

The power and control model used to understand the modus operandi of perpetrators of domestic violence is rarely applied to tactics of procurers, pimps, brothel owners, and other sex industry profiteers. This fact is likely the consequence of the success of the notion that prostitutes are sex workers who choose prostitution over other career options. The reality, however, is that the strategies of power and control used by battering husbands and boyfriends are identical to the strategies used by their counterparts in the sex industry.

The first step in the seasoning of girls and women into prostitution is isolation from family, friends, and support networks that strengthens the abuser's control. While batterers teach their wives or girlfriends that their families and friends are dangerous and untrustworthy and punish the women for any contact with them, pimps inculcate in their victims the belief that they are outlaws who exist in opposition to the hostile, judgmental, and punitive world of "straights." Emotional abuse that instills in the victims feelings of inferiority and worthlessness through derogatory name-calling and constant putdowns and criticism is a staple of batterers and pimps alike. Economic control–especially by requiring victims to turn over their earnings–is the sine qua non of pimping and pervasive in battering. Sexual abuse–both pimps and batterers often cement their control over their victims through rape–is endemic to the experience of being prostituted and battered. Likewise, intimidation and threats–to beat, to kill, to abduct her children, to harm her family members, to leave her homeless, to have her deported–are a mainstay of pimps and batterers.

DEFINING PROSTITUTION AND TRAFFICKING

The drafters of the United Nations' Convention for the Suppression of the Traffic in Persons and of the Exploitation of Prostitution of Others (hereafter, the "1949 Convention") did not find it necessary to define trafficking. They considered trafficking to be a cross-border practice of "the exploitation of the prostitution of others" and drafted a treaty that addressed both human rights violations equally. Together, as they understood it, "trafficking in persons and the exploitation of the prostitution of others" encompassed the activities of an increasingly global sex industry whose activities were "incompatible with the dignity and worth of the human person" (Marcovich, 2002). In 1979, the drafters of the Convention on the Elimination of All Forms of Discrimination Against Women (CEDAW) embraced the language of the 1949 Convention, its Article 6 requiring States Parties to "take all appropriate measures, including legislation, to suppress all forms of traffic in women and exploitation of prostitution of women."

A perceived need to define trafficking and to distinguish it from prostitution came only much later, in the 1980s. The goal was to confine both the scope of domestic and international laws addressing the sex industry and activism against it. The 1949 Convention criminalized the profit-making activities of local and global sex businesses without penalizing those exploited in prostitution. Had the Convention been equipped with implementing mechanisms that enforced its provisions, it would have posed a serious threat to sex industry businesses. An international movement to abolish prostitution, founded by Josephine Butler at the end of the Nineteenth Century, was still active in the 1980s, and feminists speaking out against the sexual exploitation of women in prostitution were beginning to join forces with the "abolitionists" to strengthen the 1949 Convention and to pass and implement national and local laws consistent with it (Barry, 1979, 1995). Media reports of the suffering of trafficking victims and the increasing globalization of the sex industry were fueling support for a campaign against the sex industry. Eager to ward off such a danger, pro-sex industry forces developed a strategy.

Ignoring or denying the harm of the sex industry was not an option, for that harm was well documented. A more pragmatic approach was to focus on the most brutal and extreme practices of the sex industry–transporting women from poor countries to rich countries using tactics of debt bondage and overt force–while legitimizing its other activities in the name of worker's rights.

The old dichotomy of Madonna-whore was replaced by a new dichotomy: sex worker-trafficked woman. In order to defend prostitution as sex work, trafficking was articulated as gender-neutral, with labor trafficking and sex trafficking collapsed under the same rubric as "trafficking in persons." Otherwise it would be too evident that the ultimate harm of sex trafficking is the decidedly gendered condition in which the trafficking victim is transported into–prostitution. "Prostitution" was stricken from the lexicon and replaced by "sex work." Similarly, "pimp," "procurer," and "brothel owner" were replaced by "business owners" or "third-party managers." The old terminology suggested that the sex industry was exploitative or worse whereas, according to the new understanding, it is about the right of individuals to make money as they choose. Indeed it is about the right to economic development. Even "trafficking" was troublesome because it implied that those who were trafficked were victims. The term "trafficking" began to be replaced with the more neutral "migration." Because there was a danger that the agents who profited from transporting women might be stigmatized as common traffickers the phrase "facilitated migration" was coined (Ditmore, 1999; Doezma, 1999; Doezma, 2001; Network of Sexwork Projects, 2002).

The battle over definitions of trafficking came to a fore in the drafting of the Trafficking Protocol to the proposed Transnational Convention Against Organized Crime. Many mainstream human rights organizations, including the International Human Rights Law Group and Human Rights Watch, influenced by the "choice" rhetoric of the sex industry's lobby, supported a definition of trafficking that required proof of force and deceit. Explicitly feminist human rights groups–most prominently the Coalition Against Trafficking in Women,

Equality Now, and the European Women's Lobby–called for a definition of trafficking that included trafficking carried out by the abuse of a position of power or a situation of vulnerability. In this international context, where developing countries grappling with the devastation wrought by the sex industry were active participants, the arguments of the pro-prostitution lobby foundered, and the more inclusive and protective definition was adopted (UN Protocol, 2000; Guide to the New UN Trafficking Protocol, 2001).

In contrast, that same year Congress passed the Trafficking Victims Protection Act, whose provisions governing the penalization of traffickers and the protection of victims were limited to cases of "severe trafficking," requiring proof that the trafficking was carried out by force or deceit. Although such a restricted definition creates an often insurmountable burden for prosecutors, who must establish beyond a reasonable doubt not only that the victim was trafficked but that she did not consent to it, the restricted definition prevailed. Two years after its passage, only four prosecutions had been brought under the new law.

PROSTITUTION OR TRAFFICKING IN WOMEN?

What is the relation if any between prostitution and sex trafficking?

The truth is that what we call sex trafficking is nothing more or less than globalized prostitution. Sex industry profiteers transport girls and women across national and regional borders and "turn them out" into prostitution in locations in which their victims are least able to resist and where there is the greatest demand for them. The demand is greatest in countries with organized women's movements, where the status of women is high and there are relatively few local women available for commercial sexual exploitation (D'Cunha, 2002a). The brothels of the United States, Canada, the Netherlands, Germany, Austria, and Australia are filled with women trafficked from Asia, Latin America, and Eastern Europe. No less than 50% of German prostitutes are illegal immigrants and a staggering 80% of Dutch prostitutes are not Dutch-born (Owen, 2002; Louis, 1999). The implications for the women's rights movements in these countries of the massive sexual exploitation of poor immigrant women, many trafficked, is staggering, but the mainstream feminist response has, for the most part, been one of indifference.

Conversely, what most people refer to as "prostitution" can also be seen as domestic trafficking. "Casual prostitution," prostitution in which a woman with apparent options enters of her own apparent volition, accounts for only about one percent of the women in the sex industry, according to Davidson (1998). The bulk of the sex industry involves pimps and other sex industry entrepreneurs controlling women and girls, often by moving them from places in which they have family and friends into locations in which they have no systems of support (D'Cunha, 1999, 2002a). Movement is also essential because customers demand novelty. In the United States there are national and regional sex industry circuits in which prostituted women and girls are rotated among cities, ensuring customers variety and sex industry entrepreneurs control (Raymond & Hughes, 2000).

Increasingly, the boundaries between local prostitution and international sex trafficking are blurred. In 2001, the Kings County District Attorney's Office in New York City busted a prostitution ring run by Russian nationals living in the United States. The ring recruited newly arrived Russian immigrant women, desperate for income, through ads in Russian language newspapers that falsely promised lucrative work. Is this prostitution or is it trafficking?

Sex trafficking and prostitution overlap in fundamental ways. Those targeted for commercial sexual exploitation share key demographic characteristics: poverty, youth, minority status in the country of exploitation, histories of abuse, and little family support. Sex industry customers exploit trafficked and prostituted women interchangeably, for the identical purpose. (There is no specific demand for "trafficked" women–any woman or girl will suffice.) The sex industry businesses in which trafficked and prostituted women are exploited are often one and the same, with trafficked and domestically prostituted women "working" side by side. Local brothels and strip clubs are usually traffickers' destinations and key to their financial success. The injuries that prostituted and trafficked women suffer are identical: post-traumatic stress disorder, severe depression, damage to reproductive systems, damage from sexual assault and beatings, and sexually transmitted diseases (Raymond, 2001; Farley, 2003).

Certainly international trafficking intensifies the dynamics of power and control that characterize domestic prostitution: the isolation of the victims; their dependence on their abusers; their difficulty in accessing criminal justice and social service systems; and their fear of exposure to the authorities. But the dynamics of trafficking and prostitution are the same dynamics, and their commonalities far overshadow their differences. In spite of efforts to differentiate and separate prostitution and trafficking, the inescapable conclusion is that the difference between the two, at best, is one of degree of, not of kind.

GOVERNMENTS RESPOND TO PROSTITUTION AND TRAFFICKING

Creating distinctions between prostitution (or "sex work") and trafficking protects business as usual in the sex industry. Those who have promoted these distinctions have for the most part been those with the greatest economic stake in the sex industry carrying on business as usual–countries, most notably the Netherlands and Germany, which legalize and tax sex industry businesses, and a pro-prostitution lobby representing a mix of Dutch- and German-funded nongovernmental organizations, libertarian groups, and sex industry interests. Their philosophy originates in the propaganda of the California-based organization, COYOTE (Call Off Your Old Tired Ethics), which took credit for coining the term "sex worker" in the early 1970s (Delacoste & Alexander, 1991). Now defunct, COYOTE represented just such a mix of libertarian activists and sex industry profiteers, organizing "Hookers Ball" celebrations of the San Francisco sex industry. COYOTE's philosophy–that prostitution is a job just like any other job and should be legitimized and legalized as such–found fertile ground in the growing sex industry centers of Western Europe, among sex industry patrons and profiteers, and among fringe groups of the Left like the British-based "Wages for Housework" and its spin offs, "Black Women for Wages for Housework" and "Wages Due Lesbians," all of which began aggressively, though with varying degrees of success, to promote COYOTE's message to social change activists. Although far more polished and less marginal than COYOTE, the contemporary adherents of the distinction between prostitution/sex work and trafficking are COYOTE's ideological heirs and their goal–the legitimization of the sex industry–is identical to COYOTE's (Ditmore, 1999; Doezema, 1999).

   If sex trafficking and prostitution were distinct and separate phenomena, and if prostitution were as innocuous as trafficking is injurious, a logical response would be to direct criminal sanctions against sex traffickers and legalize and regulate prostitution. This is the position that the Netherlands, Germany, and others following the "Dutch" example have embraced. But the Dutch and German experience–along with those of other jurisdictions that have legalized prostitution–have demonstrated just what happens when prostitution is legitimized and protected by law: the number of sex businesses grows, as does the demand for prostitution. Legalized prostitution brings sex tourists and heightens the demand among local men. Local women constitute an inadequate supply so foreign girls and women are trafficked in to meet the demand. The trafficked women are cheaper, younger, more exciting to customers, and easier to control. More trafficked women means more local demand and more sex tourism. The end result looks a lot like Amsterdam.

   Sheila Jeffreys, a professor of women's studies at the University of Melbourne, documents this phenomenon in Victoria, Australia. In 1994, prostitution was legalized in Victoria. The hope was that legalized prostitution would decrease street prostitution, diminish the health risks for prostitutes and clients, and decrease organized crime's hold over the sex industry. What happened instead was just the opposite: a massive expansion of Victoria's sex industry and an increase in sex trafficking into Victoria. The number of legal brothels escalated from 40 to 64, the "escort agencies" proliferated. A Melbourne businessman was arrested for bringing into Victoria 40 Thai women as contract workers and then confiscating their passports until they worked off their debt. A legal brothel was busted for holding 25 Asian woman in indentured servitude. Sullivan and Jeffreys (2000) observed, "Legalization was intended to eliminate organized crime from the sex industry. In fact, the reverse has happened. Legalization has brought with it an explosion in the trafficking of women . . ."

The Swedish government developed an antithetical policy response. In 1999, it passed and implemented legislation that stepped up measures against organized prostitution not only by directing strong penalties against pimps, brothel owners, and other sex industry entrepreneurs but by also instituting criminal sanctions against customers (Goldsmith, 1998). (The law also eliminated penalties against prostitutes, such as the penalty for soliciting.) After the passage of the new law, Sweden spearheaded a public education campaign warning sex industry customers that patronizing prostitutes was criminal behavior (Campaign Against Trafficking in Women, 2002). The result was unexpected. While there was not a dramatic decrease in the incidence of prostitution, sex trafficking to Sweden declined significantly. The danger of prosecution coupled with a diminished demand made Sweden an unpromising market for global sex traffickers (Winberg, 2003).

The antithetical Australian and Swedish legislative approaches to prostitution and trafficking hold important if preliminary lessons for social change activists and policy makers. Legalizing and legitimizing domestic prostitution, it appears, throws out a welcome mat to international sex traffickers. Curtailing the demand for prostitution in a destination country seems to chill sex trafficking into it. While Australia's and Sweden's experiences merit further study, they underscore the interconnection of prostitution and sex trafficking.

CONCLUSION

Prostitution and sex trafficking are the same human rights catastrophe, whether in local or global guise. Both are part of a system of gender-based domination that makes violence against women and girls profitable to a mind-boggling extreme. Both prey on women and girls made vulnerable by poverty, discrimination, and violence and leaves them traumatized, sick, and impoverished. Both reward predators sexually and financially, strengthening the demand and criminal operations that ensure the supply. The concerted effort by some NGOs and governments to separate trafficking from prostitution–to treat them as distinct and unrelated phenomena–is nothing less than a deliberate political strategy aimed at legitimizing the sex industry and protecting its growth and profitability. Unless definitions, laws, and strategies clearly identify and challenge all manifestations of local and global sex industries, the progress that we make on one front will be undone by our inaction on the others.

REFERENCES

Ananova.com. (2002). http://www.ananova.com/news/story/sm_5666031.html. May 25, 2002.
Arizona Coalition Against Domestic Violence. (2002). *What Sexual Assault and Domestic Violence Service Providers Need to Know About Sex Trafficking.*
Barry, K. (1979). *Female Sexual Slavery.* New York: New York University Press.
Barry, K. (1995). *The Prostitution of Sexuality.* New York: New York University Press.
Cambodian Women's Crisis Center. (1999). The Sale of Women and Girls to Brothels in Cambodia. In D.M. Hughes and C. Roche (eds), *Making the Harm Visible: Global Sexual Exploitation of Women and Girls.* Kingston, Rhode Island: Coalition Against Trafficking in Women. 131-133.
Cardwell, D. (2002). Officials Say Sex Trade Lures Younger Girls. *New York Times.* December 7, 2002.
Carter, V. (2002). Presentation on Panel on "Prostitution and Poverty" during 46th Session of the United Nations Commission on the Status of Women. March 6, 2002.
Council for Prostitution Alternatives. (1991). Annual Report 3.
Davidson, J. O. (1998). *Prostitution, Power, and Freedom.* Ann Arbor: University of Michigan Press.
D'Cunha, J. (1999). A Perspective on the Decriminalization of Prostitution and Reflections on Action Strategies. Presentation During Seminar, "Trafficking and the Global Sex Industry: Need for Human Rights Framework." Palais des Nations, Geneva, Switzerland.
D'Cunha, J. (2002a). Trafficking and Prostitution from a Gender and Human Rights Perspective in J. Raymond, J. D'Cunha, S.R. Dzuhayatin, H.P. Hynes, Z.R. Rodriguez, & A. Santos (eds.) (2002). A Comparative Study of Women Trafficked in the Migration Process: Patterns, Profiles and Health Consequences of Sexual Exploitation in Five Countries (Indonesia, the Philippines, Thailand, Venezuela and the United States) N. Amherst, MA: Coalition Against Trafficking in Women (CATW). Available at *www.catwinternational.org.*
D'Cunha, J. (2002b). Gender Equality, Human Rights and Trafficking: A Framework of Analysis and Action. Paper presented at Seminar to Promote Gender Equality and Combat Trafficking in Women and Children, October 7-9, 2002. Bangkok, Thailand.

Delacoste F. & Alexander, P. (eds). (1991). *Sex Work: Writings by Women in the Sex Industry.* Cleis Press.

Ditmore, M. (1999). Addressing Sex Work as Labor. Presentation During Seminar, "Trafficking and the Global Sex Industry: Need for Human Rights Framework." Palais des Nations, Geneva, Switzerland.

Diakite, F. (1999). Prostitution in Mali in D.M. Hughes and C. Roche (eds.), *Making the Harm Visible: Global Sexual Exploitation of Women and Girls.* Kingston, Rhode Island: Coalition Against Trafficking in Women: 177-180.

Doezma, J. (1999). How Existing Legal Systems Facilitate Trafficking. Presentation During Seminar, "Trafficking and the Global Sex Industry: Need for Human Rights Framework." Palais des Nations, Geneva, Switzerland.

Doezema, J. (2001). "Ouch! Western Feminists' 'Wounded Attachment' to the 'Third World Prostitute.'" *Feminist Review 67, Spring 2001. pp. 16-38.*

Duluth Domestic Abuse Intervention Project, National Training Project. Power and Control Wheel. http://www.duluth-model.org/ntppce.htm.

Dworkin, A. 1997. Prostitution and Male Supremacy. In *Life and Death* 139-151. New York: Free Press. Available at *http://www.nostatusquo.com/ACLU/dworkin/MichLawJourl.html.*

Farley, M. (2003). Prostitution and the Invisibility of Harm. *Women & Therapy* 26: 247-280. Special issue on Women and Invisible Disabilities, M. Banks and R. Ackerman (eds).

Farley, M., Baral, I., Kiremire, M., & Sezgin, U. (1998). Prostitution in Five Countries: Violence and Posttraumatic Stress Disorder. *Feminism & Psychology* 8: 415-426.

Giobbe, E. (1990). Confronting the Liberal Lies About Prostitution. D. Leidholdt & J. Raymond, (eds.), *The Sexual Liberals and the Attack on Feminism,* New York: Pergamon Press, pp. 67-81.

Giobbe, E. (1991). Prostitution, Buying the Right to Rape, in Burgess, A.W. (ed.) *Rape and Sexual Assault III: A Research Handbook.* New York: Garland Press.

Giobbe, E. (1992). Juvenile Prostitution: Profile of Recruitment, in Burgess, A.W. (ed.) *Child Trauma: Issues & Research.* New York: Garland Press.

Giobbe, E. (1993). An Analysis of Individual, Institutional & Cultural Pimping. *Michigan Journal of Gender & Law* 1: 33-57.

Giobbe, E. (1999). Presentation During Seminar, "Trafficking and the Global Sex Industry: Need for Human Rights Framework." Palais des Nations, Geneva, Switzerland.

Goldsmith, B. (1998). "Swedish sex buyers feel law's weak slap," *Reuters,* June 14, 1998.

Guide to the New UN Trafficking Protocol. (2001). CATW online website: http://www.catwinternational.org.

Hotaling, N. (1999). What Happens to Women in Prostitution in the United States. In D.M. Hughes and C. Roche (eds.), *Making the Harm Visible: Global Sexual Exploitation of Women and Girls.* Kingston, Rhode Island: Coalition Against Trafficking in Women: 239-251.

Leidholdt, D. (1993). Prostitution: A Violation of Women's Human Rights. *Cardozo Women's Law Journal* 1: 133-147.

LifeSiteNews.com (1999). Brothels Legalized in Holland.

Louis, M. (1999). Legalizing Pimping, Dutch Style. In D. M. Hughes and C. Roche (eds.), *Making the Harm Visible: Global Sexual Exploitation of Women and Girls.* Kingston, Rhode Island: Coalition Against Trafficking in Women: 192-196.

Marcovich, M. (2002). Guide to the UN Convention of 1949 on the Suppression of the Traffic in Persons and of the Exploitation of the Prostitution of Others. Coalition Against Trafficking in Women. www.catwinternational.org.

Minnesota Advocates for Human Rights. (2000). Trafficking in Women: Moldova and Ukraine. www.mnadvocates.org.

Network of sex work projects website. http://www.nswp.org.

O'Leary, C. & Howard, O. (2001). The Prostitution of Women and Girls in Metropolitan Chicago. Center for Impact Research. www.impactresearch.org.

Owen, R. (2002). Italy Divided Over Plan to Bring Back Brothels. May 9, 2002. http://www.timesonline.co.uk/article/0,,3-290855,00.html.

Parriott R. (1994). *Health Experiences of Twin Cities Women Used in Prostitution*. Unpublished survey initiated by WHISPER, Minneapolis.

Pateman, C. (1988). *The Sexual Contract*. Palo Alto, CA: Stanford University Press.

The Protection Project. (2001). Annual Human Rights Report on the Trafficking of Persons, Especially Women and Children, www.protectionproject.org.

Raymond, J. (1999). The Health Effects of Prostitution in D.M. Hughes and C. Roche (eds.), *Making the Harm Visible: Global Sexual Exploitation of Women and Girls*. Kingston, Rhode Island: Coalition Against Trafficking in Women: 59-63.

Raymond, J. & Hughes, D. (2002). Sex Trafficking of Women in the United States: International and Domestic Trends. CATW online website: http://catwinternational. org.

Raymond, J., D'Cunha, J., Dzuhayatin, S.R., Hynes, H.P. Rodriguez, Z.R., & Santos, A. (2002). A Comparative Study of Women Trafficked in the Migration Process: Patterns, Profiles and Health Consequences of Sexual Exploitation in Five Countries (Indonesia, the Phillippines, Thailand, Venezuela and the United States). N. Amherst, MA: Coalition Against Trafficking in Women (CATW). Available at *www.catwinternational.org*.

Schelzig, E. (2002). German Prostitutes Ponder Salaried Work. The Washington Post. May 13, 2002. http://www.iht.com/articles/57484.html.

Silbert, M. & Pines, A. (1982). Entrance into Prostitution. *Youth & Society*, 13: 471-479.

Silbert, M. (1983). Early sexual exploitation as an influence in prostitution. *Social Work* 28: 285-289.

Stark, C. & Hodgson, C. (2003) Sister Oppressions: A Comparison of Wife Battering and Prostitution in M. Farley (Ed.) *Prostitution, Trafficking, and Traumatic Stress*. Binghamton, NY: The Haworth Press, Inc.

Stark, E. (2000). A Failure to Protect: Unraveling the Battered Mother's Dilemma. 27 *Western State University Law Review* 29.

Sullivan, M. & Jeffreys, S. (2001). *Legalizing Prostitution Is Not the Answer: The Example of Victoria, Australia*. CATW online at http://catwinternational.org.

UN Protocol to Prevent, Suppress and Punish Trafficking in Persons, Especially Women and Children, supplementing the United Nations Convention against Transnational Organized Crime, 2000.

Vasconcelos, A. (1999). Casa de Passagem in Brazil in D.M. Hughes and C. Roche (eds.), *Making the Harm Visible: Global Sexual Exploitation of Women and Girls*. Kingston: Rhode Island: Coalition Against Trafficking in Women: 333-338.

Winberg, M. (2003). Speech by Sweden's Deputy Prime Minister at 47th Session of the United Nations Commission on the Status of Women, UN Headquarters, New York City, March 5, 2003.

*HEALING
FROM PROSTITUTION
AND TRAFFICKING*

Emotional Experiences
of Performing Prostitution

Lisa A. Kramer

SUMMARY. Survey data obtained from 119 women who were prostituting in escort agencies and on the street in Phoenix, Arizona provide insight into women's emotional experiences of turning tricks. Results indicate that women experience a range of negative emotions while performing sex acts with customers including feelings of sadness, worthlessness, anger, anxiety, and shame. Far less frequently, emotional experiences of turning tricks were described as involving feelings of excitement and desirability. In addition to experiencing acts of prostitution as overwhelmingly emotionally unpleasant, if not traumatic, women feel more negatively about themselves after entering prostitution and would strongly prefer to leave prostitution for a different occupation with similar earnings. Findings from this study suggest that while some women may enter prostitution to support a drug or alcohol habit, they also use these substances once in prostitution to detach emotionally and to cope with fears of being hurt in prostitution. Practical impli-

Lisa A. Kramer, MS, is at Department of Sociology, Arizona State University, Tempe. She can be contacted at P.O. Box 2327, Monterey, CA 93492 (Email: Kramerla@osd.pentagon. mil).

Special thanks go to Kathleen Mitchell for her invaluable assistance in administering the surveys used in this study and to Melissa Farley for her insightful suggestions concerning earlier drafts of this manuscript.
Printed with permission.

[Haworth co-indexing entry note]: "Emotional Experiences of Performing Prostitution." Kramer, Lisa A. Co-published simultaneously in *Journal of Trauma Practice* (The Haworth Maltreatment & Trauma Press, an imprint of The Haworth Press, Inc.) Vol. 2, No. 3/4, 2003, pp. 187-197; and: *Prostitution, Trafficking, and Traumatic Stress* (ed: Melissa Farley) The Haworth Maltreatment & Trauma Press, an imprint of The Haworth Press, Inc., 2003, pp. 187-197. Single or multiple copies of this article are available for a fee from The Haworth Document Delivery Service [1-800-HAWORTH, 9:00 a.m. - 5:00 p.m. (EST). E-mail address: docdelivery@haworthpress.com].

http://www.haworthpress.com/store/product.asp?sku=J189
10.1300/J189v02n03_10

cations of these findings for therapists, social workers, and substance abuse counselors are discussed.

In recent decades, prostitution has become a topic of debate. In contrast to anecdotal research that portrays prostitution as an empowering form of work, social scientists have proffered evidence that individuals are incapable of selling sexual services without experiencing emotional pain and psychological harm. Some authors conceptualize prostitution as exemplifying the objectification and commodification of women's bodies (Farley & Barkan, 1998) and view prostitution as oppressive to women and destructive to their sexuality (Barry, 1979). Research suggests that many women in prostitution have been victims of sexual and physical assault as children or adolescents, and that the decision to enter the sex industry reflects childhood trauma (Seng, 1989; Simons & Whitbeck, 1991). While there is substantial empirical evidence lending credibility to these claims concerning the unfortunate experiences of women prior to, and during prostitution, it is conceivable that individuals enter prostitution for other reasons, and experience prostitution positively.

In contrast to research that frames prostitution as inherently unhealthy and reflective of individual and social dysfunction, others advocate the conceptualization of "sex work" as a legitimate employment option, chosen freely by the women who do it (Bell, 1987; Delacoste & Alexander, 1987). Some authors reject the conceptualization of prostitutes as victims, and minimize the significance of sexual and physical abuse in childhood as precursors to prostitution. Activists and researchers who seek to legitimize prostitution often claim that social stigma is responsible for emotional harm that might result from selling sexual services. Sex work advocates furthermore propose that when women in prostitution do encounter harm, the injury is physical rather than emotional, and results from a lack of legal protection. It is claimed that prostitutes do not necessarily suffer emotionally from the work they do (Chapkis, 1997), and that the labor required of the prostitute is no more intrinsically damaging to the sex-worker than acting is to the actress (Delacoste & Alexander, 1987).

Little research explores the emotions women experience while performing prostitution. In one study that explored psychological distress associated with prostitution, 68% of 130 prostitutes met criteria for a diagnosis of post-traumatic stress disorder (Farley & Barkan, 1998). The high rate of PTSD was believed to result from acts of prostitution as well as violent experiences outside of prostitution, including childhood abuse and violence encountered in adulthood (which many prostitutes have endured). Another study found a strong relationship between prostituting and emotional distress when prostituting women were compared to a non-prostitute control group (El-Bassel & Schilling, 1997). Women in prostitution scored higher than the control group on several measures of psychological distress including depression, anxiety, and paranoid ideation. The authors concluded that psychological distress among women in prostitution results from the dangerous and degrading circumstances surrounding their work. Other researchers have asserted both that prostitution is emotionally traumatic, and that prostitutes use drugs to cope with the psychological pain of turning tricks. Young, Boyd, and Hubbell (2000) found that prostituting women were more likely to use drugs than a control group, and used drugs specifically to increase feelings of confidence, control, and closeness to others, and to decrease feelings of guilt and sexual distress. These authors concluded that while women may enter prostitution to fund substance use, they also increase their drug use to deal with negative emotions caused by performing prostitution.

This study was conducted in an effort to better understand women's emotional experiences of performing prostitution, their feelings about themselves since entering prostitution, and the extent to which they manage their emotions through substance abuse while turning tricks.

METHODS

The women completing surveys for this investigation were included because they were more accessible to the researcher than other women engaging in prostitution. Survey respondents were women incarcerated for minor offenses (including drug offenses, petty theft, and solicitation of prostitution) at the time they completed the questionnaires, and women working in an escort agency who were provided surveys by the owners or managers.

Sixty-four percent of the 119 respondents were participating in a voluntary support group for prostitutes. Twenty-five percent of the surveys were obtained from women in jail for prostitution or minor offenses who had not attended the voluntary group meetings. The remaining 11% were in escort prostitution, and were recruited through chain referral or snowball sampling procedures–methods commonly employed with difficult to access populations (Biernacki & Waldorf, 1981; Watters & Biernacki, 1989). The managers of several escort agencies distributed the surveys to the women at the request of an individual who previously prostituted and who assisted with data collection.

Survey items were developed from a review of prostitution literature (e.g., Barry, 1979; Bell, 1987; Chapkis, 1997; Delacoste & Alexander, 1987; El-Bassel &

Schilling, 1997; Hoigard & Finstad, 1992; Miller, 1986; Miller, 1995; Potterat, Rothenberg, Muth, Darrow, & Phillips-Plummer, 1998; Prince, 1986; Seng, 1989; Simons & Whitbeck, 1991; Young, Boyd, & Hubbell, 2000) and through information gleaned from 15 pilot interviews with women working in street and escort prostitution. Social service providers contributed to the survey design as did healthcare professionals and law enforcement personnel. Subsequently, 17 questionnaires were piloted. The surveys contained 103 items, requested no identifying information, and took approximately 40 minutes to complete.

Demographic variables included age, sexual orientation, ethnicity, marital status, educational background, age of entry into prostitution, length of time in prostitution, types of prostitution engaged in, and type of prostitution engaged in for the longest period of time. Types of prostitution included phone sex, pornography photographs or videos, Internet pornography, dancing/stripping, streetwalking, massage parlor, escort, or "other."

Several items asked the women to indicate the extent to which they use drugs or alcohol to numb out or to cope with fear while turning tricks. Respondents were also asked to indicate the extent to which they used drugs or alcohol to detach emotionally while turning tricks and the extent to which it was necessary to be high to turn tricks. Response options for these survey items were "never," "sometimes," "often," and "always." Responses of "often" or "always" are reported here.

Respondents were asked to indicate if their feelings toward themselves had changed since entering prostitution, if their enjoyment of sex with partners outside of prostitution had changed, and to describe their emotional experiences of turning tricks. The women were asked to indicate the extent to which they push away their true emotions while turning tricks and to indicate the extent to which turning tricks involved acting. We asked if she would leave prostitution for a different job with similar earnings. Lastly, the women were asked to list five words that described their feelings while turning a trick. Percentages reported in this paper were calculated using the number of respondents for each item (versus the total number of study participants).

RESULTS

Sample Characteristics

Respondents were 119 women aged 18 to 56. Because most of the surveys were administered at an adult jail, no respondent reported being younger than age 18. The average age was 33 (SD 8.0). Seventy-seven percent were heterosexual, 20% were bisexual, and 3% were lesbian. The sample was somewhat ethnically diverse with 59% white European American, 18% African American, 15% Latina American, and 3% Native American women. Forty-seven percent of the women were single, 41% were separated or divorced, 10% were married, and 3% were widowed. Seventy-four percent of respondents had a high school diploma or GED. Forty percent had completed some college. Further information on sample characteristics is available from the author.

Prostitution Experiences

Age of entry into prostitution ranged from 13 to 47 years. The average age of entry was 23 (SD 7.7). Twenty-one percent entered prostitution before age 18, 45% entered between the ages of 18 and 25, and 22% entered prostitution between 26 and 34 years of age. Twelve percent of these respondents entered prostitution at age 35 or older. Length of time in prostitution ranged from 1 month to 42 years; the average length of time in prostitution was 8.7 years.

Seventy-eight percent of respondents reported involvement in street prostitution, 41% percent reported involvement in escort prostitution, and 32% indicated that they had worked in strip club prostitution. Twenty-eight percent had engaged in pornography (i.e., still photographs, videotaping, and/or the Internet). Fifteen percent had worked in massage parlors, and 12% had performed phone sex. Sixteen percent of the women surveyed reported that they had engaged in other types of prostitution; these included a "naked maid service" and "bar prostitution." Forty-one percent of respondents indicated that they had performed prostitution at the street level as well as one or more forms of indoor prostitution (e.g., stripping, massage parlor, escort, etc.). While some types of prostitution do not involve physical sex acts with customers, all of the women in this study had engaged in prostitution in which sex acts had occurred. Sixty-six percent reported that they were involved in street prostitution (as compared with other types of prostitution) for the longest period, and 33% had worked in indoor prostitution the majority of the time (in strip clubs, in massage parlors, and as escorts).

Substance Use to Cope with Emotions

Fifty-nine percent of respondents indicated that they used drugs while turning tricks to numb out and 28% reported using alcohol to numb out. Seventy percent of respondents reported using substances to detach emotionally while turning tricks. Forty-four percent indicated that they use substances to cope with fear while turning tricks. Fifty-four percent indicated that it was necessary to be high to go through with turning a trick.

Self-Esteem and Feelings About Sexuality

Two items asked respondents to indicate if their feelings about themselves had changed since entering prostitution. Seventy-seven percent of respondents indicated that their self-esteem had decreased since entering prostitution while 15% of respondents stated that their self-esteem had improved since entering prostitution. Sixty-five percent of the women indicated that their enjoyment of sex in their personal lives had diminished since entering the sex industry, while 16% reported more enjoyment of sex with partners outside of prostitution since entering prostitution.

Emotional Experiences While Performing Prostitution

Seventy-three percent of respondents indicated that turning tricks involved pushing away their true emotions, and 75% of respondents indicated that turning a trick involved acting.

On a Likert scale ranging from pleasurable to painful, respondents were asked to rate their experiences of turning tricks. Scores of 1, 2, and 3 on the scale represented varying degrees of "pleasure" and scores of 5, 6, and 7 represented varying degrees of "pain"; a score of 4 was considered neutral. Fifty-two percent of respondents reported that turning tricks was physically painful and 76% reported that turning tricks was emotionally painful. By contrast, 19% of respondents indicated that prostitution was physically pleasurable and 13% indicated that turning tricks was emotionally pleasurable.

Sixty percent of respondents reported that sex acts during prostitution were painful while 13% indicated that sex acts during prostitution were pleasurable. Thirty-three percent indicated that sex in their personal life was painful, while 54% indicated that sex in their personal life was pleasurable. Finally, 65% indicated that sex outside of prostitution was less enjoyable since entering prostitution and 16% indicated that sex outside of work was more enjoyable since entering prostitution. Ninety-four percent of the women stated that they would leave prostitution for a different job with similar earnings.

Respondents were asked to "list five words that describe your feelings while turning a trick." The 458 responses to this item were organized by theme.

Table 1 summarizes the women's negative emotions while turning tricks, in rank order of frequency. Turning tricks results in feelings of sadness and distress (14%), undesirability/unattractiveness (14%), anger/resentment (13%), detachment/disconnection (11%), fear (8%), anxiety (6%), shame/guilt (6%), pain (4%), degradation/humiliation (3%) and nausea (3%). Nine percent were other negative emotions. Of the categorized responses, 90% were negative.

TABLE 1. Negative Emotional Experiences During Prostitution

	N	Percent of Categorized Responses (n = 394)
Sad / Distraught Sad / sadness (21), lonely / loneliness (7), depressed / depression (6), empty / emptiness (4), hopeless / hopelessness (4), helpless (3), unhappy (3), powerless (2), bad, broken-hearted, distraught, lost, not loved, and upset	56	14%
Undesirable / Unattractive Dirty / feel dirty / filthy / unclean (18), worthless / worthlessness / no self worth / cheap / low down / lower than dirt / trash (10), ugly (7), gross / nasty / scum (5), disgusting / disgusted in myself (4), stupid / dumb (4), bad esteem / low esteem / I hate myself (3), being a nobody, fake, hoe, and whore	55	14%
Angry / Resentful Angry / anger / mad (22), disgusted / irritated / disgruntled (11), hate / hateful / hatefulness / hatred (11), bitchy (2), mean (2), loathing and resentment	50	13%
Detached / Disconnected Numb / numbness (20), detached / unattached / disconnected (6), blank (3), dead (2), none / feelingless / I don't feel a thing / nothingness (5), not there (2), dreaming, out of touch, spaced, turned off, and non-existent	43	11%
Fearful / Scared Afraid / scared / fear / fearful / fearing disease / frightened / paranoid (33)	33	8%
Anxious / Tentative Anxious / anxiety / nervous (16), stress (2), butterflies, insecure, pressure, suspicious, uneasy, and worried	24	6%
Ashamed / Guilty Ashamed / shame / shameful / shame of what I have done (12), guilt / guilty (4), greedy / selfish (3), embarrassed (2), and disgrace	22	6%
Painful / Hurting Hurt / hurting (7), pain / painful / pain at times (8)	15	4%
Degraded / Humiliated Degraded / degrading (3), used (2), cheated, disrespect for me, disrespect for my honey, disrespected, and humiliated	10	3%
Sick / Nauseous Sick / nauseated / nauseous / sick to stomach / feel like puking (10)	10	3%
Other Negative Emotions Disgust (10), bored / boring (6), confused / confusion (4), cold / coldness (2), tired / tiredness (2), abused due to addiction, didn't like me, disappointment, diseases, disturbed, doubting, exhausted, hard, horrible, hungry, and not right	35	9%
Total Negative Responses	353	90%

TABLE 2. Positive Emotional Experience During Prostitution

	N	Percent of Categorized Responses (n = 394)
Satisfied / Desired Happy / having fun / amused (6), power / powerful (6), excited / excitement / exciting (5), content / gratification / successful / "job well done" when over (4), enjoyable / pleasure / pleasurable (4), sexy / wanted (4), confident (2), safe / secure (2), eager, free from life, good, great, horny, grateful, respected, and where I belong	41	10%

TABLE 3. Emotional Responses During Prostitution That Were Not Categorized as Negative or Positive

	N	Percent of All Responses (n = 458)
Uncategorized Responses Impatient / in a hurry / hurried / hurry / rushed (10), in charge / in control / control / controlling / in control of man (8), high (5), relief / relieved / relieved by money (3), acting / pretending (2), alone (2), alert, asleep, black, careful, careless, closure, curious, demanding for drugs, don't care, disbelief, drugs, focus, hyper, intriguing, manipulating, money, my job, okay, one stop service shop, out of control, overwhelmed, playing with me, quiet, ready to leave, rush, sarcastic, serious, sometimes happy, smug, steady, swallow, take a shower, thinking hard, and weird	64	14%

Ten percent of categorized responses were positive and included feelings of amusement, satisfaction and desirability (Table 2). Fourteen percent of all responses were not categorized as negative or positive (Table 3).

DISCUSSION

Responses of 119 women in eight different types of prostitution indicated that performing prostitution was a negative and/or traumatic experience 90% of the time. Seventy-three percent of respondents indicated that turning tricks involved pushing away their true emotions, 52% reported that turning tricks was physically painful, and 76% reported that turning tricks was emotionally painful. Seventy-seven percent of respondents indicated that their self-esteem had decreased since entering prostitution. Like other research that suggests that women who engage in prostitution experience sexual dysfunction with their chosen partners (Farley, 2003), 65% of women in this study reported a decrease in sexual pleasure with sexual partners outside of prostitution. Ninety-four percent of women surveyed indicated that they would prefer to leave prostitution for a job with similar earnings.

Our findings suggest that while some women may enter prostitution to support a drug or alcohol habit, once in prostitution, women use substances to self-medicate and to manage their fears of being hurt. Fifty-nine percent of respondents indicated that they used illicit drugs while turning tricks to "numb out" and 70% of women reported using substances to detach emotionally while turning tricks. Fifty-four percent of respondents indicated that it was necessary to be high to go through with turning a trick.

Emotionally positive experiences of prostitution were reported 10% of the time. Our findings suggest that while prostitution is experienced as negative and/or traumatic by most women all of the time, it is not unpleasant all of the time, for all women. It is possible that differences in emotional experiences of prostitution reflect differences in time spent in prostitution, differences in the amount of violence suffered, or differences in the meaning attributed to prostitution. Because the women's emotional responses to prostitution were overwhelmingly negative, it was not possible to compare emotional responses to different types of prostitution. No single respondent described prostitution as eliciting only positive emotions; the 41 positive emotional descriptions of prostitution came from 17 women, who also described prostitution as eliciting negative and unpleasant emotions. Nonetheless, it is possible that some individuals in prostitution may construe selling sex acts as a form of rebellion, and that they may have economic alternatives to prostitution, and thus experience prostitution more positively.

We found that women prostituted in more than one type of prostitution simultaneously or sequentially. Some have suggested that it may be misleading to categorize women as "indoor" or "outdoor" prostitutes (Raphael & Shapiro, 2002). Forty-one percent of our respondents performed prostitution both on the street and in some type of indoor prostitution. Sixty-six percent reported that they were involved in street prostitution (as compared with other types of prostitution) for the longest period, and 33% had worked in indoor prostitution the majority of the time.

There are some limitations to this study. Caution must be exercised in interpreting findings from any sample of respondents whose inclusion in a study is related to the ability of the researcher to gain access to them. Additionally, 16% of all responses to the question concerning emotions while turning a trick were not categorized as either positive or negative due to the ambiguity of the responses. The value of open-ended questions may outweigh the disadvantages of being unable to draw quantitative conclusions about some responses in terms of their negative or positive tone. The voices of women in prostitution are not often heard, and the researcher wanted every response recorded.

Women who are striving to leave prostitution can benefit from counseling that improves their understanding of the way in which prostitution evolved as a viable option for them. Findings of this study suggest that the conditions under which prostitution is performed, feelings experienced while performing sex acts, and the impact of prostitution on self-esteem and sexuality are additional topics that can be explored in a long-term counseling relationship. For substance-abusing women, it appears that achieving insight into the role that drugs and alcohol may have played in coping with negative emotions while turning tricks, may be an essential aspect of recovery.

In addition to addressing mental health issues, women who are striving to leave prostitution can benefit from services that assist them in overcoming economic and educational disadvantages, and which promote the development of living skills. Women in prostitution often have limited educational backgrounds and erratic or nonexistent employment histories. These women may need substantial assistance to reenter the workforce. Finally, women who have left prostitution may also need support to secure safe and affordable housing. Women are often denied access to public housing because of a history of substance abuse, and are denied access to private housing due to laws that allow landlords to refuse rental space to people with criminal records (Holsopple, 2000).

REFERENCES

Barry, K. (1979). *Female sexual slavery*. New York: Avon Books.

Bell, L. (1987). *Good girls/bad girls: Feminists and sex trade workers face to face*. Toronto: The Seal Press.

Biernacki, P. & Waldorf, D. (1981). Snowball sampling: Problems and techniques of chain referral sampling. *Sociological Methods and Research, 10*, 141-163.

Brewis, J. & Linstad, S. (2000). The worst thing is the screwing: Consumption and the management of identity in sex work. *Gender, Work and Organization, 7*: 84-97.

Chapkis, Wendy. (1997). *Live sex acts: Women performing erotic labor*. New York: Routledge.

Delacoste, F. & Alexander, P. (1987). *Sex work: Writings by women in the sex industry*. Pittsburgh: Cleis Press.

El-Bassel, N. & Schilling, R. (1997). Sex trading and psychological distress among women recruited from the streets of Harlem. *American Journal of Public Health, 87*, 66-70.

Farley, M. (2003). Prostitution and the Invisibility of Harm. *Women & Therapy, 26*(3/4): 247-280.

Farley, M. & Barkan, H. (1998). Prostitution, violence, and posttraumatic stress disorder. *Women and Health, 27,* 37-49.

Hoigard, C., & Finstad, L. (1992). *Backstreets: Prostitution, Money and Love.* University Park: University of Pennsylvania Press.

Holsopple, K. (2000). The Women's Recovery Center: Survivors' initiative to help prostituted women heal. *Pakistan Journal of Women's Studies, 7,* 29-37.

Miller, E. (1986). *Street woman.* Philadelphia: Temple University Press.

Miller, J. (1995). Gender and power on the streets: Street prostitution in the era of crack cocaine. *Journal of Contemporary Ethnography, 23,* 427-452.

Nagle, J. (ed.). (1997). *Whores and other feminists.* New York: Routledge.

O'Neill, M. (1995). Prostitution and feminism: Toward a politics of feeling. Cambridge: Polity Press.

Pheterson, G. (ed.). (1989). *A vindication of the rights of whores.* Seattle: Seal Press.

Potterat, J., Rothenberg, R.B., Muth, S.Q., Darrow, W.W., & Phillips-Plummer, L. (1998). Pathways to prostitution: The chronology of sexual and drug abuse milestones. *The Journal of Sex Research, 35,* 333-340.

Prince, D. (1986). A psychological profile of prostitutes in California and Nevada. Doctoral dissertation. United States International University.

Raphael, J., & Shapiro, D. (2002). Sisters speak out: The lives and needs of prostituted women in Chicago. Chicago, IL: Center for Impact Research.

Seng, M. (1989). Child sexual abuse and adolescent prostitution: A comparative analysis. *Adolescence, XXIV,* 665-675.

Simons, R.L., & Whitbeck, L.B. (1991). Sexual abuse as a precursor to prostitution and victimization among adolescent and adult homeless women. *Journal of Family Issues, 12,* 361-379.

Young, A.M., Boyd, C., & Hubbell, A. (2000). Prostitution, drug use, and coping with psychological distress. *Journal of Drug Issues, 4,* 789-800.

Watters, J.K., & Biernacki, P. (1989). Targeted sampling: Options for the study of hidden populations. *Social Problems, 6:* 416-30.

Dissociation Among Women in Prostitution

Colin A. Ross
Melissa Farley
Harvey L. Schwartz

SUMMARY. The authors summarize four studies on dissociation among women in prostitution, and discuss clinical aspects of the relationship between trauma, dissociation and prostitution. Dissociative disorders are common among those in escort, street, massage, strip club and brothel prostitution, and are frequently accompanied by posttraumatic stress disorder, depression, and substance abuse. These in turn are linked to high rates of childhood physical and sexual abuse, and to violent victimization while in prostitution. The existing data suggest that almost all who are in prostitution suffer from at least one of the following types of disorders; dissociative, posttraumatic, mood or substance abuse. Further research to refine and replicate these findings is warranted.

Colin A. Ross, MD, is affiliated with Ross Institute for Psychological Trauma, 1701 Gateway, Suite 349, Richardson, TX 75080-3644. He can be reached at: (rossinst@rossinst.com).

Melissa Farley, PhD, is at Prostitution Research & Education, Box 16254, San Francisco, CA 94116-0254. She can be contacted at (mfarley@prostitutionresearch.com).

Harvey L. Schwartz, PhD, is in private practice of psychotherapy. He can be contacted at 257 Connecticut Avenue, San Francisco, CA 94107.

Melissa Farley could not have completed her research without the generous participation and support of clients and staff at PROMISE, San Francisco; Council for Prostitution Alternatives, Portland; SOS (Sisters Offering Support), Honolulu; DIGNITY House, Phoenix; Genesis House, Chicago; Exodus, Chicago; and YANA (You Are Never Alone), Baltimore. Thank you.

Printed with permission.

[Haworth co-indexing entry note]: "Dissociation Among Women in Prostitution." Ross, Colin A., Melissa Farley, and Harvey L. Schwartz. Co-published simultaneously in *Journal of Trauma Practice* (The Haworth Maltreatment & Trauma Press, an imprint of The Haworth Press, Inc.) Vol. 2, No. 3/4, 2003, pp. 199-212; and: *Prostitution, Trafficking, and Traumatic Stress* (ed: Melissa Farley) The Haworth Maltreatment & Trauma Press, an imprint of The Haworth Press, Inc., 2003, pp. 199-212. Single or multiple copies of this article are available for a fee from The Haworth Document Delivery Service [1-800-HAWORTH, 9:00 a.m. - 5:00 p.m. (EST). E-mail address: docdelivery@haworthpress.com].

http://www.haworthpress.com/store/product.asp?sku=J189
10.1300/J189v02n03_11

Dissociation among women in prostitution has been examined in four studies: from Winnipeg, Canada (Ross, Anderson, Heber, & Norton, 1990), from Vancouver, Canada (Cooper, Kennedy, & Yuille, 2001), from Istanbul, Turkey (Yargic, Sevim, Arabul, & Ozden, 2000), and from several cities in the United States (Farley, 2003). This report summarizes the findings from these four studies and calls for further research regarding the psychological harm resulting from prostitution in general. The reader is referred to Farley and Kelly (2000) for a recent review of the medical and social sciences literature on prostitution, and to Ross (1997, 1999, 2000) and for a review of the literature on pathological and non-pathological dissociation.

According to the trauma model of dissociation (Ross, 1997, 1999, 2000), pathological dissociation is a core element of the response to chronic, severe childhood trauma which includes physical, sexual, emotional, and verbal abuse, neglect, loss of primary caretakers through death, divorce, addiction, mental illness or imprisonment, family chaos and violence, violence outside the home, medical and surgical trauma, and severely disturbed family dynamics. Traumatic events include war, famine, poverty, hunger, endemic disease, and natural disasters. These events interact with biological endowment and with other compounding and restorative influences in the environment in a complex fashion.

In clinical populations, pathological dissociation is only one element of the trauma response, and is accompanied by extensive co-morbidity including anxiety, mood, substance abuse, psychotic, eating and personality disorders. Since women in street and brothel prostitution report high rates of childhood trauma in addition to violence while prostituting (Farley & Kelly, 2000; Farley, Baral, Kiremire, & Sezgin, 1998), one would predict elevated levels of pathological dissociation and of other forms of co-morbidity. One would make the same prediction for other types of prostitution, including exotic dancers and pornographic film actors.

FOUR RESEARCH STUDIES OF DISSOCIATION AMONG WOMEN IN PROSTITUTION

The Winnipeg, Canada Study

In the Winnipeg, Canada study, we interviewed three groups of 20 women each: multiple personality patients, women in street prostitution, and exotic dancers. Women were approached while working on the street and were interviewed without permission or interference by their pimps. Their average age was 24.5 years (*SD* = 5.3), and they had an average of 1.2 children (*SD* = 0.9). The exotic dancers were interviewed (without permission or interference by their employers) in the dining room of the hotel where they were stripping. All were female, their average age was 22.9 years (*SD* = 2.2), and they had an average of 0.6 children (*SD* = 0.8). The racial backgrounds of the respondents were not recorded.

Research participants completed the Dissociative Experiences Scale (DES), (Bernstein & Putnam, 1986; Waller, Putnam & Carlson, 1996) and the Dissociative Disorders Interview Schedule (DDIS, Ross, 1997). The DES is a widely used self-report measure of dissociation that yields a score from zero to one hundred. The DDIS is a structured interview that permits DSM-IV diagnoses of somatization disorder, major depressive disorder, borderline personality disorder, and each of the five dissociative disorders (i.e., psychogenic amnesia, psychogenic fugue, depersonalization disorder, dissociative disorder not otherwise specified, and dissociative identity disorder–previously known as multiple personality disorder). It also inquires about substance abuse, psychotic symptoms and history of childhood physical and sexual abuse.

In the Winnipeg study, the DSM-III-R version of the DDIS was used; therefore DSM-III-R nomenclature for the dissociative disorders was reported. Rates of reported childhood sexual abuse were: multiple personality patients, 80%; women in street prostitution, 55%; and, exotic dancers, 65%. Rates of reported childhood physical abuse were: multiple personality patients, 75%; women in street prostitution, 40%; and exotic dancers, 50%. There were no statistically significant differences between the three groups on rates of childhood physical and sexual abuse.

Rates of major depressive disorder were: multiple personality patients, 85%; women in street prostitution, 60%; and exotic dancers, 60%. Rates of borderline personality disorder were: multiple personality patients, 60%; women in street prostitution, 35%; and exotic dancers, 55%. Rates of substance abuse were: multiple personality patients, 55%; women in street prostitution, 80%; and exotic dancers, 40%. None of the differences between groups on rates of these disorders were statistically significant.

The multiple personality patients all had a dissociative disorder by definition. Among the 20 respondents in street prostitution there were 7 diagnoses of psychogenic amnesia, 3 diagnoses of depersonalization disorder and one diagnosis of multiple personality disorder. Among the exotic dancers, there were 5 diagnoses of psychogenic amnesia, 4 diagnoses of depersonalization disorder and 7 diagnoses of multiple personality disorder. The exotic dancers were questioned carefully to determine that they were not referring simply to stage names when endorsing diagnostic criteria for multiple personality disorder.

The average DES scores were: multiple personality patients, 39.3; women in street prostitution, 13.2; and exotic dancers, 17.6. The mean DES score for the general population of Winnipeg is 10.8 (Ross, 1997). The DES scores of the patients were significantly higher than those of the women in street prostitution or in exotic dancing.

The Vancouver, Canada Study

In the Vancouver, Canada study, 33 women primarily in street prostitution were given the DES and an unstructured interview. The interviews were conducted at a safe house for prostitutes in the Downtown Eastside of Vancouver. Their average age was 35.2 years ($SD = 7.8$), two thirds were Native American, and one third were (white) European-American. Ninety-seven percent of these respondents reported lifetime sexual abuse, much of which had occurred while in prostitution. They reported an average of 16.2 episodes of sexual victimization prior to entering prostitution. Ninety-seven percent reported drug or alcohol dependence. Their average DES score was 32.6, which is in the range of dissociative disorder not otherwise specified.

The Istanbul, Turkey Study

The Turkish investigators interviewed 50 women in prostitution and 50 non-prostituting women with the DES and DDIS. They were asked additional questions about trauma. The women were interviewed at a legal brothel in Istanbul. Demographic data were not available and the researchers did not state whether the women were interviewed alone or in the presence of pimps.

DSM-IV nomenclature for the dissociative disorders was reported. Rates of childhood trauma among the women in brothel prostitution were: physical abuse, 48%; sexual abuse overall, 20%; incest, 8%; emotional abuse, 34%; and family violence, 64%. Rates of psychiatric disorders among the women in prostitution were: depression, 50%; alcohol abuse, 46%; other substance abuse, 20%; and borderline personality disorder, 8%. Rates of dissociative disorders were: dissociative amnesia, 20%; dissociative fugue, 4%; depersonalization disorder, 18%; dissociative identity disorder, 18%; and dissociative disorder not otherwise specified, 12%. The average DES score was 19.5 in contrast to 8.2 among women who were not prostituting. Rates of trauma and psychiatric disorders were far higher among those in prostitution than among the control respondents.

The United States Study

Farley (2002) interviewed 37 women who had previously prostituted, but who had been out of prostitution for at least 1.5 years, with some having left prostitution as long as 15 years before the time of the interview. Each of the women had prostituted in various combinations of escort, massage, brothel, strip club, and street prostitution. The women were interviewed in 5 cities in the United States. As part of a clinical interview, they were asked questions about childhood trauma and about experiences in prostitution. The DES was also administered. The women's mean current age was 38.9 years. In order of frequency of race/ethnicity, 46% were (white) European American, 24% were African American, 11% were Native American, and 19% identified as Armenian/Portuguese, Italian, Japanese, Samoan, Biracial, or Multicultural.

Eighty-seven percent of these interviewees reported a history of childhood sexual abuse, with an average of 3 perpetrators of sexual abuse. With respect to violence in prostitution, 97% had been physically assaulted while prostituting, 92% had been raped in prostitution, and 73% had pornography made of them while in prostitution. The mean DES score of the 37 women was 24.1. Sixteen percent were in the normal adult range of dissociative response. Twenty-two percent of the women had DES scores of 30 or above, indicative of abnormal levels of dissociation, with 16% at 50 or above, a score which Bernstein and Putnam (1986) suggest is indicative of a dissociative identity disorder diagnosis. An identical mean DES score (24.1) was found in a 1999 study of dissociative responses of treatment-seeking French rape survivors, with 33% of the DES scores of this sample of rape survivors higher than 30 (Darves-Bornoz, Degiovanni, & Gaillard, 1999).

CONCLUSIONS

The evidence is clear: Those in prostitution have experienced extremely high rates of childhood trauma, violent victimization while in prostitution, substance abuse, and psychiatric disorders. While there are some cultural variation and sampling differences, the overall pattern is consistent (Cooper et al., 2001; Farley, Baral, Sezgin, & Kiremire, 1998; Hoigard & Finstad, 1986; Nadon, Koverola, & Schludermann, 1998; Phoenix, 1999; Ross et al., 1990; Silbert & Pines, 1981; 1982; 1983; 1984; Yargic et al., 2000).

Results of the Winnipeg study dispel some misconceptions about prostitution. It has long been assumed that street prostitution is the most harmful type of prostitution. With the exception of substance abuse (which was higher among those in street prostitution), the Winnipeg study found that childhood trauma preceding strip club prostitution (where the exotic dancers worked) was greater than that reported by those in street prostitution. Furthermore, the dissociative and other psychiatric symptoms of women prostituting in strip clubs exceeded those of women in street prostitution.

The low rate of childhood sexual abuse in the Turkish sample reported here (8%) might not be representative of overall rates among women prostituting in Turkey. Farley et al. (1998), for instance, found a rate of reported childhood sexual abuse of 34% in a sample of 50 Turkish women in prostitution. This percentage may also be lower than is actually the case because of the hostile setting in which the research took place. The women described their histories of abuse to researchers after having been transported by police from brothels to an STD clinic. Nevertheless, the Yargic (2000) and Farley (1998) data suggest that childhood sexual abuse is not the only pathway into prostitution. In some cultures, poverty and normalized sexual exploitation may also be critical factors in channeling women into prostitution. Other traumatic events such as childhood physical abuse direct women toward prostitution, as do economic, political, and cultural factors that are beyond the scope of this discussion.

Dissociation is a core element of the response to both acute and chronic childhood trauma. Dissociative disorders, anxiety disorders, substance abuse and depression are common among those in prostitution. High levels of interpersonal violence are directed at women in prostitution, which compounds the psychological problems stemming from childhood trauma. Preliminary results from the U.S. study suggest that dissociative symptoms persist many years after exit from prostitution (Farley, 2002).

Those who are diagnosed with dissociative identity disorder, on average, meet lifetime criteria for another ten to fifteen psychiatric disorders (Ross, 1997). One would therefore expect that women in prostitution would meet criteria for many different psychiatric disorders if assessed with a structured interview that made a wide range of Axis I and II diagnoses. The dissociation, substance abuse and depression are probably accompanied by high rates of eating, sleep, impulse control, anxiety and personality disorders, as well as posttraumatic stress disorder and sexual dysfunction.

Future research on prostitution should interview women from a range of locations where prostitution takes place: street, escort prostitution agencies, strip clubs, pornography studios, and telephone and Internet prostitution. Research should include women, men, the transgendered, adults and children in a range of cultures and countries. Standardized measures should be used to document symptoms and DSM-IV diagnoses, including the dissociative disorders and pathological dissociation as measured by the DES (Waller, Putnam, & Carlson, 1996).

Based on the data and our clinical experience, we predict that future research will demonstrate that entry into prostitution as a child, and/or long-term employment/exploitation in prostitution, cause severe trauma and severe mental health problems. Such data might help to form public policy, and would inform intervention programs for those in prostitution.

CLINICAL OBSERVATIONS AND THEORY REGARDING DISSOCIATION IN PROSTITUTION

Prostitution has been described as one type of slavery (Barry, 1979). Writing about the psychological trauma of being enslaved, W. E. B. DuBois (1903/1961) described a

> double-consciousness, this sense of always looking at one's self through the eyes of others, of measuring one's soul by the tape of a world that looks on in amused contempt and pity. One ever feels this twoness . . . two souls, two thoughts, two unreconciled strivings, two warring ideals in one dark body whose dogged strength alone keeps it from being torn asunder. (p. 16-17)

Dissociation permits psychological survival, whether the repeated trauma is slavery, military combat, incest, or prostitution. Dissociation is an elaborate escape and avoidance strategy in which overwhelming human cruelty results in fragmentation of the mind into different parts of the self that observe, experience, react, as well as those that do not know about the harm. Given the burden of lifetime trauma experienced by women in prostitution, the extended use of dissociation is easy to understand. One survivor proposed that we view the many parts of her self as "a small army fighting for the rights of women" (Dworkin, 2002, p. 211).

Paradoxically, although the dissociative adaptation protects the person from the emotional impact of trauma, it increases the risk of further victimization since the survivor tends to dissociate in response to actual danger cues that are similar to the original trauma. For example, even though she knows she is about to be betrayed, hit, or raped, she may not be able to mobilize other, healthier defensive strategies.

Like other dissociative trauma survivors, many in prostitution have encapsulated personified internal child parts of the self, prostitute ego states, adult protectors and a pantheon of other identities. The psychological device of splitting the self into parts serves many functions. These parts of the self are variously present, absent, and co-conscious, each with varying combinations of amnesia, depersonalization and derealization for the prostitution when they are in other social settings (Kluft, 1987). A primary function of dissociation is to handle the overwhelming fear, pain and to deal with the encounter with systematized cruelty that is experienced during prostitution (and earlier abuse), by splitting that off from the rest of the self. Dissociation also reduces internal conflict and cognitive dissonance. The dissociative solution to prostitution is an extreme version of the denial that occurs daily in all sectors of society: Bad things are ignored, or we pretend they will go away, or we call them by another name (Schwartz, 2000, p. 122).

An understanding of the internal logic and structure of the dissociative disorders is useful for the understanding and treatment of a majority of those in prostitution. Dissociation occurs on a continuum from normal daydreaming to dissociative identity disorder (DID), in which discrete parts of the self are amnestic for each other. In our clinical experience, most of the women in prostitution we have interviewed do not meet formal criteria for dissociative identity disorder (DID). Those who dissociate would likely be diagnosed as having dissociative disorder not otherwise specified (DDNOS), a less severe form of dissociation than DID, in which there are alterations of integrated consciousness, but with fewer discrete personified parts of the self.

Drugs, alcohol, and other addictive behaviors potentiate dissociation, and they obscure the reality of prostitution from the dissociated person. The high rates of depression among prostituted women tell us, however, that none of these strategies fully shield the traumatized person from despair, demoralization, and hopelessness. Shutting down the naturally-occurring trauma response to prostitution requires disconnection and internal fragmentation. A woman who prostituted at a strip club described an increasing degree of fragmentation, and consolidation of distinct identities: "I turn into a totally different personality [at the club] . . . and it's getting to where it's really hard to find Sandra again. I'm becoming this other person completely."

Another woman described a dissociative response to prostitution, which had its origin in childhood sexual assault:

> Prostitution is like rape. It's like when I was 15 years old and I was raped. I used to experience leaving my body. I mean that's what I did when that man raped me. I went to the ceiling and I numbed myself because I didn't want to feel what I was feeling. I was very frightened. And while I was a prostitute I used to do that all the time. I would numb my feelings. I wouldn't even feel like I was in my body. I would actually leave my body and go somewhere else with my thoughts and with my feelings until he got off me and it was over with. I don't know how else to explain it except that it felt like rape. It was rape to me. (Giobbe, 1991, p. 144)

A third woman described both her depression and the origins of her prostitution in childhood trauma:

> . . . all I knew was how to be raped, and how to be attacked, and how to be beaten up, and that's all I knew. So when he put me in the game [pimped her] I was too down in the dumps to do anything. All I knew was the abuse. (Phoenix, 1999)

A gradual depersonalization resulting from stripclub prostitution was eloquently summarized by this person:

> You start changing yourself to fit a fantasy role of what they think a woman should be. In the real world, these women don't exist. And they stare at you with this starving hunger. It just sucks you dry; you become this empty shell. They're not really looking at you. You're not you. You're not even there. (Farley, 1998, unpublished interview)

Dissociative symptoms are frequently somatic in nature (Nijenhuis, 1999). A woman who was prostituting in a massage parlor made clear the process of dissociating those parts of her body that were being sold in prostitution:

> The first time a guy tried to feel up my breasts, I got really angry and wouldn't let him. Pretty soon, I wised up. I figured I wasn't working here [at the massage parlor] for my health. So the next time a guy tried to feel me up I let him. . . . Now I let most customers feel me up some. I've learned not to be there when they touch me. When they touch my breasts I tell myself they're not really touching me . . . And sometimes I wonder how I can let the men do that. I wonder what there is left for me. I wonder where I am. (Edelstein, 1986, p. 63)

A woman who worked in peep show prostitution (where there was no physical contact between herself and customers) described how prostitution seeped into her relationship with her partner, and the somatic dissociation contributing to that process:

> At work, what my hands find when they touch my body is 'product.' Away from work, my body has continuity, integrity . . . Last night, lying in bed after work, I touched my belly, my breasts. They felt like Capri's [her peep show name] and they refused to switch back. When [her partner] kissed me I inadvertently shrunk from his touch. Shocked, we both

jerked away and stared at each other. Somehow the glass had dissolved
and he had become one of them. (Funari, 1997, p. 32)

Although prostitution provides only an illusion of power, control and mastery, these illusions can be compelling. The lack of physical safety, lack of alternatives for equal pay, and lack of equal social and economic resources
preclude her having any real control in the prostitution transaction. Still, the illusions of love, money, and power in prostitution have a culturally-sanctioned
appeal. Many women with dissociative disorders who have been prostituted
appear to be re-enacting and mastering some aspects of childhood trauma.
Sometimes women feel that in prostitution they are in control of when sex acts
(which are often tantamount to rape) take place, with whom, and where, and
furthermore, they are paid for it. One woman said that at age 17, she felt safer
and more in control turning tricks on the street than she did at home with her
stepfather raping her (Farley, 2003). The prostitution appears to place her in a
position of control. Another woman said

> From my incest experiences, I learned that sex was associated with deg-
> radation, humiliation, powerlessness and pain. . . . By turning tricks, I
> was re-enacting my trauma. . . . The encounters I had as a prostitute were
> 'secret' like my incest experience; they were degrading, and in the end, I
> was abandoned. My father would just leave me there after sexually mo-
> lesting me and act like nothing happened the next day. (Williams, 1991,
> p. 111)

In order to survive the brutal commodification of their sexuality in prostitution, women dissociate, and appear to accept the view of themselves as sexual
commodities. Healing from prostitution is a lengthy process of re-connecting
all parts of the self. As one woman said:

> That was probably one of the hardest things to get over–re-attaching with
> feelings and re-attaching with myself and my physical body. . . . The goal
> of [the program she participated in] is to slowly take every shattered
> piece of your life and build you back up. (Hartman, 1999, p. 2)

In the dissociative disorders, there is a failure of protective behavior, a failure to recognize (and occasional misperception of) cues for interpersonal conflict and danger, and a learned mistrust of her own intuition. The therapeutic
relationship and other social supports begin to rebuild the battered self-esteem
of the survivor, and in the early phase of therapy, even before the dissociation
is addressed, there is an urgent need for teaching basic self-care such as eating,

sleeping, exercise, cessation of self-injurious behaviors, learning to trust her own instincts, and learning to separate the internal voice which promotes self-care from the self-sabotage voice internalized from perpetrators.

Unless screening questions are asked, prostitution will remain invisible. Just as clinicians screen for sexual abuse and substance abuse history, prostitution history should be addressed at intake, and also at a later point in treatment after a therapeutic relationship is established, since an initial denial of prostitution is not unusual. The questions "have you ever exchanged sex for money, drugs, housing, food, or clothes?" and "have you ever worked in the sex industry: for example, dancing, escort, massage, prostitution, pornography, phone sex?" are routine in the authors' intake inquiry.

Treatment approaches that are used by those who work with battered and raped women are also applicable to prostituted women. The first goal must be to establish physical safety. Thus both client and therapist agree on the goal of ultimately leaving prostitution. Only after that has occurred (often by locating safe housing) can the initial stage of therapy proceed, in which chemical dependence, acute and chronic PTSD, and dissociative symptoms are addressed. This goal of physical safety may take longer to achieve when neither therapist nor patient are aware of the prostitution until later in therapy.

Another goal of therapy is to enable the different parts of her self to see the past, present and future from a whole person perspective, rather than from the perspective of insulated, separate identities. For example, by prostituting, she exposes her body to the same treatment it received from pedophiles in childhood. Not only is prostitution similar to incest, but the converse is also true: to incestuously assault a child is to prostitute her. Yet the dissociated part of the self who prostitutes may not be aware of the harm to the body, which is often itself dissociated as a separate part of the self.

The therapist working with survivors of prostitution must be vigilant regarding countertransference. The therapy cannot proceed unless the therapist has an ongoing means of addressing his/her own reactions to the survivor's trauma (Elsass, 1997; Herman, 1992; Schwartz, 2001). Therapists who work with survivors of extreme violence, such as prostitution, are well advised to obtain supervision, not only to address their own symptoms of vicarious traumatization, but to ensure that these responses do not interfere with the survivor's healing. A range of responses to extreme trauma are common in therapists working with survivors–from minimization, avoidance, denial and under-diagnosis to outrage, overreaction, and over-politicization of the treatment setting. The possibilities of therapist voyeurism and other sexual exploitation of the survivor must be carefully monitored.

Clinicians treating prostitution survivors for dissociative and other trauma related symptoms must be familiar with

. . . not only memory and its vicissitudes but also about the dynamics of incestuous families, of perpetrators and perpetrator groups, of coercive thought-reform [as used by pimps and possibly others in her life] and its social influences, of complicity, collusion, and collaborationism, about the psychobiology of trauma and dissociation, and about the relationship between the abusive power arrangements in the culture [such as the abuse of power which occurs in the john-prostitute transaction] . . . (Schwartz, 2000, p. 212)

The purpose of this paper has been to review four studies of dissociation in those in prostituted women, and to present some clinical and anecdotal evidence that suggests that dissociation is a common psychological defense in response to the trauma of prostitution. For more extensive literature on treatment of dissociative disorders, the reader is referred to Herman (1992), Ross (1997), or Schwartz (2000). The high rates of childhood trauma, depression, posttraumatic stress disorder, and dissociation among the prostituted indicate that they are often struggling with previous trauma, or are mired in the unresolved consequences of childhood trauma. This cycle is compounded by the beatings, rapes, verbal abuse and other forms of trauma that are intrinsic to prostitution. Public policy should take into account the pervasive trauma in prostitution.

REFERENCES

Barry, K. (1979). *Female sexual slavery.* New York: New York University Press.
Belton, R. (1992). Prostitution as traumatic reenactment. Paper presented at 8th Annual Meeting of International Society for Traumatic Stress Studies, Los Angeles, CA. October 22, 1992.
Bernstein, E.M., & Putnam, F.W. (1986). Development, reliability, and validity of a dissociation scale. *Journal of Nervous and Mental Disease* 174: 727-735.
Cooper, B.S., Kennedy, M.A., & Yuille, J.C. (2001). Dissociation and sexual trauma in prostitutes: Variability of responses. *Journal of Trauma and Dissociation* 2: 27-36.
Darves-Bornoz, J.M., Degiovanni, A., & Gaillard, P. (1999). Validation of a French version of the Dissociative Experiences Scale in a rape-victim population. *Canadian Journal of Psychiatry* 44(3): 271-275.
DuBois, W.E.B. (1961). *The souls of black folk.* New York: Fawcett. (Originally published 1903).
Dworkin, A. (2002). *Heartbreak: The political memoir of a feminist militant.* New York, Basic Books.
Edelstein, J. (1986). In the massage parlor. In F. Delacoste & P. Alexander (Eds.). *Sex work: Writings by women in the sex industry* (p.p. 62-69). Pittsburgh, PA: Cleis Press.

Elsass, P. (1997). *Treating victims of torture and violence.* New York: University Press.

Farley, M. (2003). Prostitution and the invisibility of harm. *Women & Therapy* 26(3/4): 247-280.

Farley, M., & Barkan, H. (1998). Prostitution, violence against women, and post-traumatic stress disorder. *Women and Health 27:* 37-49.

Farley, M., & Kelly, V. (2000). Prostitution: A critical review of the medical and social sciences literature. *Women & Criminal Justice 11 29-64.*

Farley, M., Baral, I., Kiremire, M., & Sezgin, U. (1998). Prostitution in five countries: Violence and post-traumatic stress disorder. *Feminism and Psychology* 8: 405-426.

Funari, V. (1997). Naked, naughty, nasty: Peepshow reflections. In J. Nagle (ed.). *Whores and other feminists.* New York: Routledge.

Giobbe, E. (1991). Prostitution: Buying the right to rape. In A. Burgess (Ed.), *Rape and sexual assault III: A handbook.* New York: Garland Press.

Goodman, L. & Fallot, R. (1998). HIV risk-behavior in poor urban women with serious mental disorders: Association with childhood physical and sexual abuse. *American Journal of Orthopsychiatry*, 68: 73-83.

Hartman, A. (1999). Survivor pursues real recovery. *The StopLight.* 1901 Portland Ave. S. Minneapolis, MN 55404.

Herman, J.L. (1992). *Trauma and Recovery.* New York: Basic Books.

Hoigard, C., & Finstad, L. (1986). *Backstreets: Prostitution, money and love.* University Park, PA: Pennsylvania State University Press.

Kluft, R.P. (1987). The simulation and dissimulation of multiple personality disorder. *Journal of Clinical Hypnosis* 30: 104-118.

Nadon, S.M., Koverola, C., & Schludermann, E.H. (1998). Antecedents to prostitution: Childhood victimization. *Journal of Interpersonal Violence, 13,* 206-221.

Nijenhuis, E.R.S. (1999). *Somatoform dissociation: Phenomena, measurement, and theoretical issues.* Assen, The Netherlands: Van Gorcum.

Phoenix, J. (1999). *Making sense of prostitution.* London: MacMillan Press.

Ross, C.A. (1997). *Dissociative identity disorder: Diagnosis, clinical features, and treatment of multiple personality.* New York: Wiley.

Ross, C.A. (1999). Dissociative disorders. In T. Millon, P.H. Blaney, & R.D. Davis, (Eds). *Oxford Textbook of Psychopathology* (pp. 466-481). New York: Oxford University Press.

Ross, C.A. (2000). *The trauma model: A solution to the problem of comorbidity in psychiatry.* Richardson, TX: Manitou Communications.

Ross, C.A., Anderson, G., Heber, S., & Norton, G.R. (1990). Dissociation and abuse among multiple personality patients, prostitutes, and exotic dancers. *Hospital and Community Psychiatry*, 41, 328-330.

Schwartz, H. (2000). *Dialogues with forgotten voices: Relational perspectives on child abuse trauma and treatment of dissociative disorders.* New York: Basic Books.

Silbert, M.H., & Pines, A.M. (1981). Child sexual abuse as an antecedent to prostitution. *Child Abuse and Neglect 5:* 407-411.

Silbert, M.H., & Pines, A.M. (1982). Entrance into prostitution. *Youth and Society* 13: 471-500.

Silbert, M.H., & Pines, A.M. (1983). Early sexual exploitation as an influence in prostitution. *Social Work* 28: *285-289.*

Silbert, M.H., & Pines, A.M. (1984). Pornography and sexual abuse of women. *Sex Roles* 10: 857-868.

Waller, N.G., Putnam, F.W., & Carlson, E.B. (1996). The types of dissociation and dissociative types: A taxometric analysis of dissociative experiences. *Psychological Methods* 1: 300-321.

Williams, J.L. (1991). *Sold Out: A Recovery Guide for Prostitutes Anonymous.* P.O. Box 3279 North Las Vegas, NV, 89036 USA.

Wood, Marianne. (1995). *Just a prostitute.* Queensland: University of Queensland Press.

Yargic, L.I., Sevim, M., Arabul, G., & Ozden, S.Y. (2000). Childhood trauma histories and dissociative disorders among prostitutes in Turkey. Paper presentation at Annual Conference of the International Society for the Study of Dissociation. San Antonio, Texas.

Providing Services
to African American Prostituted Women

Vednita Carter

SUMMARY. This article describes the history and dynamics of African/African American women in prostitution beginning with the arrival of the African woman to America, her life and the obstacles she faced living in America. We discuss treatment philosophy and services offered by Breaking Free, a Minneapolis organization offering services to African American prostituted women.

PROSTITUTION AND SLAVERY

For 200 years, thousands of Africans were kidnapped or purchased and transported to the Western Hemisphere to be used as slaves. During transport on the slave ships, slaves suffered extreme levels of abuse. African women and girls were forced to be naked, providing their captors with easy access to their bodies at all times. Once they arrived in the United States, the degradation continued as men, women, and children were routinely auctioned off to the highest bidder. Women stood on auction blocks, forced to undergo the humiliation of auctioneers and potential buyers poking and fondling their body parts, forcing them to bend and squat on command, without regard for their humanity. Unrestrained by law or custom, slave owners raped and impregnated enslaved

Vednita Carter is at Breaking Free, 770 University Avenue W, St. Paul MN (Email: vcarter@breakingfree.net)
Printed with permission.

[Haworth co-indexing entry note]: "Providing Services to African American Prostituted Women." Carter, Vednita. Co-published simultaneously in *Journal of Trauma Practice* (The Haworth Maltreatment & Trauma Press, an imprint of The Haworth Press, Inc.) Vol. 2, No. 3/4, 2003, pp. 213-222; and: *Prostitution, Trafficking, and Traumatic Stress* (ed: Melissa Farley) The Haworth Maltreatment & Trauma Press, an imprint of The Haworth Press, Inc., 2003, pp. 213-222. Single or multiple copies of this article are available for a fee from The Haworth Document Delivery Service [1-800-HAWORTH, 9:00 a.m. - 5:00 p.m. (EST). E-mail address: docdelivery@haworthpress.com].

http://www.haworthpress.com/store/product.asp?sku=J189
10.1300/J189v02n03_12

Black women with impunity. In addition to serving the objective of satisfying their sexual desires, the slave owners deliberately used enslaved women and girls to generate income as breeders. Many of the biracial female children that resulted from these rapes were sold to brothels as young as ten years of age. Called "fancy girls," they were given food, blankets, and a place to sleep in exchange for performing sex acts each day with numerous strangers. The legacy of physical, sexual, and psychological abuse continues to have lasting, scarring effects on the lives of many African-American women.

After 1863, many freed slaves fled to the north in search of employment, guided by the hope that they might find true freedom. The options for African-American women were discouraging, at best, as they routinely found themselves in domestic servitude in white households. Women who did not find jobs as servants were forced to sell their bodies in order to provide necessities for their families—food, clothing and housing. Many women continued to be brutalized, raped and murdered as they searched for the illusive freedoms promised in the Emancipation Proclamation.

The turn of the century brought little change in the economic realities of African Americans. By 1910, African-American people continued to be exploited by racist practices that severely restricted access to employment, and low pay for the few jobs that were available. Black Americans were systematically forced to take menial, subservient employment to survive. The inevitable outcome of these practices has been that many African-Americans have been kept in a state of poverty and dependency—undereducated, with limited horizons.

PROSTITUTION TODAY

Today, much prostitution occurs in the streets and in the clubs of U.S. cities, in poor, urban communities populated by African-Americans and other people of color. Middle-class men, predominantly of European descent, drive through these neighborhoods for the purpose of finding a girl or woman to buy and use for sexual gratification.[1] Like slave women on the auction block, African-American women are displayed on the streets or in stripclubs, surveyed like cattle, and selected to perform at the orders of a stranger. They are routinely berated and shouted at while being sexually assaulted, and are often slapped, beaten, and shoved out of cars. It is not difficult for thoughtful people to see the connections between slavery and prostitution.

Some have said that prostitution is tolerated in the Black community. This is not true. Prostitution is no more tolerated by African-American women and girls than slavery was tolerated by their ancestors. The system of prostitution functions now as the system of slavery did then. Women in African-American communities are disproportionately targeted for the abuse and violence of prostitution, stereotypically marked as sexually insatiable or deviant. At the same time, the racist assumption that prostitution is somehow acceptable in African-American communities creates a nearly insurmountable barrier of shame and perceived rejection to women used in prostitution, effectively silencing them from speaking about their experiences and feelings. African-American women used in prostitution are harmed by racist stereotypes, and simultaneously rendered silent or invisible. It is through this paradoxical dynamic that Black women are held in the bondage of slavery.[2]

The racist stereotyping of African-American women as sex-crazed or animalistic perpetuates all forms of violence against Black women without consequences for the perpetrators. In addition, law enforcement practices disproportionately target African Americans for harassment, arrest, imprisonment and fines. For example, several studies have shown that African-American women arrested for prostitution in the Minneapolis area were charged higher court fines, and given longer jail and probationary sentences than white women.[3]

Black women are more likely to be trapped in the pattern of arrest, incarceration and fines, and probation. This, and other forms of systemic racism, create barriers between Black women and most social institutions, except for those that perpetuate the cycle of poverty and despair–corrections, welfare, and the underground economy of drugs and prostitution. The most fundamental needs, such as housing for their families, are often beyond the reach of African-American women, due to past criminal histories and eviction notices.

PROSTITUTION AND HEALTH

People of color are more likely to suffer from chronically poor health than their white peers. The insidious stress caused by numerous expressions of systemic racism combines with conditions that create poor health. Racism restricts socioeconomic opportunities and mobility, limits access to and bias in medical care, and is the basis for residential segregation (which often limits access to social goods and services). All of these contribute to significant disparities in the health of African-Americans. For example, according to data collected at the Minnesota Department of Health and the Center for Disease Control (2000), African-American girls in the 15 to 29 age group have the highest rate of HIV/STD infection in the United States.

A lack of attention to reports of violence and sexual abuse has resulted in repeated failures of the health care system to provide adequate services to African-American girls and women in general, and specifically for those used in prostitution. Access to services which are widely available to others is extremely limited to prostituted women. Fear of arrest and fear of the general contempt with which they are treated, make it difficult for women to seek out the meager services that are available (Nelson, 1993). A 1994 study by Parriott found that African-American prostituted women were at greater health risk in several categories than their European-American counterparts.

Based on intake interviews at Breaking Free and based on street outreach, we estimate that there are between 6000 and 8000 prostituted women in Minnesota. A profile of women used in street prostitution has been developed from data in Breaking Free's Annual Report (2000). Women used in street prostitution are between 14 and 45 years old; two-thirds are women of color (primarily Black and Latina), and have been in prostitution for an average of six years. Three-quarters are single and unemployed; most live in poverty. In addition, 90% of these women have STDs due to the inconsistent use of condoms and high number of sexual exchanges. Ninety percent abuse drugs or are chemically dependent, primarily to combinations of alcohol, heroin, and crack cocaine; 76% report that they have exchanged sex for crack. Sixty percent have experienced physical and/or sexual violence prior to prostitution.

Preventive health services which are readily available to many, are not available or easily accessible to prostituted Black women in Minneapolis and St. Paul. Lacking health insurance coverage, hospital emergency rooms provide the only health care and other services that most of these women receive. Poverty prevents women in these circumstances from filling prescription medications, except for the partial prescriptions dispensed by emergency room physicians. This crisis care does not meet immediate needs or address the numerous long-term health problems of these women.

SERVICES FOR AFRICAN-AMERICAN PROSTITUTED WOMEN

In order to provide adequate services to African-American prostituted women, providers must better understand the dynamics of prostitution, and the many complex issues that prostituted women and girls face on a daily basis. The services that Black women need may seem to be the same as those required by white women however, because of the repeated and sustained harms of racism, the needs of African-American women are significantly different. Service providers must identify and understand:

1. the relationship between slavery and prostitution
2. the major barriers created by numerous racist systems and practices that bring women into prostitution and keep them trapped

3. issues of child abuse; the average age of entry into prostitution is fourteen years old
4. the complex influences of poverty and homelessness
5. the prevalence of multiple health-related conditions, including depression, post-traumatic stress disorder, drug and alcohol addictions, HIV/AIDS and other STDs, diabetes and high blood pressure, and
6. the cultural and social barriers that exist within Black communities that make it difficult to discuss and deal with prostitution.

African-American women are more likely to seek services if there are Black women visibly employed in the offices of service providers. African-American women share a common historical and cultural background that can bridge the gap between African-American service providers and prostituted women. In other words, the strength of common racial and cultural identity creates the basis for a sustained, trusting relationship in which the difficult and painful work of rebuilding a life can take place.

BREAKING FREE–A SERVICE MODEL

Breaking Free is an Afro-centric social service agency with offices in predominantly African-American neighborhoods in St. Paul and Rochester, Minnesota. Eighty percent of the staff are African and African-American, half are survivors of prostitution. All of the members on the governing board are people of color; eight are African-American. The main office in St. Paul is located in a large house that has been converted into 10 office spaces, a reception area, a large meeting room, a youth center and a large kitchen. A drop-in center is being added to provide crisis services to women and girls who come in directly from the streets, without restrictions regarding their sobriety, health status, or cleanliness.

Breaking Free provides several services to assist women escaping prostitution. These services include:

Women's Program. This is the gateway to other services provided by Breaking Free. After an initial intake assessment is completed, a plan is established and enacted. Most women enter this program in a state of extreme crisis, often lacking basic needs such as shelter and food, and in need of immediate medical attention for the treatment of illness, injury and/or addiction.

Sisters of Survival. Once the emergency conditions are addressed, the women begin a 10-week, intensive education group to examine prostitution as a slave-based system, the impact prostitution has had on their lives, and issues related to addiction and recovery. This is a closed group.

Journey to Success. This program involves on-going group meetings for women who have successfully completed the 10-week program. Topics include relationship issues, building self-esteem, money management, and health care.

Building Strong Families. This group meets twice monthly to deal with women's relationships with their families. Facilitated by a female African-American psychologist with expertise in family relationships, the women learn how to improve their parenting skills, and to understand and effectively deal with the impact of prostitution on the lives of other family members.

Relapse Prevention Group. A chemical dependency counselor from a local treatment center works closely with women in this weekly group to discuss and deal with addictions.

Health Program. Working with a local health clinic, women in this group are offered physical examinations, lab testing when appropriate, family planning services, and a variety of other essential medical services. As transportation is often a major barrier to health care, women are transported by the clinic's van at no cost. Breaking Free also provides education and information regarding HIV/AIDS and other STDs, maternal alcohol abuse (FAS/FAE), breast and cervical cancer, and diabetes.

Internship Program. This program allows women who may have never held a real job to become employable. Breaking Free has formed contractual partnerships with local businesses willing to hire women in this program, regardless of their criminal records or lack of employment history. Breaking Free covers the cost of up to six months of employment. Women who successfully complete internships are then hired on a permanent basis. During this probationary period, a case manager is assigned to monitor progress and mediate as needed between the employer and the intern.

Youth Program. These participants are referred to Breaking Free by the courts and homeless shelters, some are self-referred. Many are unable to return home; others refuse because home is where the abuse first began. Minnesota law requires that services are provided with great care, and Breaking Free is sometimes limited as to the ways in which we can provide services. Some of these girls are minors and not independent from their parents/families. In some of these cases, the youth are encouraged and taken through the steps of the reunification process. In other cases Child Protection Services must be involved in solving the complex problems of these young girls.

Housing Program. Breaking Free currently operates three apartment buildings which provide homes to thirty-seven women and their children. Two locations are in St. Paul, one is in Rochester. Twelve of the women have minor children, and at least sixteen of the women have never had their own homes. Lack of adequate, safe housing affects 60% of Breaking Free's clientele. Helping prostituted African-American women locate safe housing presents a formidable challenge. Due to the intergenerational cycle of abuse and neglect, most of the women who live in the supportive housing complexes have never learned the basic skills required to live independently.

Case Example

Joline, a thirty-year-old African-American woman, was ordered by the county's criminal justice system to attend Breaking Free. Appearing in court for prostitution-related charges was a pattern that had begun when she was 16 years old. She had been active in prostitution since the age of 15.

Joline was physically and sexually abused at home by her father, who began molesting her at the age of 5 years. By the time she was 11, he began to penetrate her. Because of the sexual abuse, she ran away at age 14. While on the run, she met a man twice her age who turned her out into prostitution, and introduced her to addictive drugs.

Joline had her first child at the age of 16; at age 20, she had 3 children. Each of her children became wards of the state soon after they were born. The pimp died of a drug overdose when Joline was 27. Although he was physically, sexually, and mentally cruel and abusive to her, she felt that part of her died with him. She felt that he was the only one who truly understood her and loved her. She continued in prostitution, eventually coming to feel that she had nothing to live for.

When Joline first came to Breaking Free, she was given an intake assessment, during which multiple acute and chronic health conditions were revealed, none of which had ever been diagnosed or treated. The only time Joline had seen a physician was during pregnancy or in a medical emergency, for example, after being beaten by her pimp or someone else. We also discovered that Joline had never spoken to anyone about the physical or sexual abuse in her childhood, and that she had given little thought to the impact of prostitution on her life. She used drugs and alcohol on a daily basis to cope with the unbearable circumstances in her life. She had also become physically self-destructive, cutting her arms and legs with a knife.

Joline's story is in many ways typical of the clients at Breaking Free, trapped in a cycle of constant retraumatization. Because Breaking Free provides comprehensive services that address the complex network of traumatic, destructive influences that afflict African-American women in prostitution, Joline began to make major strides toward building a normal life. She was first referred to a health care clinic for treatment provided by individuals trained to understand the particular needs of prostituted women who receive no regular health care. She was tested for hepatitis C and HIV. A mental health evaluation revealed bipolar disorder, for which she was immediately treated. Once medicated, her volatile moods and extreme behaviors subsided considerably.

Joline also began to participate in the chemical dependency program where, in addition to receiving medical treatment, she began to address the underlying causes for her addictions and to learn the skills she would need to avoid relapse. She came to understand how her addictions went hand-in-hand with prostitution, keeping her trapped. In the Women's Program support group meetings, Joline was able to talk freely about prostitution. She came to understand how the dynamics of prostitution specifically applied to her as an African-American woman, how prostitution is about slavery and survival rather than lifestyle choices. Although she was able to speak about the abuses in her childhood during group sessions, Joline was also referred to a child sexual abuse specialist.

Joline was homeless and had never had her own housing when she came to Breaking Free. She had no income and she had a criminal record. These factors made it extremely difficult for her to secure permanent housing. Breaking Free was able to move Joline into its permanent supportive housing program. In this program, Joline began to see a case manager on a regular weekly basis. Together, they created a plan to structure her life into a normal routine of self-care. Her case manager ensured that she took her medications and reminded her about appointments. Breaking Free provided furniture, household goods and food until Joline was able to earn an income to provide for herself.

Joline continues to work hard, struggling to overcome the numerous obstacles in her life. She is self-supporting, drug-free, and has made tremendous progress in all areas of her life.

CONCLUSION

At Breaking Free, we believe that prostitution is the last piece of the puzzle in the battered women's movement. Health and social systems have begun to identify the causes and effects of domestic violence. We must now be willing to do the same with prostitution. Like other victims of sexual assault, Black women and girls used in prostitution need and deserve assistance to overcome the trauma of commercial sexual exploitation. It is often difficult for Black women to escape prostitution because it often requires that she abandon her home, flee from an abusive husband, boyfriend or pimp who has coerced her into turning tricks for his benefit. Black women must receive appropriate forms of support and advocacy in order to establish new lives for themselves and their children.

The African-American community and their allies must recognize the shackles of slavery that still bind Black women. African-American churches must recognize that women used in prostitution, pornography, and stripping are victims, rather than "bad women." Black men need to unlearn the lessons which are the legacy of white slave masters–that Black women are not "bitches" and "whores." *Black women are not the property of white men on plantations, and they are not the property of Black men in the 'hood.*

All Black Americans need to educate themselves about how history has shaped their identity as African-Americans since the day the first African was thrown onto American shores and forced into bondage and sexual slavery. Only then will Black Americans all be able to effectively reject the toxic propaganda that has distorted their collective identity. And only under these conditions will prostituted African-American women understand their worth. This fight against sexual slavery is the key to dismantling systems of dual oppression–of racism and sexism. Internalized oppression must be externalized. Only then can it be ended.

NOTES

1. In every Southern U.S. city in the 1920s and 30s, the red-light district was on the "other side of the tracks" in the black ghetto, where young white boys routinely "discovered their manhood" with the help of the "two dollar whore" Carmen & Moody, 1985, pp. 184-185.

2. See Iris Marion Young's definition of cultural imperialism as a paradoxical oppression in which the oppressed are marked by stereotypes which identify them as deviant while concurrently rendering them invisible. I. M. Young, 1995, p. 81.

3. In 1996, 47% of the arrests were of white offenders while 36% were Black offenders. On the other hand, in 1997, 38% were listed as white offenders and 45% were Black offenders. In both cases for the data as a whole, this means that the majority of

arrests were of people of color with a larger margin in the first seven months of 1997 than was the case in 1996. (Commercial Sexual Exploitation Resource Institute, 1998 , pp. 32-34).

REFERENCES

Breaking Free Annual Report. (2000). Prostitution in Hennepin county, a review of the criminal justice system. Unpublished report. Minneapolis: Breaking Free.

Carmen, A. & Moody, H. (1985). *Working Women: The Subterranean World of Street Prostitution.* New York: Harper & Row.

Commercial Sexual Exploitation Resource Institute (1998). Prostitution in Hennepin County, a Review of the Criminal Justice Response Between 1/96-7/97. Minneapolis: Commercial Sexual Exploitation Resource Institute.

Minnesota Department of Health and Center for Disease Control (2002). Populations of Color in Minnesota, Health Status Report. Minneapolis: Minnesota Department of Health.

Nelson, V. (1993). Prostitution: Where Racism & Sexism Intersect. *Michigan Journal of Gender and Law*, 1: 81-89.

Parriott, R. (1994). Health experiences of Twin Cities women used in prostitution: Unpublished survey initiated by WHISPER, Minneapolis, MN.

Young, I.M. (1995). Five faces of oppression. In D. Harris (Ed.), *Multiculturalism From the Margins.* Westport: Bergin & Garvey.

The Importance of Supportive Relationships Among Women Leaving Prostitution

Ulla-Carin Hedin
Sven Axel Månsson

SUMMARY. This article discusses the role of social support in women's breakaway from prostitution. We present results of a study based on qualitative interviews with 23 Swedish women who left the sex trade during 1985-95. The article describes the women's exit in terms of a salutogenic process in which different factors interact. Critical factors in this process are the women's supportive relationships and their ability to mobilize both informal and professional support providers. Another important factor appears to be the woman's own capacity to change her coping strategies and actively work with her relational problems in different ways. We found that women's break with prostitution does not necessarily lead to good health and development–these presuppose extensive work on relationships and social networks. There are three main components to this work; working through traumatic experiences, repairing and mastering previously close relationships and building a new heterogeneous social network. On a theoretical level the study is closely linked to research which addresses processes of change, turning points,

Ulla-Carin Hedin, PhD, and Sven-Axel Månsson, PhD, are Associate Professors of Social Work at Göteborg University in Sweden.

They can be contacted at the Department of Social Work, Göteborg University, PO Box 720, SE 405 30 Göteborg, Sweden (E-mail: Hedin@socwork.gu.se and Sven-Axel.Mansson@socwork.gu.se).

Printed with permission.

[Haworth co-indexing entry note]: "The Importance of Supportive Relationships Among Women Leaving Prostitution." Hedin, Ulla-Carin, and Sven Axel Månsson. Co-published simultaneously in *Journal of Trauma Practice* (The Haworth Maltreatment & Trauma Press, an imprint of The Haworth Press, Inc.) Vol. 2, No. 3/4, 2003, pp. 223-237; and: *Prostitution, Trafficking, and Traumatic Stress* (ed: Melissa Farley) The Haworth Maltreatment & Trauma Press, an imprint of The Haworth Press, Inc., 2003, pp. 223-237. Single or multiple copies of this article are available for a fee from The Haworth Document Delivery Service [1-800-HAWORTH, 9:00 a.m. - 5:00 p.m. (EST). E-mail address: docdelivery@haworthpress.com].

role changes and exit behavior. It is also linked to the study of social networks and social support; informal support providing as well as professional support interventions.

THE BREAKAWAY THEORY

This article is based on a qualitative study that examines women's break from prostitution. One of our goals has been to focus on the way in which relationships make possible the break from prostitution. We view it in terms of an interactionist perspective, that is, we ask questions about the woman's interaction with her personal social network and her need for professional help during the course of the break. Three central questions in this regard are:

(1). Which persons closest to the woman have positively influenced the course of the breakaway?

(2). Which relationships and strategies have been important for the woman's constructing a new life?

(3). What kinds of social work and psychotherapy are needed to support and strengthen the woman's own capacities and efforts?

We conducted qualitative interviews with 23 women who had left the sex trade between 1985 and 1995. Half of the women were referred to us via a special social outreach program within the social services in Göteborg, Sweden,[1] and the other half were recruited on a national basis via newspaper advertisements. In 1995, their ages ranged from 20 to 58 years. Seventy percent of the 23 women had been involved in the sex trade for more than five years, 34% for more than ten years. Fifty percent of the women had been involved only in street prostitution, the others worked in brothels, sex clubs, escort services, or in combinations of different types of prostitution. The time span between the breakaway and the interview varied widely. Seventy-five percent of the women had left prostitution more than three years prior to the interview. Only 25% had stopped prostituting more recently (Hedin & Månsson, 1998).[2]

The interviews took place in a social service agency in Göteborg or in the woman's home, lasted between 2-5 hours and were conducted by one of the authors. Some of the women wished to speak to another woman about their experiences of traumas and violence during prostitution, others preferred a male interviewer. The function of the interview seemed to depend upon the amount of time which had elapsed between the breakaway and the interview. For those who had recently left prostitution, the interview was clearly therapeutic, an opportunity to work through various feelings and experiences. For those who had broken away several years prior to the interview, it seemed to be a way to understand the context and meaning of their lives. We characterize the interviews as life story interviews since they cover the whole life course of the individual, from the early childhood years and on.

In order to understand and analyze women's breaks with prostitution, we derived ideas and inspiration from a theory regarding the exit process from harmful situations developed by sociologist Helen Fuchs Ebaugh (1988) which was based on qualitative studies of 173 people who differed in the nature of their breakaways. Her analysis described the consecutive phases of a breakaway, which was affected by an individual's inner drives, their relationships with others, and external events which accelerate or freeze the course of the breakaway. She noted that social and structural conditions, such as options for job or profession change, the possibility of moving to another region in the country and responses of close relatives, all affected the process of the breakaway.

Based on Fuchs Ebaugh's theory, we suggest that the break with prostitution can be described as a process that includes four phases:

(1). *Preliminary stages of the breakaway*, when the woman is thinking about quitting, seeking alternatives to the sex trade and trying various strategies in order to distance herself from prostitution and to locate the resources and points of support needed for another life.

(2). *The turning-point*, when the woman is in the process of deciding to actually break away. This can happen quickly and dramatically or it can be a more gradual process.

(3). *The post-breakaway marginal situation*, when the woman finds herself dangling between two life patterns, living in a state of uncertainty and ambivalence. Here she encounters a number of challenges.

(4). *Building a new life*, when the women develops new roles through work, studies or parenthood. Gradually, old injuries are repaired and a new life gradually develops.

The course of the breakaway can be described as a *salutogenic process*, in which a range of factors interact and move the process forward (Antonovsky, 1987). These include critical events, structural and relational factors, as well as the woman's individual strengths. We focus here on relational factors and on how they interact with the women's inner strengths. Below we will discuss the women's relationships with different categories of people in their social networks, which either promote or prevent the women's break with prostitution.

PREVIOUS RESEARCH ABOUT WOMEN'S ENTRY
INTO PROSTITUTION

Many women in prostitution come from working class and poor families with multiple social problems (Larsson, 1983; Davis, 1993; Karlsen, 1993). The women's relationships to their mothers were severely conflicted, and positive attachments to a male caregiver were minimal. The women felt unwanted, unnoticed or rejected, sometimes throughout their childhoods. Many had lived periodically with relatives, in foster homes or in residential care. Many girls entered prostitution when they were on the run from foster homes or institutions, lacking money and shelter (Larsson, 1983; Høigård & Finstad, 1986; Earls & David, 1990; Karlsen, 1993).

Another group of studies found that female prostitutes were victims of childhood physical and sexual abuse, which contributed to entry into prostitution. Silbert and Pines (1982, 1983), for example, investigated street prostitution in San Francisco, and found that 62% of the women had been physically abused as children and 60% had been sexually abused by a relative or family friend. These results have been replicated in other parts of the world by other researchers (Davis, 1993; Vanwesenbeeck, 1994; Farley & Kelly, 2000).

A third area of research investigated individual events and factors that over the long term promote entry into prostitution. The step into prostitution is seen as the consequence of a long process of exposure to violence, psychological abuse, stigmatization, and estrangement prior to entry into the sex trade. The notion of a drift into prostitution is central to this model and reflects a social psychological process. During this process, internal and external contextual factors interact (Whitbeck, Hoyt, & Ackley, 1997; Vanwesenbeeck, 1994; Hedin & Månsson, 1998).[3]

FAMILY OF ORIGIN

The women we interviewed grew up in relatively stable family situations, in that most have lived at home with one or both parents and siblings. Only a few women reported growing up primarily outside the family or with foster home or institutional placements (Larsson, 1983; Karlsen, 1993). However, 75% described a childhood filled with many problems. The maltreatment varied from isolated events to chronic exploitation. Fathers, brothers and other relatives were the perpetrators. The women also expressed feelings of bitterness toward their mothers, who failed to discover the abuses and who could not or did not try to protect their daughters. Sexual abuse in childhood or early adolescence was a common background factor for many women who enter prostitution or who become addicted. The women coped with the trauma of sexual abuse and subsequent symptoms of PTSD via drug and alcohol use.

A consistent theme in the interviews was problematic relationships with parents. We heard many painful descriptions of childhood emotional rejection. The mothers, with problems of their own, were not able to take an active interest in their daughters. Mental illness, substance abuse, or destructive conflicts stood in the way of attention and love. Some women described other problems such as punishment bordering on physical assault, the early death of a beloved father, or severe poverty. These childhood backgrounds have been corroborated by other research (Davis, 1993). Nonetheless, 25% of the women reported happy childhoods, with love and attention from parents.

When the women began to think about leaving the sex trade, they initiated new contact with the most trusted person in the family. At this point, the women talked openly about prostitution and clearly sought help. It is striking how this search for help broke down barriers and created opportunities for new relationships. In these instances, the family member understood the gravity of the situation and provided immediate emotional, practical, and instrumental support (Vaux, 1988; Hedin, 1994). This person became a coordinator of all sorts of additional support from the family network (Hedin & Månsson, 1998).

During the turning point itself and for a time afterwards, the women were emotionally and practically dependent on their primary support people. Some women described how this person protected them from attacks and criticism from others in the family network. This renewed contact brought up past difficulties and conflicts. On this point the women's stories diverge and we discerned several patterns. In some cases, the woman and her parents had changed and matured and were thereby able to form a new relationship. In other cases, a key person in the network, a sibling, or partner served as intermediary and arbitrator. In still other cases, we saw lingering conflicted relationships–earlier maltreatment and betrayals were impossible to work through. Even when these difficulties were not overcome, there seemed to be a silent agreement to try to preserve the reestablished, though fragile, contact.

Some of our interviewees described being stuck in the family network since the break with prostitution. They had not gone to work, begun studies, or made new contacts. Although the family offered crucial support during crises, in the long run, it did not provide opportunities for stimulation and development. Our results here are similar to other research such as that investigating women's situations following divorce or life crises. Several studies found that women with more diverse social networks had better mental health (Hirsch, 1980; Wilcox, 1981; Vaux, 1988).

Twenty-five percent of the women were able to leave prostitution without any contact with their families. For them, family relationships were too weak and conflict-ridden. They chose others such as partners or social workers as primary support providers. In many cases, women have described how support from professionals was a bridge to renewed contact with the family. The social workers in our study worked with the women in reconstructing and strengthening her own network (Hessle, 1995). This support was seen by the women as invaluable, and it sometimes was the determining factor regarding whether or not she could get out of prostitution (Larsson, 1983; Ljökjell, 1994).

RELATIONSHIPS WITH PARTNERS

The women's family histories failed to provide them with adequate models for close relationships. Sexual exploitation, emotional rejection, and parents' relationship problems all had a negative effect on their self-confidence and ability to form attachments. The women described great insecurity and low self-esteem, in combination with a strong desire for secure and affirming relationships during their teenage years, when they began to make contact with men. Their life stories contained numerous examples of poor choices of partners. This "weakness," as the women often described it, is a consistent theme that resurfaced in connection with later attempts to break away from prostitution. Desperation and uncertainty led them to throw themselves headlong into new relationships with men. In some cases, the women ran straight into the arms of pimps who perceived their vulnerability and exploited that. They then failed to escape at that point and were forced to continue in the sex trade for several years at an even more grueling pace, mentally and physically exhausting themselves. This torment occurred before they finally succeeded in breaking away.

In other patterns of escape from prostitution, some women spoke of men they met in connection with the breakaway who were different from earlier relationships. These men provided practical and instrumental support, for example, offering refuge from drug dealers or pimps, or connections to housing and new jobs. Through these men, the women sometimes accessed new social networks. We view these as transitional relationships, which have a particular function in contributing to the breakaway (Hessle, 1995). Here, the women used her partner in order to better cope with difficulties and acute crises. Our interviews show that these relationships can run various courses. In some cases, the relationship solidified and strengthened over time. In other cases the partners separated.

The majority of our interviewees left the sex trade with the help of relatives and social workers. They worked through their experiences of violence and their relationship problems later on in psychotherapy, only after this point starting a new partnership. They then chose men who were different from previous partners and who were more committed to the relationship. These relationships that were initiated during the women's rehabilitation have often worked out well and sometimes led to stable marriages or partnerships.

THE IMPORTANCE OF CHILDREN

Some of the women in our study had children prior to their involvement in prostitution. These women report that one of the most important reasons for prostituting was to support their children. They describe a stressful double life: They have taken "business trips" to other cities and left their children in the care of others. They often felt the need to lie about such trips. In the short-term, prostitution provided a good income, but it also resulted in constant worries about the children and the fear of being discovered and stigmatized by those around them.

Thirty percent of our interviewees had their children immediately after the breakaway. This often meant that the women's relationships with their parents improved when the maternal grandparents became involved with the grandchild. The women required practical and material support from their parents during the child's infancy. Research on female substance abusers notes a similar process of improved relationships with the family of origin after having children (Trulsson, 1998).

A few women experienced the total collapse of their worlds when their children were taken away from them by social welfare authorities. Additional problems such as drug abuse or psychological problems led to an inability to cope with the double life of prostitution and childrearing. Women addicted to drugs have sometimes lost custody of their children.[4] These women were especially dependent upon professional support. They needed social workers who offer stability and who can support their relationships with the children in the foster home–relationships that are often fragile and charged with conflict. On the other hand, the loss of custody of children marked a definite turning point in some women's prostitution histories. The struggle to regain custody sometimes was a motivating factor for a long-term process of change (Trulsson, 1998).

Women who became pregnant in connection with the breakaway found in the pregnancy a longed-for opportunity to escape prostitution and build a new life. Upon discovering the pregnancy, some women immediately left the sex trade, while others remained in prostitution for a short time. The emotional adjustment associated with the arrival of the child's birth sometimes made it impossible for the woman to remain in the sex trade. Many women told us that having a child filled their lives with new meaning. Someone needed them and required their care and attention. At the same time, the women were quite fragile in the marginal situation following the breakaway. Several described great difficulty during their child's infancy when they needed considerable support and help from their networks in order to cope with the stress. When the child matured to pre-school age, the situation tended to stabilize and the women were able to develop in their role as parents.[5]

REPAIRING RELATIONSHIPS AND FORMING NEW ATTACHMENT

Relationships with friends were profoundly affected by the women's numerous changes in lifestyle and group affiliation. Upon entering the sex trade, the women gradually lost contact with former friends and schoolmates. In prostitution, they developed strong ties to the prostitution subculture.[6] In most cases, quitting prostitution brought about a break with all contacts in that social environment. Still, some women maintained contact with women friends from prostitution. These relationships provided a kind of security, in that someone else understood how things were. These contacts tended to diminish with time and to finally come to an end.

After the breakaway, most women's networks consisted of family members and social workers or health professionals. The initial security of this network was eventually replaced by feelings of impatience and insufficiency. The women struggled to broaden their circles, make new friends, and repair old networks. This was a rapid process for some women, often connected to beginning studies or a new job. For others, however, this took a considerable amount of time–especially for women who found themselves unemployed following the breakaway or unable to identify with a new social role from which they can form new relationships. These women were caught in permanent marginal situations. Such experiences often lead to relapse (Biernacki, 1986; Svensson, 1996; Kristiansen, 1999; Hedin, 2002).

While there are many external hindrances that can obstruct and prolong the woman's path toward a new life, there are also appreciable internal barriers. Biernacki (1986) studied the path of drug addicts out of that lifestyle, and found that the two most important difficulties to be overcome on the way towards a "normal," non-abusive life were the doubts and negative attitudes of others and the addict's own feelings of shame and guilt. This is also the case for former prostitutes. The general trend seemed to be that although women felt intense anxiety prior to the breakaway–anxiety about not being admitted into or accepted in new social contexts and environments–in fact, they were able to develop friendships, new roles, and social identities.

During the breakaway, the women often find themselves between two worlds, the one they want to leave and the one they want to join. Both worlds fill them with ambivalence and insecurity. Sometimes, the women strove to repair earlier, positive relationships, in which the foundations of trust, understanding, and communication already existed. At first, the women needed to mobilize support from others, but in the long-run, mutuality was an important aspect of their ongoing relationships (Hessle, 1995).

At other times, our interviewees worked to transform previously destructive relationships. Here, they struggled to change both the internal views of relationships and the relationships themselves. Sometimes this involved distancing, setting limits, expressing her own needs, and claiming her own identity, or accepting differences. In order to develop better strategies for changing relationships, most women needed psychotherapy.

THE NEED FOR PSYCHOTHERAPY

Sixty percent of our interviewees received psychotherapy during the course of the breakaway. These were both short-term contacts and long-term relationships. We previously described the effectiveness of brief mental health intervention (Hedin & Månsson, 1998). Here, we address longer-term mental health support.

The prostituted women underscored the difficulty of obtaining sufficient help during the preliminary stages of the breakaway. They had trouble clearly expressing their needs. Another obstacle was a general lack of knowledge in the field of mental health about what prostitution was like. The women's cries for help were often not acknowledged. Several staff members dismissed women's anxiety and requests for help with naive comments, which led women to prolonged periods of doubt and uncertainty. Some women also told us about "john-like behavior" from male professionals when they sought help. Male physicians or psychologists, for example, invited them to dinner or night clubs when they asked for medical treatment or psychotherapy. These unethical and unprofessional behaviors made the women feel even more powerless and unworthy of help.

Relationships with the staff at the special social program ("the prostitution group," see footnote 1) were particularly meaningful to the women. Even if contacts with the social workers were initiated on the street by giving out a business card, these were a reminder to the women that someone was willing to help them. The women at first withdrew but some returned later during a crisis. In many instances this outreach person became a key support person during the breakaway, along with family members. Following the break with prostitution, the women were vulnerable, exposed, and in need of various forms of assistance such as crisis sessions, psychotherapy, and resource mobilization.

Psychotherapy was initiated a few years later in the rehabilitation process, once the women established some stability and had the psychological resources necessary for a more in-depth treatment. Their experiences in prostitution blocked emotional development. Forty percent of our interviewees participated in long-term psychotherapy during some phase of the breakaway.

Over time, the therapy relationship resulted in the social worker's becoming a person of great importance in the woman's network (Hessle, 1995). In dialogue, and via the experience of being seen for who she is, she develops a sense of new meaning to her life and the hope that change is worthwhile. The dialogue seems to affect her self-image and allows her to view herself differently (Ljökjell, 1994).

Women's break with prostitution does not inevitably lead to good health and personal development. Former prostitutes reported health problems which may or may not be symptomatic of PTSD. They reported frequent headaches, difficulty sleeping, difficulty concentrating, and eating disorders (Vanwesenbeeck, 1994; Kleber & Brom, 1996). After the breakaway, some women were caught in marginal situations between the two worlds. They were isolated with few social ties. It is necessary to change not only former coping strategies, but to work on relationships and networks at both the intra-psychological and interpersonal levels (Vanwesenbeeck, 1994). Her internalized view of relationships must be altered, and she must also improve existing relationships. There are several components to this relationship work: working through traumatic experiences experienced in childhood, adolescence or in prostitution, changing destructive relationships in her primary social network, for example, with parents and siblings. Other components of this work include improving self esteem, developing new interests, constructing a new identity, and improving her ability to set limits.

A majority of prostituted women experienced maltreatment and sexual abuse during childhood and adolescence.[7] Upon entering the sex trade the women encountered destructive relationships in which they were exposed to violence, threats and degradation that mirrored childhood trauma. Even those women who grew up in better family environments were not spared the destructive events in prostitution. Fifty-five percent of our interviewees experienced severe violence. They had been severely beaten, raped, or had threats against their lives These acts were usually committed by johns or by pimps who were afraid of losing control over the woman. These events caused mental and physical symptoms that can be classified as post-traumatic stress disorder (Farley & Barkan, 1998; Farley & Kelly, 2000). However, many women minimized the dangers and the harm in prostitution.

Prostitution leads to long-term problems with intimacy and sexuality. In order to protect their psychological integrity, and defend themselves against the customer's violation, women learn to dissociate so that they do not experience physical and emotional pain. But a psychological price is paid for this emergency protection. After the breakaway, it is difficult for women to do away with their body armor and to feel pleasure, especially sexual pleasure. "A devastated sex life is part of the price of prostitution" (Høigård & Finstad, 1986). Most of Høigård and Finstad's interviewees reported difficulty in feeling desire or pleasure. They could not cope with sexual relationships outside of prostitution, experiencing them as dull and disgusting. Almost 70% of the women in our study reported similar problems.

Another consequence of the sex trade is contempt for men which is resistant to change and makes it difficult for women to establish positive relationships with men. Healing from traumatic experiences of abuse and violence almost always requires psychotherapy. Some felt that body therapy was helpful in reducing somatic dissociation, and in addressing physical symptoms caused by chronic traumatic stress. Traumatic memories which had been repressed surfaced as a result of body therapy. A combination of body therapy and psychotherapy has proven to be most effective. At Umeå University in northern Sweden, body awareness training in small groups of eight women with a leader, along with individual or group psychotherapy helped women to process traumatic events (Pennebaker, 1995; Kleber & Brom, 1996). This method of treatment has been effectively used with sexually assaulted women who were not in prostitution, (Mattsson et al., 1997, 1998).

BUILDING A DIVERSE SOCIAL NETWORK

Fractured relationships and incomplete social networks were common among women in prostitution (Høigård & Finstad, 1986; Karlsen, 1993). In prostitution, the women had limited social contacts and only with a few psychologically important people, such as a partner or a female friend. Friends and family members were kept at a distance because they might ask questions or might see behind the mask. The women tried to avoid people from their pasts and were ashamed of the stigma of being a prostitute (Pheterson, 1985).

A heterogeneous social network, including a new social identity, and repaired social network, are important in the breakaway from prostitution (Hirsch, 1980; Wilcox, 1981; Vaux, 1988). The women need not only attachments to psychologically important people, but also new social relationships. Women who remained marginalized lacked close relationships that stimulated and supported change (Biernacki, 1986). Thirty percent of the women in our study had children soon after the breakaway. Parenthood, education and new jobs facilitated new relationships.

CONCLUSION

Supportive social relationships are crucial for the break from prostitution. This finding is consistent with previous research, for example, in breaking away from drug addiction. The internal and interpersonal problems that contributed to entry into prostitution are still there after the breakaway. During prostitution, these problems are increased by violence and other traumatic events. After the breakaway the woman is in urgent need of supportive relationships in both informal social networks and in formal professional relationships with therapists. She must change coping strategies and escape destructive relationships in order to build a new life. Social work with former female prostitutes should not operate from an overly narrow, individually directed perspective. We must carefully acknowledge the harm these women have experienced in prostitution, and offer them psychotherapy to work through earlier traumatic experiences. But we should also support the reparation and regeneration of social networks that are necessary in their new lives.

NOTES

1. With a population of 500,000, Göteborg is the second largest city in Sweden. In Göteborg, as well as in the two other major cities in the country, specially designed social support programs for prostitutes have been in operation since the late 1970s. The main purpose of the programs has been to help women leave prostitution. Over the years, the "prostitution groups" as they are called (mainly consisting of social workers), have developed different strategies and methods of outreach work, treatment, and resource mobilization.

2. See Hedin and Månsson 1998 or an article in English Månsson and Hedin (1998): Breaking the Matthew effect–on women leaving prostitution, paper presented at the 93rd Annual Meeting of American Sociological Association in San Francisco, August 1998.

3. In our study external factors were lack of jobs, money and lodging, lack of social support and interest from parents, exploitation and violence from "boyfriends" and contacts with female friends already "working" in the sex trade. The internal factors were feelings of being rejected from parents, feelings of depression, and low self esteem. These feelings made an impact on the woman's coping strategies and made her weaker or inable to fight for herself against the external factors. This social psychological process has to be studied in detail, if we will be able to prevent young women from going into prostitution.

4. In our study four women were drug abusers when entering prostitution. Some also started to use drugs as means to being able to perform sex acts for clients (cf. Høigård & Finstad, 1986). The majority of our interviewees did not have drug problems. On the contrary, some women emphasized that you have to be sober and on guard to avoid violence from clients.

5. This stabilization seems to occur when the child became 3-6 years old and the woman grew into the parental role (Trulsson, 1998).

6. Cf. the description of the network and social life spheres of the drug addict's world in Svensson 1996.

7. A total of 43% of the women in our study reported childhood sexual abuse. We regard this figure as rather low according to other research (Vanwesenbeeck, 1994; Farley & Kelly, 2000).

REFERENCES

Antonovsky, A. (1991). *Unravelling the Mystery of Health*. New York: Jossey-Bass Inc.

Biernacki, P. (1986). *Pathways from heroin addiction. Recovery without treatment*. Philadelphia, Temple University Press.

Cutrona, C. (1996). Social Support in Couples, Thousand Oaks, California: Sage.

Davis, N.J. (1993). *Prostitution. An International Handbook on Trends, Problems, and Policies*, London: Greenwood Press.

Earls, Ch. & David, H. (1990). Early Family and Sexual Experiences of Male and Female Prostitutes. *Canada's Mental Health*, December 1990: 7-11.

Farley, M. & Barkan, H. (1998). Prostitution, Violence, and Posttraumatic Stress Disorder. *Women & Health*: 27(3): 37-49.

Farley, M. & Kelly, V. (2000). Prostitution : A critical review of the medical and social sciences literature. *Women & Criminal Justice*. 11 (4): 29-64.

Fuchs Ebaugh, H.R. (1988). *Becoming an Ex, the Process of Role Exit. Chicago: University of Chicago Press*.

Hedin, U.C. (1994). Social Support at the Workplace in the Event of Illness Göteborg. Dissertation submitted for degree in Department of Social Work, Göteborg University, Sweden. (Swedish title: Socialt stod pa arbetsplatsen vid sjukdom.)

Hedin, U.C. & Månsson, S.A. (1998). Vägen ut–om kvinnors uppbrott ur prostitutionen (*The way out-on women leaving prostitution*). Stockholm: Carlsson bokförlag.

Hedin, U.C. (2002). Uppbrott från missbruk–rekonstruktion och socialt stöd (Exit from drug abuse–reconstruction and social support) i Leissner & Hedin: Könsperspektiv på missbruk (*Gender perspective on addiction*), Stockholm: Bjurner & Bruno.

Hessle, S. (1995). Sociala nätverk i kris, utveckling och fördjupning. Nätverksstudier på Barnbyn Skå med psykosocialt utsatta familjer (*Social networks in crisis and development. Studies in social networks of underprivileged families*). Stockholms universitet, Inst för socialt arbete rapport nr 74/1995.

Hirsch, B. (1980). Natural support systems and coping with major life changes. *American Journal of Community Psychology* 8: 159-172.

Høigård, C. & Finstad, L. (1986). Bakgater: om prostitusjon, penger og kjaerlighet. (*Backstreets–on prostitution, money and love*) Oslo: Pax förlag.

Karlsen, C. (1993). Mödre og engler? En evaluering av to tiltak for prostituerte i Oslo (*Mothers and angels? An evaluation of two social projects for prostitutes in Oslo*) Oslo: Forskningsavdelningen vid Diakonhjemmet, rapport 4/93.

Kleber, R.J. & Brom, D. (1997). *Coping with Trauma. Theory, Prevention and Treatment*, Lisse: Swets & Zeitlinger.

Kristiansen A. (1999). Fri från narkotika–Om kvinnor och män som har varit narkotikamissbrukare (Free from drugs–About women and men leaving drug abuse). Department of Social Work, Umeå University.

Larsson, S. (1983). Könshandeln. Om prostituerades villkor (*The sex trade. On the living conditions of prostitute women*). Stockholm: Skeab förlag.

Ljökjell, T.R. (1994). Kvinnor med prostitutionserfaring i möte med ett hjelpetiltak. En brukerundersökelse ved Prosentret. (*Prostitutes' encounter with a social program. An investigation at the prostitution center in Oslo*). Institutt for kriminologi, Universitet i Oslo.

Månsson, S.A. & Hedin, U.C. (1998). Breaking the Matthew Effect–on women leaving prostitution, paper presented at the 93rd Annual Meeting of American Sociological Association in San Francisco, August 1998.

Mattsson, M., Wikman M., Dahlgren, L., Mattson, B., & Armelius, K. (1997). Body awareness therapy with sexually abused women. Part 1. Description of a treatment modality. *Journal of Bodywork and Movement Therapies* 1 (5): 280-88.

Mattsson, M. et al. (1998). Wilkman, M., Dahlgren, L., Mattson, B., & Armelius, K. Body awareness therapy with sexually abused women Part 2. Evaluation of body awareness therapy in a group setting. *Journal of Bodywork and Movement Therapies* 2 (1): 38-45.

Pennebaker, J.W. (ed). (1995). *Emotion, Disclosure & Health*. Washington DC: American Psychological Association.

Pheterson, G. (1986). *The Whore Stigma: Female Dishonor and Male Unworthiness*, the Netherlands: Dutch Ministry of Social Affairs and Employment.

Silbert, M. & Pines, A. (1982). Victimization of Street Prostitutes, *Victimology* 7 (1-4): 122-133.

Silbert, M. & Pines, A. (1983). Early Sexual Exploitation as an Influence in Prostitution. *Social Work*, July-August 1983.

Svensson, B. (1996). Pundare, jonkare och andra–med narkotikan som följeslagare (*Speed freaks, junkies and others–with narcotics as companions*). Stockholm: Carlssons Bokförlag.

Trulsson, K. (1998). Det är i alla fall mitt barn! En studie om att vara missbrukare och mamma skild från barn, (*After all it is my child! A study about being a drug addict and a mother separated from her child*). Stockholm: Carlssons Bokförlag.

Vanwesenbeeck, I. (1994). *Prostitutes' Well-Being and Risk. Amsterdam: Amsterdam University Press*.

Vaux, A. (1988). *Social Support, Theory, Research: and Intervention. New York: Praeger.*

Whitbeck, L., Hoyt, L., & Ackley, K. (1997). Abusive Family Backgrounds and Later Victimization Among Runaway and Homeless Youth. *Journal of Research on Adolescence* 7: 375-392.

Wilcox, B.I. (1981). Social support in adjusting to marital separation. A network analysis. In B.H. Gottlieb (Ed). *Social networks and social support.* Beverly Hills: Sage.

PEERS:
The Prostitutes' Empowerment, Education and Resource Society

Jannit Rabinovitch

SUMMARY. This paper describes the philosophy of PEERS (Prostitutes' Empowerment, Education and Resource Society) in Victoria, British Columbia, Canada. PEERS was developed, managed, and staffed by prostitution survivors. PEERS' programs are culturally relevant, responding to the disproportionately high participation of Aboriginal women and youth in prostitution in Canada. PEERS offers services to those in the sex trade regardless of whether they wish to leave or stay in prostitution. Eighty-six percent of the people who use PEERS services eventually leave the sex trade and move on to further training, education or other employment. The paper further discusses the need for community liaisons, and the triumph as well as the stress of public disclosure of prostitution in one's life.

PROSTITUTION IN CANADA

If you are trying to transform a brutalized society into one where people can live in dignity and hope, you begin with the empowering of the most powerless. You build from the ground up. (Rich, 1994, p. 158)

Jannit Rabinovitch, a PEERS founder and board member, can be contacted at PEERS, 211-620 View Street, Victoria, BC V8W 1J6 Canada (Email: jrabinovitch@shaw.ca). Printed with permission.

[Haworth co-indexing entry note]: "PEERS: The Prostitutes' Empowerment, Education and Resource Society." Rabinovitch, Jannit. Co-published simultaneously in *Journal of Trauma Practice* (The Haworth Maltreatment & Trauma Press, an imprint of The Haworth Press, Inc.) Vol. 2, No. 3/4, 2003, pp. 239-253; and: *Prostitution, Trafficking, and Traumatic Stress* (ed: Melissa Farley) The Haworth Maltreatment & Trauma Press, an imprint of The Haworth Press, Inc., 2003, pp. 239-253. Single or multiple copies of this article are available for a fee from The Haworth Document Delivery Service [1-800-HAWORTH, 9:00 a.m. - 5:00 p.m. (EST). E-mail address: docdelivery@haworthpress.com].

http://www.haworthpress.com/store/product.asp?sku=J189
10.1300/J189v02n03_14

Prostitution exists in every city in Canada (Lowman, 1997). Across a range of different types of prostitution, annual median income in Victoria is $18,000. Most women are employed in more than one type of prostitution over time (Carter & Walton, 2000; Benoit & Millar, 2001).

In Victoria, prostitution takes place on the street, in escort agencies, massage parlors, bawdy houses, brothels, bath houses, bars, and night clubs. There are few intrinsic differences between different types of prostitution. Exotic dancers report that the physical contact between dancer and customer during a lap dance at a strip club sometimes includes oral sex, penetration with fingers, and intercourse. These acts may be perpetrated despite the wishes of the lap dancer. Exotic dancers, like women in other types of prostitution, may move from one kind of prostitution to another (Maticka-Tyndale, Lewis, Clark, Zubick, & Young, 2000).

A number of medical problems have been connected to prostitution (Rechsteiner, 1999). Most of those who have been in prostitution for some time experience symptoms of sexual trauma. Mental health problems include depression, suicide attempts, panic attacks, traumatic stress, sleep disorders, flashbacks, and migraines (Smith, 1996; Rechsteiner, 1999; Benoit & Millar, 2001). People in prostitution commonly feel isolated, alienated, suicidal, are alcohol or drug dependent, have eating disorders, self-mutilate, have difficulty concentrating, have gynecological problems, and sexual dysfunction. Many addicted prostitutes were not involved in substance abuse before entering prostitution. Only about half of those in prostitution have drug and alcohol addictions (Benoit & Millar, 2001; James, 1977).

The average age of entry into street prostitution in Canada has been estimated at 14 (Committee of the Capital Regional District, 1997). A Canadian survey of 229 youth found that 80% turned their first trick before age 18, with some children as young as 8 years (Badgley, 1984). Aboriginal youth are overrepresented in prostitution and they enter the sex trade at progressively younger ages (Kingsley & Mark, 2000, Assistant Deputy Minister's Committee, 2001).

Having begun prostitution as children, many people in the sex trade do not have access to educational institutions or social services (Benoit & Millar, 2001; Rabinovitch, 1996). Many have not completed junior high school, have not had the experience of going to the library or a museum, and may not have had a job other than prostitution. They are isolated from the rest of the community (Kingsley & Mark, 2000; Assistant Deputy Ministers' Committee on Prostitution and Sexual Exploitation of Youth, 2001).

The sex trade in Canada, as elsewhere, is dangerous. Those in prostitution are 60 to 120 times more likely to be beaten or murdered than other groups of Canadians (Lowman, 1997). Because prostitutes are often viewed as subhuman, the consequences of perpetrating harm against them are minimal. The language used to refer to people in the sex trade (whores, trash, sluts, ho's) justifies their treatment as less than human. This prejudicial treatment of women in prostitution has included law enforcement.[1]

MISSION AND PHILOSOPHY OF PEERS

PEERS' mission is to support people currently and formerly in the sex trade. As an agency, PEERS is committed to maintaining a staff made up of a mix of people who have recently exited and people who have some distance from their time in prostitution. Many of the staff are former PEERS' clients.

Staff who are exiting the sex trade need room for that process to take place. PEERS' staff and Board recognize that the skills needed to survive in the sex trade differ from the skills needed to develop programs and services in a social service agency and that the process of transition will be different for everyone. Working at PEERS is a training opportunity and in many ways the hiring of recent survivors is harm reduction. No one is expected to excel when they begin. Because of the emotional stress of the work, all PEERS' staff are encouraged to engage in frequent debriefings.

PEERS is based on a harm reduction approach to prostitution. Harm reduction is a pragmatic approach which involves setting up a hierarchy of goals, with immediate goals as steps on the way to risk-free behaviour or sometimes, abstinence (Riley & O'Hare, 2002). Harm reduction has recently gained popularity in Australia, Britain, Canada, and the Netherlands as a response to the spread of AIDS among injection drug users. Decreasing the negative consequences of a given activity is the priority of harm reduction, which recognizes that abstinence may be neither a realistic nor a desirable goal for some, especially in the short term. As a result, anyone in the sex trade who arrives at PEERS is welcomed–even if all they want at the time is a bus ticket or a condom.

Making connections and building relationships have proven to be crucial first steps in moving out of prostitution. Those who come to PEERS know they will not be judged. PEERS' staff have learned from personal experience the importance of supporting people wherever they are in their process. It is a complicated balancing act, however. Some women refuse to visit PEERS because they see a bias toward leaving the sex trade. This impression is reinforced as most people who come to PEERS, regardless of their original intention, decide to eventually leave prostitution. Many of the staff provide role models for this option. The three-month pre-employment program exemplifies the harm reduction approach. Women are encouraged to come to the program even if they are still using drugs and prostituting. The only requirement is to show up and participate while they are present in the program. Such open access permits women to come to the program who do not believe that they are ready or able to make a significant change in their behaviour. One woman came because she heard there were free bus tickets, which she planned to sell. She then discovered a world of possibility for herself, completed the program, and eventually became a PEERS staff member. Some clients are referred by law enforcement agencies and are required as a condition of their parole or probation to work at PEERS. Some women referred in this way have continued as volunteers.

PEERS began in 1995 with a small group of dedicated volunteers, most of whom were survivors of prostitution, many quite recently exited. The group incorporated and received some funding for participating in research projects during 1996. PEERS was granted $200,000 in 1997 from the provincial government for the development of an agency that would provide training and employment for survivors of prostitution and programs and services for sex workers. Over the years the core operating grant of $200,000 has been maintained (not without much effort) and additional program dollars have been received for several time limited projects. The federal government, through Human Resources Development Canada, Justice Canada, and Health Canada, have supported projects such as pre-employment, youth employment and training, men at PEERS, national fetal alcohol prevention, Aboriginal and public education. As well, PEERS has received support from a number of private foundations for its work. Currently, a group of business leaders are meeting to discuss how the local community can economically support PEERS in a more substantial way.

Almost all of the staff are survivors of the sex industry. Working at PEERS is a stepping stone out of the trade and into mainstream employment for many. Over 60 women (and a few men) have been employed at PEERS, most receiving social assistance at the time they became employed. In addition, 250 women and men have participated in the various employment training projects PEERS has offered over the years. Of these, 86% have moved on either directly into employment, further training or education, or into a treatment program for alcohol and drug misuse, or into mental health services. For some the process takes less than one year while for others it may take several years before they make the decision to enter into one of PEERS more structured programs. Currently PEERS has fifteen full-time staff each being paid $18/hour and receiving extended medical benefits. For many this is their first regular employment.

Megan Lewis, a founder of PEERS, speaks eloquently about her experience as both a client and staff member:

There were so many things that we didn't know how to do. Sometimes we knew we didn't have a clue and tried to muck it together anyway. Record keeping was a good example of this. We didn't keep any records. We didn't think that it was important. Then we were told that we should really be keeping some records . . . [But] [w]hat is important to keep and what isn't? How do you file something so that you can find it again? . . . These were skills that we simply didn't have. I think that there is the assumption that if you tell some one what to do or even how to do it, then they'll know how to just pick up the ball and run with it. But there is so much negotiation in doing small tasks that people aren't even aware of. I will use my history as an example (as I have for the last six years). I never filed anything in my life until I started working for PEERS . . . I was never in school at a level that I had to organize any paper. People start learning to organize paper through doing little bits of it at school . . . Then they get a job somewhere and move into their own apartment . . . Eventually they have bank statements, tax returns, book club memberships, car payments, and checking accounts. Maybe they go to post secondary school. They have papers and research to organize, classes to keep separate . . . Then, if they are thrust into a brand new agency, creating a simple filing system is not a trying chore. The basic understanding of what goes on is there.

The other problem to organize was time. In order to organize your time like the rest of the world, you have to know a couple of things. Here's an example of some of the questions you have to think about if you have stuff to do and an appointment. (a) What time is it now? (b) How long is it going to take you to get there? (c) What is the mode of transportation and do you have the means? (d) Is it more important to be on time or to finish what you are doing and will the person you're meeting care? (e) How long will you be there?

I would take something on, only to find that I had no idea even how to start it. Often I would sit there for hours looking at blank pages trying to figure out exactly what it was I was supposed to do. Then, when I finally just started it, the work was of poor quality, not reflecting my intelligence but certainly reflecting my level of competency.

I wasn't used to following through over the long term, and I found it very difficult to stick with a task until it was done unless it was a very short-lived task. This isn't to say that I had no attention span. It was just that I had no experience or confidence to keep going back to the same task. It was always a bit of a shock to me when I would check on a task only to find that there was still more to do.

We also had to negotiate tasks and projects. I used to just do one task until it was finished so that I was assured of getting it done. This proved to be unwieldy, as I had to put so many things on hold in order to finish the first task, that I would have 17 other things waiting for me when I finally finished . . . I would take on so much that there was no way I could complete it in the allotted time, or I would get scared of it all and avoid it . . . We didn't know how to decide how much time you should spend on a task . . . Other people just didn't do it at all, or would lose track of what they were supposed to have done and it would disappear. There were some staff who were excellent at keeping things organized but for most of us it was a challenge.

[My] transition from working in [prostitution] to working at PEERS is a long and interesting one. I was at an extreme point in my life. On the one hand, I was severely depressed. I had left the trade 10 months before, and I had just attempted suicide. On the other hand, I found the idea of PEERS very exciting and it gave me a sense of future that I didn't otherwise have. I also found it very scary. I was constantly feeling like I was faking it. Like I was just bluffing people about what I was capable of and what I wasn't. Part of the difficulty in working out who I was, was that I didn't have all the tools to pull off a new identity. I had to pretend. I had to pretend that I had it all together, that I knew why I did what I did. I had to pretend that we, at PEERS, knew best.

I found it very difficult to attend meetings where there were many bureaucrats. I didn't understand their language or manner of speaking. It wasn't that I didn't know what the words they were saying meant, but the way they used them was confusing to me. I was accustomed to people saying what they meant in clear terms. If you disagreed with someone, you said so; you didn't sound like you were agreeing with them. It took me a long time to understand and analyze what people were saying. It didn't take as long to realize I was being patted on the head by many of them.

At first I thought that the bureaucrats were really supportive. I remember wondering why I was ever scared to tell people about my sex trade history, these people were so nice. Then I started to notice that mostly I was there as a token . . . and that I wasn't taken as seriously as originally I thought. I don't think anyone really ever forgets that you were a hooker.

I began buying more conservative clothing. I was careful to hide my tattoos at meetings, I changed the tone and pitch of my voice . . . I still felt like a fraud or like I was faking it, but this time I felt like it was for the greater good–like my faking would actually get the agency somewhere. Eventually it became more natural and now I switch from one to the other without thinking about it, depending on whom I am with. (Rabinovitch & Lewis, 2001, pp. 16, 20-21)

COMMUNITY INVOLVEMENT

Prostitution is a separate and hidden culture with its own values, cultural norms, and language. It is important to anticipate the differences between survivors and community supporters, otherwise there can be clashes of culture and background. Non-survivor staff do not take on leadership roles in the organization, acting instead as supportive advisors. Community supporters develop egalitarian relationships with women currently or formerly in the sex trade. Community supporters who are not survivors bring a diverse range of experience and ideas, and are not dismissed as 'do-gooders.'

PEERS' staff have carefully developed relationships with other agencies and speak eloquently and with passion about the sexual exploitation of children and youth and the pervasiveness of the sex trade. Table 1 illustrates some of the ways people from PEERS have worked in the community.

TABLE 1. PEERS' Activities with Various Community Partners

Community Partners	Activities Shared with Community Partners
Feminist Organizations	- speak at Take Back the Night - speak & have information table at International Women's Day - volunteer opportunities at local women's centre
Anti-Poverty Groups	- access to photocopying before PEERS had a reliable copier - information about programs & services for people living in poverty - provide welfare advocacy training for PEERS staff
Youth Services	- peer counsellor training at local YM/YWCA youth outreach program - counsellors on their staff provided supervision to PEERS counsellors during PEERS' first year
AIDS Agency	- hire PEERS' volunteers & staff - act as mentors for new PEERS staff - share information on harm reduction & philosophies of care - provide condoms, clean needles & other harm reduction equipment - create Bad Date Sheet that details violent clients of sex workers - assist PEERS staff in doing workshops for participants & staff
Homeless Women's Services	- donate space for Prostitute's Anonymous meetings & support group - provide letters of support for various projects & funding proposals - partner with PEERS staff in working with street level sex workers - invite PEERS staff to do weekly drop-in workshops with women - partner with PEERS staff to do advocacy & support for mutual clients
Ex-Offender Programs	- provide free labour for office renovations using men in their programs who are required to do community volunteer hours

TABLE 1 (continued). PEERS Activities with Various Community Partners

Community Partners	Activities Shared with Community Partners
Aboriginal Friendship Centre	- jointly address Aboriginal over-representation in the sex trade
	- work with PEERS staff to deliver workshops, hold healing circles
	- refer women to PEERS programs
Post-Secondary Institutions	- partner with local community college to incorporate retail & hospitality certifications into training programs
	- partner with local community college in offering a four week pre-employment course for PEERS participants
	- PEERS staff tell their stories to Nursing & Social Work classes
	- place School of Social Work practicum students at PEERS
	- provide work experience for university writing student
	- partner with a Sociology professor to conduct research
Media	- donate advertising in weekly paper that has a double page of escort ads
	- extensive coverage of activities & events in local daily newspaper
	- support & coverage by local monthly mainstream magazine for women
	- local TV station sponsors fund raising events
Community Partners	Activities Shared with Community Partners
Municipal Government	- PEERS staff participate in activities sponsored by the City
	- city staff recognize PEERS staff as having significant expertise
	- request assistance in the project design, potential interviewers, project advertising & dissemination of the report for City sponsored research on sexually exploited youth
	- address sexual exploitation of youth through regional committee with city councillors, police, Ministries of Attorney General, Children & Families, School Districts, parent groups, & other local agencies
Police	- attend regular PEERS/Vice Squad meetings to discuss incidents between police & sex trade workers; develop an enforcement strategy focussing on women's safety, targeting violent tricks & pimps
School Districts	- present to Parent Advisory Council in order to reassure parents that the presentation would not glamorize the sex trade
	- official endorsement from School Board
	- speak to junior & senior high school classes about the sex trade, recruitment strategies, & an accurate description of the experience
Elected Officials	- maintain relationship with both provincial Member of the Legislative assembly & federal Member of Parliament to keep them informed
Regional Health Authority	- work closely with street nurses, part of the public health program
	- receive medical support, condoms & needles for distribution
Collaborative Research	- report on multi-disadvantaged street women's health needs funded by Community Health Promotion Centre, University of Victoria, 1996
	- consultation with survivors of childhood sexual exploitation funded by the Ministry of Women's Equality, 1996
	- gender analysis of sex trade funded by Status of Women Canada, 2000
	- in collaboration with University of Victoria, research on health impact of sex trade work funded by the BC Health Research Foundation, 2001

Those in the sex trade have stated that they need supportive housing (Smith, 1996; Rabinovitch, 1996; Committee of the Capital Regional District, 1997; Carter & Walton, 2000; Benoit & Millar, 2001), counselling and mental health support (Smith, 1996; Benoit & Millar, 2001), general healthcare (Rechsteiner; 1999; Benoit & Millar, 2001) and a range of services for drug and alcohol addiction (Smith, 1996; Carter & Walton, 2001). Most who come to PEERS were in the sex trade for ten to fifteen years before leaving and had attempted to leave an average of six times (Benoit & Millar, 2001). Crucial ongoing supports are advocacy and mentoring opportunities, access to employment bridging programs and meaningful employment, life skills training, vocational training, internships, up-grading, and post-secondary education and long term support programs (Benoit & Millar, 2001; Carter & Walton, 2000; Rabinovitch, 1996).

PEERS offers a three-month life skills training program for people still involved in prostitution and/or addicted to drugs or alcohol. Employment and training for people exiting the trade include a six month youth internship program, volunteer speakers bureau, administrative support volunteers, and employment at PEERS (Rabinovitch & Lewis, 2001).

PEERS provides educational programs about youth and adult prostitution, myths and stigmas associated with the sex trade, the risks and dangers of prostitution, recognizing common pimp recruitment methods, long term effects of prostitution, where to go for support, and how to support a loved one who is prostituting. We offer a list of myths and facts about prostitution as a way to begin discussions (see Table 2).

TABLE 2. Myths About Prostitution

1.   There is no chance that your daughter, sister, mother, brother, father or cousin is ever or ever will be a prostitute.
2.   Prostitutes love sex. They are nymphomaniacs.
3.   Male prostitutes are all gay.
4.   Prostitutes are diseased and are responsible for the spread of HIV/AIDS.
5.   Female prostitutes have magical sexual secrets that 'normal' women just can't do.
6.   Prostitutes are all big money makers and are very rich.
7.   Prostitutes are all poor and destitute.
8.   Prostitutes want and need to be rescued.
9.   Prostitutes all work for the Mafia, pimps, or biker gangs.
10.   Prostitutes have no morals and can't be trusted.

TABLE 2 (continued). Myths About Prostitution

11. Prostitutes are all drug addicts.
12. Prostitutes all work on the street or out of sleazy bars.
13. Prostitutes are all mean and tough.
14. You can tell a prostitute by what she/he's wearing.
15. Prostitutes all come from broken homes.
16. Once a prostitute, always a prostitute.
17. All prostitutes make lousy parents and abuse their kids.
18. Prostitutes fight amongst one another and will kill each other for twenty-five cents.
19. Prostitutes are indiscriminate about who they sleep with. They will do anything for money.
20. You can't rape a prostitute.
21. Prostitutes like to be degraded.
22. It's okay to beat up prostitutes. They have no feelings.
23. Prostitutes are not part of your community.
24. All women fantasize about being a prostitute.
25. You can't be a 'real' man unless you have been with a prostitute. (PEERS, 1999, p. 4)

THE NEED FOR HOUSING

For many of the women who come to PEERS, finding a place to stay is a daily struggle that precludes their ever moving beyond a crisis mode. In order to participate in PEERS programs, they need someplace to live that is affordable and that includes ongoing staff support. In 2001, PEERS' Place opened, providing housing for 14 women. The women who moved into PEERS' Place were in extreme economic need, usually homeless, addicted, and prostituting.

THE NEED FOR CULTURALLY RELEVANT SERVICES

The Canadian sex trade is grim evidence of the ongoing struggles of Aboriginal peoples in Canada. The century of policies that removed children from Aboriginal families via the residential school system undermined family structures, resulting in fractured and dysfunctional families.

Aboriginal youth are recipients of the pain and trauma of residential schools, as well as racism, forced adoption, and cultural fragmentation. To attempt an understanding of the commercial sexual exploitation of Aboriginal children and youth without this wider context is to invalidate the harms of colonial practices which continue today (Kingsley & Mark, 2000).

There is consensus among community organizations and service providers in Canada that First Nations' youth participation in the sex trade is disproportionately high and is increasing (Kingsley & Mark, 2000). Estimates of the proportion of sexually exploited youth who are First Nations varies considerably across regions/communities, from about 14% to 60% (Assistant Deputy Minister's Committee, 2001). While First Nations comprise only 2-3% of Canada's population (Statistics Canada, 2001), in some communities the numbers and proportion of Aboriginal youth in the sex trade is staggering. In Winnipeg, for example, all of the visible sexually exploited youth on the street are from First Nations (Kingsley & Mark, 2000).

The disproportionately high percentage of First Nations in the sex trade is not limited to children and youth; 52% of 100 women prostituting in Vancouver's Downtown Eastside were First Nations, compared to 1.7-7% of Vancouver's population (Farley & Lynne, 2003), and 15% of 201 respondents from Victoria BC identified as Aboriginal, Inuit, or Metis (Benoit & Millar, 2001). This figure is substantially higher than the percentage of Aboriginal people in Victoria, which was 2% in 1996 (Statistics Canada, 2001).

Recognizing the disproportionate number of Aboriginal youth and women in prostitution, and acknowledging their unique needs, PEERS Board and staff hired a First Nations survivor to coordinate the development of community workshops that highlight the experiences of Aboriginal women in prostitution. An Indigenous Community Empowerment Vision workshop attempts to overcome resistance within the Aboriginal community to acknowledging the over-representation of Aboriginal women in the sex trade. The goals of the workshop are to generate a sense of awareness of and responsibility for community members in the sex trade. "We owe it to our ancestors, Nations, children and selves to work together and reclaim our lost community members" (Tallefer & Moore, 2002, p. 1).

THE PSYCHOLOGICAL IMPACT OF PUBLIC DISCLOSURE OF PROSTITUTION

Disclosure of having worked in the sex trade is a complex issue. Hearing a personal story has a powerful impact on the listener. At the same time, the effect of regular public speaking about one's traumatic history in prostitution can become one's primary identity, eclipsing other facets of personality and life experience. As one woman stated,

> Talking about it all the time put those of us who were the founders of PEERS at risk because of the stress. It can be like trying to sober up and being in a bar every day. For me, it was too much. At the beginning . . . I

had an inflated sense of what I could do. Then I just crashed. Started using drugs and working [in prostitution]. I relapsed for six months. (Rabinovitch & Lewis, 2001, p. 24)

Megan Lewis, the first survivor/Director of PEERS, shaped the structure of the organization. In the following excerpts, she describes the effects of disclosure of a history of prostitution, as well as the challenges of beginning work at PEERS and the development of a new identity.

Many of us . . . prior to employment at PEERS . . . were poverty stricken and unsure of our futures. When we began to be paid, there was a feeling of abundance . . . [Our] safety and security rested on our telling our stories over and over again. There was a direct causal link.

Mostly it was an exhilarating experience. Speaking gave me a chance to separate from my story and understand it in an objective manner, almost like looking at some one else's life and analyzing it. However, it also meant that I could objectively pick it apart for the juicy bits to feed the waiting public. Sometimes it felt like I was being trotted out, the token hooker. We used to joke about it, but there was a truth to it. Fact is, you need some one who will tell their story and tell it well. Some one who can elicit emotion in the people who are listening and that someone has to have experience.

After I'd speak, lots of people I never knew and were never a part of my life would come up to me and tell me how proud they were of me. What a good job they think I'm doing and how brave I am to speak. It was very weird. I didn't like it.

The thing about living in the 'ex-sex worker' identity is that it gave me a defined place to get myself together. I didn't have to stretch myself about a lot of things because I didn't have to think about who I was. I knew I was an ex-prostitute. Because I wasn't sure of where I was, I always felt like I was on constantly shifting sand. It wasn't until much later that I actually did some soul searching to find out who and what I was.

Disclosing your history over and over does a couple of things. First, because your history is used as a story, it becomes almost a dissociative activity. You distance from your story and this, among other things, can lead to questioning the validity of it. Because you end up using small pieces of your story to illustrate things and to use as examples, you end up giving weight to parts of your history that would not otherwise be weighted. This also can make you feel fraudulent. It's as if the story becomes so far away from your own perceptions of what your life was like that it doesn't feel true. The above two things together have led several people into feeling like the telling of their story was fraudulent in some way or like they were 'prostituting' their stories. No grey area of what is a choice, what is not, what were the good parts, what was not so good. It all gets boiled down to the Cole's Notes of my life.

Second, the constant and regular talk/work/energy of one per-spective or aspect of your life turns this into your primary identity. On the one hand, it allows one to deeply explore one's sex trade history; on the other, it dismisses the variety and complexity of life. I think it does a dis-service after a time. I also think that it needs reclaiming after one stops working on the one issue. Becoming so immersed in this identity allows one to explore thoroughly and exhaustively their sex trade history. There are constant revisions to our story being made as another layer of insight is revealed. Often this is coupled with . . . [l]ots of questioning, clarifying, and comparing to other experiences and perspectives . . . [H]ow our story is seen by peers makes a difference.

Eventually I needed to dig through my old life and find the pieces that got no attention for the five years I was with PEERS. I felt that I would become trapped in my 'story' if I didn't (Rabinovitch & Lewis, 2001, pp. 24-25).

CONCLUSION

Myths and stereotypes about prostitution abound, as does a sense of hope-lessness for many when approaching this complex issue. PEERS offers a model of how to provide programs and services for prostitutes and survivors of prostitution developed by survivors of prostitution themselves. In order to work successfully with this traditionally "service resistant population," it is important to recognize the value of a peer-driven approach. PEERS is commit-ted to supporting all who seek their services, whether they are entrenched in the culture of prostitution, exploring other options, or actively looking for sup-ports to exit. PEERS was created in 1995 and continues to be effective today because the staff have been where the clients are now. Service resistant clients come to PEERS because they feel safe. They know they won't be judged.

The strengths of the women and men who survive the sex industry must be recognized and allowed to develop. Listening to their expertise is a critical first step in the development of effective strategies. Personal choice is an important aspect of PEERS' philosophy. PEERS' mission states both, "We respect those involved in prostitution and we work to improve their safety and working con-ditions," and "We assist individuals who desire to leave the sex industry and strive to increase public understanding."

Along with personal choice must come access to needed supports and re-sources required to make any choice realistic and available. A significant part of the success of the training programs at PEERS is that they were designed and are implemented by women who have been through the process of exiting prostitution themselves. Working closely with community supporters PEERs is able to offer what the people who come to PEERS want and need. As a result, most of those who come to PEERS eventually leave prostitution and move on to training, education, or alternative employment.

Traditional service delivery models don't work when addressing prostitution. The PEERS model illustrates an effective approach to supporting what many perceive as a hopeless situation. PEERS provides programs and services to women and men who have been alienated and isolated from mainstream society for a very long time. Many of the people who access PEERS' programs and services are reluctant to access any agency services. They come to PEERS because it is different. That difference needs to be understood, documented, and replicated.

NOTE

1. A week before Christmas in 1981, Kim Wrebeky was hitchhiking to a friend's house. A man picked her up, violently assaulted and raped her, and left her for dead. She survived providing the police a five-page statement. They charged the offender, Clifford Olson, until they found out that in her past, Kim had been prostituted. Then the case was dropped because as a prostitute, no one believed her. Clifford Olson eventually murdered eleven children. He is now confined in a maximum security institution serving a life sentence.

REFERENCES

Assistant Deputy Minister's Committee on Prostitution and Sexual Exploitation of Youth. (2001). Sexual Exploitation of Youth in British Columbia. Victoria: Ministry of Attorney General, Ministry for Children and Families, and Ministry of Health.

Badgley, R. (1984). Sexual Offences Against Children. Report of the Committee on Sex Offenses Against Children and Youths. Ottawa: Department of Supply and Services.

Benoit, C. & Millar, A. (2001). Dispelling Myths and Understanding realities: Working Conditions, Health Status, and Exiting Experiences of Sex Workers. Victoria: Prostitutes Empowerment, Education and Resource Society.

Carter, C. & Walton, M. (2000). Is Anyone listening? A Gender Analysis of Sex Trade Work. Victoria: Prostitutes Empowerment, Education and Resource Society.

Committee of the Capital Regional District. (1997). Report of the Sexually Exploited Youth Committee. Victoria: Capital Regional District.

Farley, M. & Lynne, J. (2003). Prostitution in Vancouver: Violence and the Colonization of First Nations Women. *Fourth World Journal.* Available online at http://www.cwis.org/fwj/index.htm.

James, J. (1977). Prostitutes and Prostitution. Deviants in a Hostile World. General Learning Press.

Kingsley, C. & Mark, M. (2000). Sacred Lives. Canadian Aboriginal Children and Youth Speak Out about Sexual Exploitation. Vancouver: Save the Children Canada.

Lowman, J. (1997). Rates of Homicide: Comparing Prostitute and Non-Prostitute. Retrieved March 2001 from the World Wide Web: http://users.uniserve.com/~lowman/violence/5.htm.

Maticka-Tyndale, E., Lewis, J., Clark, J. P., Zubick, J. & Young, S. (2000). Exotic Dancing and Health. Women and Health, 31(1), 87-108.

Prostitutes' Empowerment, Education & Resource Society (PEERS). (1999). PEERS Information Package. Victoria: Prostitutes' Empowerment, Education and Resource Society.

Rabinovitch, J. (1996). Creating an Atmosphere of Hope for All Children and Youth: Teen Prostitutes Speak Up and Speak Out. Victoria: Prostitutes' Empowerment Education and Recovery Society.

Rabinovitch, J. & Lewis, M. (2001). Impossible, eh? The Story of PEERS. Vancouver: Save the Children Canada.

Rechsteiner, R. J. (1999). Access to Healing: An Inquiry into Equitable Health Care for Sex Trade Workers. Masters Thesis in Master of Arts in Leadership and Training. Victoria Canada: Royal Roads University.

Rich, A. (1994). *Going There and Being Here. Blood, Bread and Poetry: Selected Prose, 1979-1985.* New York: W. W. Norton and Company.

Riley, D. & O'Hare, P. Harm Reduction: Policy and Practice. Retrieved August 20, 2002 from the World wide Web: http://www.canadianharmreduction.com/facts.php.

Smith, B. (1996). Report on the Health Needs of Multi-Disadvantaged Street Women. Victoria: Community Health Promotion Centre, University of Victoria.

Statistics Canada. (2001). Population by Aboriginal Group, 1996 Census, Census Metropolitan Areas. Retrieved May 27, 2002 from the World Wide Web: www.statscan.ca/english/Pgdb/People?Population/demo39b.htm.

Tallefer, A. & Moore, M. (2002). Indigenous Community Empowerment Vision. Victoria: Prostitutes' Empowerment Education and Resource Society.

Been There Done That:
SAGE, a Peer Leadership Model
Among Prostitution Survivors

Norma Hotaling
Autumn Burris
B. Julie Johnson
Yoshi M. Bird
Kirsten A. Melbye

SUMMARY. Women in prostitution and those in the process of exiting prostitution experience many barriers to social services traditionally encountered by other marginalized populations, including discrimination, alienation, stigmatization, victim-blaming and inaccessibility to social services. Compounding these problems are the wariness and distrust that result from years of sexual and emotional trauma. Standing Against Global Exploitation (The SAGE Project) is a human rights non-profit survivor-run drug, mental health, and trauma treatment center that offers

Norma Hotaling, HED, founder of SAGE, can be reached at SAGE Project, Inc., 1271 Mission Street, San Francisco CA 94103 (Email nhsage@sageprojectinc.org).

Autumn Burris, AA, is Administrative Director of Sage Project (Email: autumnsage@sageprojectinc.org).

B. Julie Johnson, PhD, can be contacted at Sage Project.

Yoshi M. Bird, JD, is Co-founder of the SAGE Volunteer Legal Advocacy Program (Email: womanrebel@aol.com).

Kirsten A. Melbye, MHS, is affiliated with Community Substance Abuse Services, San Francisco Department of Public Health.

Printed with permission.

[Haworth co-indexing entry note]: "Been There Done That: SAGE, a Peer Leadership Model Among Prostitution Survivors." Hotaling et al. Co-published simultaneously in *Journal of Trauma Practice* (The Haworth Maltreatment & Trauma Press, an imprint of The Haworth Press, Inc.) Vol. 2, No. 3/4, 2003, pp. 255-265; and: *Prostitution, Trafficking, and Traumatic Stress* (ed: Melissa Farley) The Haworth Maltreatment & Trauma Press, an imprint of The Haworth Press, Inc., 2003, pp. 255-265. Single or multiple copies of this article are available for a fee from The Haworth Document Delivery Service [1-800-HAWORTH, 9:00 a.m. - 5:00 p.m. (EST). E-mail address: docdelivery@haworthpress.com].

job training and placement and other forms of advocacy to women, girls, men, and transgender survivors in the San Francisco sex industry. SAGE has developed a survivor-centered model of peer counseling and harm reduction. SAGE trains and employs survivors of prostitution at all levels of management, development, and service provision in order to build trust and empathy among its clients and staff.

INTRODUCTION

The critical importance and effectiveness of community-based peer counseling programs has been documented for a number of marginalized populations, including immigrants, refugees, survivors of state-sponsored violence, homeless persons, drug-addicted persons, HIV-infected individuals, and Vietnam veterans (Becker, Lira, Castillo, Gomez, & Kovalskys, 1990; Breton, 1999; Egendorf, 1975; Martin-Baro, 1988; Figley, 1978; Lifton, 1978; Turner, 1996; Lykes, 1993). In these populations, it is important to avoid traditional intervention models that position service providers as clinically neutral authority figures. Client-created programs in which providers address the social, political, and economic contexts of clients' difficulties tend to be most effective. Supportive partnerships between professional and poor women, gender-specific social action, and community-based programs, have been identified as crucial elements of successful women's programs (Wetzel, 2000).

Early examples of non-traditional service delivery are the rap groups formed in the 1970s for Vietnam veterans (Egendorf, 1975; Figley, 1978; Lifton, 1978; Turner, 1996). Lifton found that traditional psychoanalysis with Vietnam veterans was ineffective because it alienated clients by reinforcing the social denial veterans encountered when trying to communicate their experience. An emphasis on individual pathology did not allow veterans themselves to define their own experiences. One veteran who attended these groups and later became a psychotherapist wrote that the rap group "confirms as nothing else does that we carry a legacy of the war in our memories, that we exist as veterans despite the denials within and around us" (Egendorf, 1975).

When working with traumatized, politically disenfranchised and stigmatized individuals, service providers must avoid traditional therapeutic neutrality and clearly support those they work with. They must promote systemic, as well as individual, solutions and community-based interventions (Becker, Lira, Castillo, Gomez, & Kovalskys, 1990; Martin-Baro, 1988).

Women in crisis are receptive to nontraditional intervention. Describing group work with immigrant and refugee women, Breton (1999) explained that they often face language differences, cultural dissonance, social invisibility and isolation, loss of supportive social networks, and sometimes domestic violence when accessing traditional mental health services. She noted, "One of the most critical barriers for immigrant and refugee women is the use . . . of professional practice paradigms that fail to recognize . . . oppression when working with people of low status and low power . . ." Rap groups identify structural obstacles to group empowerment, and may be more flexible than traditional intervention paradigms in tailoring solutions to individual needs and community resources.

Many of the problems facing women in prostitution are the same as those addressed in other marginalized populations: finding affordable housing, financial planning, creating safe environments and relationships, escaping and healing from the emotional and physical effects of violence, trauma, and engaging in treatment for drug/alcohol addictions, and resuming educational or vocational training. Like Vietnam veterans, women in prostitution must overcome public denial about the truth of their experiences. The social denial of harm results in self-contempt and an acceptance of toxic stereotypes about prostitution. Social denial of the reality of prostitution has on the one hand glamorized and romanticized prostitution, while at the same time viewing the women as criminal, sexually deviant, socially inept, and/or mentally deficient.

Women trying to escape prostitution, already traumatized by lifelong physical and sexual violence, routinely endure listening to jokes about "whores" and "hookers"–jokes that diminish, belittle, or even idealize their pain. Many SAGE participants clearly state that their experience of prostitution was not that of a victimless crime or a sexual act carried out by two equal and consenting partners. Rather, many women characterize their prostitution as exploitation based on an extreme power difference: men who use disposable income to buy sex acts from women and girls who need the money for survival.

In addition to having some experiences in common with war veterans, immigrant women, and non-prostitute survivors of rape and domestic violence, women involved in or escaping prostitution suffer unique harms as well as barriers to health services. By the time women enter SAGE, many have experienced prolonged sexual, physical, and emotional violence. Between 75-95% of girls in prostitution have histories of sexual exploitation and abuse (Hughes, Sporcic, Mendelson, & Chirgwin, 1999).

In a pilot study initiated by Norma Hotaling and Melissa Farley in 1994, 82% of those surveyed had been physically assaulted since entering prostitution, 68% had been raped in prostitution, and 49% had pornography made of them in prostitution. These data are included in an international study of violence in prostitution from 5 countries (Farley, Baral, Kiremire, & Sezgin, 1998). However, some health and social services may fail to recognize prostitution as a source of harm (Boyer, 1995; Greenman, 1990). Due to their unique situations, survivors of prostitution urgently need client centered intervention methods designed specifically to meet their needs. In the following, we describe a program that was designed by persons who are most familiar with the lives of individuals involved in prostitution: survivors themselves.

A PEER SUPPORT MODEL FOR INTERVENTION IN THE LIVES OF WOMEN IN PROSTITUTION: THE SAGE PROJECT

I am very out about being a transgender, former prostitute, addict, and HIV positive, because any one of those issues can be something that people find hopelessly debilitating. SAGE is what gave me the courage to be out about all these aspects of my life. I came through the court referral program. I was happy to get out of jail but I was really annoyed about being court-mandated to a treatment program. I had given up on ever being clean because I had tried and failed so many other times. I just wanted to keep turning tricks, smoking crack, and drinking vodka. So I just thought I would do my hours and go back to the life I thought I was choosing. I thought I was choosing that life out of a clear head, but instead I was choosing it from my history of trauma. When I heard counselors here talking about smoking crack and turning tricks and seeing that they had recovered from histories of trauma like mine, I began to realize that treatment for trauma had been the missing piece in all the other attempts at recovery. At SAGE, they gave me healthcare, treatment, hope, encouragement, love, and support. Instead of just doing the hours and returning to my former life, I have completed over 80 hours of counseling, have almost four and a half months in recovery from both drugs and trauma, and someday I want to be a counselor at SAGE.

–Chris

Standing Against Global Exploitation (The SAGE Project, Inc.) is a human rights organization formed in 1992 that has been continuously managed and staffed by prostitution survivors. In addition to community education programs, SAGE offers intensive drug and mental health treatment, case management, emergency intervention, job training and placement, and career development and support. To address the physical, emotional, and sexual trauma experienced by the majority of clients, counselors offer acupuncture, art therapy, massage, healing touch, movement, drama, and medical care for sexually transmitted diseases and infections resulting from unprotected sex with partners, johns, pimps, and through sexual assault. The agency provides emergency transitional housing, substance abuse and mental health treatment, individual counseling, vocational training and placement and group support to overcome histories of low self-esteem, trauma, exploitation, abuse, shame, guilt, and anger. The organization serves over 275 individuals each week and as a result of SAGE's assistance, over 1,500 women, girls, and transgender individuals have exited the criminal justice system, entered treatment, gained education and skills, and most have made exit plans or left prostitution.

SAGE has a diverse staff whose characteristics and experiences mirror their clientele. Most clients arrive with a profound lack of self-esteem and disempowering behaviors–dropping out of school, substance abuse, re-enactment of previous traumas and abuse in relationships, dependency on exploitative relationships, and extreme confusion about who to trust. Most of the staff were former clients and have an intimate knowledge of the trauma suffered by prostitution survivors. Most staff have criminal histories and were formerly homeless. Their involvement in the sex industry included stripping, escort services, massage parlors, phone sex, pornography, sadomasochism, bondage, sex trafficking, involvement with pimps, acting as pimps/madams, and being sexually abused, photographed, or statutorily raped as children in child prostitution.

Clients who seek treatment at SAGE frequently find that they knew staff when they were on the streets using drugs and prostituting. The experiences of staff allow them to relate sensitively and compassionately to the client's experience of exchanging sex acts for as little as $5, the inability to think of oneself as human but instead a collection of mechanical parts, the compartmentalization of experiences and body parts and the complex dynamics of the pimp/madam-prostitute relationship.

Because of the shame and social stigma associated with prostitution, survivors and those involved feel a greater trust for those who have had similar experiences. "You don't understand" disconnects survivor from the non-survivor (or "straight") counselor. Staff who have lived through recruitment into prostitution and later identified their recruiters/pimps as such will more quickly recognize the same behavior patterns in a client. It may take years for women, especially adolescents, to understand that they are being pimped.

Pimps/madams routinely present themselves as "friends" and/or "lovers" to women and girls whose vulnerability they recognize and exploit–runaways, victims of previous abuse, poor women with low self-esteem (Gamache & Giobbe, 1990). For those attempting to leave their pimps and madams, some may think it impossible because of the intense brainwashing and traumatic bonding to the perpetrator. Peer staff support and educate clients while providing refuge from the exploitative relationships.

Peer support counselors know firsthand the overwhelming obstacles. Many women return to the sex industry as a result of untreated trauma, financial need, substance abuse or other ongoing problems in their lives. Concurrently, if they leave SAGE, they are always welcome to return without bias, and when they do, their return is celebrated. One client noted that there has "never been a time I don't feel welcome [at SAGE]."

SAGE counselors serve as role models for clients. Many women who come to SAGE have never made money other than through prostitution. When clients see that others just like themselves have achieved the goals of living independently and outside of the sex industry, they begin to believe they, too, can accomplish this. Clients see women who were once just like themselves now holding jobs, pursuing their education, having safe homes, owning cars, reuniting with children, establishing healthy relationships, having healthcare and health insurance, paying taxes, having fun, and otherwise enjoying the basics of life which most people consider "normal."

SAGE staff use a nonjudgmental harm reduction model which allows every woman the chance to be helped to some degree. The goal of this approach is to reduce the harm resulting from the survival strategies of homeless and prostituting women. An abstinence standard is not imposed on clients, since abstinence is unrealistic when the person has few if any alternatives to using. Incremental steps are used, based on the client's own plan and timetable. For those involved in and exiting prostitution, harm reduction may include strategies to reduce, change or eliminate drug and alcohol use; reduce violence and risks of re-traumatization; employ safer sex practices with customers; decrease destructive self-soothing behaviors while simultaneously increasing healthier ones; develop networks of safe people, community resources, and partnerships; manage prescribed medication; prevent disease, death, incarceration, and isolation; and develop stable primary health care for participants and their children.

Consistent with a model of harm reduction, women are not required to leave the sex industry in order to receive services. All women are welcomed, whether or not they are currently prostituting, using drugs, or living with a pimp. There is no fee for treatment; thus, services are available to indigent and poor women. SAGE counselors attempt to meet women "where they are." Although counselors seek to help women develop exit plans, these are implemented only when the clients elect to do so. Exit planning is an ongoing process, which involves financial planning and plans for escape from pimps. Since many women in prostitution are also battered women, counselors develop safety plans to reduce immediate physical danger. Clients are also offered food, shampoo, and personal care articles to help them make it to the next day.

SAGE counselors tailor each client's treatment to her stage of recovery and readiness for change. The first stage, crisis intervention and stabilization, typically lasts two to four months, and focuses on medical care, safe housing, protection from pimps or other perpetrators, food, and necessities for survival. The second stage, integration/skill-building/education, lasts one to six months, and includes anger management classes, individual and group therapy, and emotional skill-building to re-integrate into the world outside of prostitution. The final stage consists of on-site vocational training and placement, which can last up to six months or more.

Collaborative relationships with other agencies allow staff to direct clients–in their preliminary ventures into the "straight" world–to vocational counselors, educators, therapists, and potential employers. SAGE counselors work with community agencies such as family planning clinics, self-defense programs, free medical clinics, and body awareness groups. Comprehensive and diverse programs are absolutely essential, as no two women in prostitution need exactly the same services. In the 1994 pilot project by Norma Hotaling and Melissa Farley, 88% reported that they wished to leave prostitution, 78% wanted a home or safe place, 73% wanted job training, 67% needed drug or alcohol treatment, 58% wanted health care, 50% wanted support from other prostitution survivors, 49% wanted self-defense training, 43% needed legal assistance, and 34% wanted childcare (Farley et al., 1998).

Networking and collaboration are crucial in SAGE's work. Following their participation as clients and then staff at SAGE, some women may go on to work in other community agencies. SAGE counselors offer training to others on prostitution-related issues such as heroin overdose, sexual exploitation and violence, domestic violence, sexual assault, use of acupuncture and drug/alcohol detoxification, addiction, and homelessness. A group of therapists specializing in the treatment of trauma utilizing Eye Movement Desensitization Reprocessing (EMDR) provide countless hours of pro-bono therapy through the EMDR Humanitarian Assistance Program. This collaboration offers personal healing support for staff as well as serving as a tool for professional development. EMDR supports the clients as they move through their treatment at SAGE.

It has been the experience of SAGE clients that some agencies insist that the prostitution survivor address issues which are the agency's priority, rather than the survivor's. For example, drug treatment programs, domestic violence programs and homeless shelters treat drug addiction as the core issue instead of a symptom of and coping behavior for lifelong histories of abuse, violence, and resulting trauma. SAGE is committed to the client-centered approach that combines and integrates trauma recovery, education, and drug treatment.

Another component of a peer support model is building positive relationships. Seeing the staff interact in healthy, respectful, professional ways models positive relationships for clients. Staff solidarity helps to make the program safe for clients. New clients witness the camaraderie among staff, among clients, and between staff and clients—and eventually participate themselves.

Both staff and clients are encouraged to express their emotions. It's clear that staff really care about each other and about clients. One client commented that the staff "really love you—open arms and just love you. That's what kept me here."

Unfortunately, many women and girls involved in prostitution have learned to mistrust other women. The envy, jealousy, competition, and anger among women in the society at large is condensed and acted out on the streets, especially in pimp-controlled environments. Many women on the streets see others as "taking business away," which endangers someone whose pimp establishes and violently enforces a financial quota: "Don't quit until you've got $1500." Additionally, for many clients, mistrust of women began early in life when they were sexually abused and not protected or even blamed by their mothers. Regaining trust in women is a primary step for SAGE clients.

Clients are able to witness and build positive relations, thus countering the devastating alienation that, according to most survivors, divides them from themselves and from others in their community. For many women, dissociation and numbing out began in early childhood and continues in adulthood through prostitution. They hide feelings of profound rage, suicidality, psychological paralysis and in some cases, homicidality, while showing sweetness, sexiness, and interest to demanding customers. The individualized, lengthy, and difficult process of identifying and uncovering true feelings is the challenge of SAGE counselors. The peer support groups at SAGE are non-confrontational. Women who come to SAGE have already survived so much traumatization that they cannot tolerate pressure and confrontation. When clients feel unconditional support from others who have "been there," they begin to believe they, too, can recover.

Women who choose to exit prostitution need constant affirmation and assurance that their lives and their safety are worth the often overwhelming effort. When someone has been bartered and sold like a used car, or has been made to stay in a motel room while men file in and out taking turns sexually exploiting or raping her, she needs to repeatedly hear that she is a valuable human being who can make a difference in the world. Some clients have been told they are simply not worth protecting; they are toss-aways and/or they are responsible for their own victimization and abuse. This kind of thinking becomes ingrained. They need to be told again and again that they are not just "junkies," "whores," or "criminals." SAGE staff focus on clients' strengths, knowing that in the world of prostitution, survival is a testament to one's capabilities.

Seeing a woman who was on the streets a few years ago and who is now a counselor, coordinator of services, or working in administration–can be a real inspiration. SAGE provides staff with opportunities for higher education, coaching, mentoring, peer support, on-site training, and specialized training. The staff have training in substance abuse, cultural competency, domestic violence, the psychological impact of trauma, and peer counseling. Many are pursuing drug treatment certification. Certification validates the counselor professionally, in her eyes as well as the client's. Striving for degrees and certification–learning professional terminology, for example–allows SAGE staff to join other substance abuse treatment providers in a collegial way. It also counters the myth that women and girls involved in prostitution are toss-aways and incorrigibles who are not worth wasting resources on for rehabilitation.

A CASE STUDY OF COMPASSIONATE INTERVENTION: THE SAGE CIRCLE

SAGE counselors have regular meetings where staff and clients share their feelings openly. The expression of genuine emotions is an experience often missing from the lives of prostitution survivors, whose pleasure and pain is suppressed, disguised, or manipulated as a regular part of their exploitation. A circle at SAGE contrasts the dark side of women's experience in prostitution and instead celebrates coming together, recognizing the connection staff and clients at SAGE experience as women, healers, counselors, employees, and team members.

One circle was used to support a staff member who was dealing with fears about being a new mother. Another circle celebrated the life and deeply mourned the death of one of SAGE's founding staff. On September 11, 2001, clients and staff shared in a circle to offer safety and hope during the national tragedy. The day was spent sitting in a circle and sharing with others those things that offered safety and offering healing energy to individuals affected by the September 11 events. The circle allowed women to come together and link experiences and feelings of safety and security in their everyday lives to events and problems in the outside world.

CONCLUSION

The delivery of services in an empowering, compassionate, non-shaming, and non-judgmental way is crucial to women's recovery from prostitution. The peer education model created by and for survivors of prostitution at SAGE has been successful because it offers tools to live as independently as possible and promotes healing and a life free from abuse. The SAGE staff create a mentoring relationship with clients to help them develop their own treatment plans.

By decreasing or eliminating barriers traditionally encountered by marginalized populations to social services, including discrimination, alienation, stigma and victim-blaming, individuals are afforded the opportunity to heal, create safety and financial independence, build community, expand choice. They are therefore more able to contribute to their own lives, as well as the lives of their families and to society as a whole. Since the peer education model is most effective when integrated into the structure of healthcare, domestic violence or sexual violence programs–existing agencies are advised to seek out organizations with peer-support models and to include them as central, rather than peripheral, to treatment programs. Peer education is an effective treatment and support model that is not only helpful but is necessary for those with histories of exploitation and violence.

REFERENCES

Becker, D., Lira, E., Castillo, M. L., Gomez, E., & Kovalskys, J. (1990). Therapy with victims of political repression in Chile: The challenge of social reparation. *Journal of Social Issues* 46: 133-49.

Boyer, D. (1995). *Survival sex in King County: Helping women out.* Report to Seattle Women's Commission.

Breton, M. (1999). The relevance of the structural approach to group work with immigrant and refugee women. *Social Work with Groups* 22(2/3): 11-29.

Egendorf, A. (1975). Vietnam veteran rap groups and themes of postwar life. In D.M. Mantell & M. Pilisuk (eds.) *Journal of Social Issues: Soldiers in and after Vietnam* 31(4): 111-124.

Farley, M., Baral, I., Kiremire, M., & Sezgin, U. (1998). Prostitution in Five Countries: Violence and Posttraumatic Stress Disorder. *Feminism & Psychology* 8 (4): 405-426.

Figley, C. R. (Ed.) (1978). *Stress Disorders Among Vietnam Veterans: Theory, Research and Treatment.* New York: Brunner/Mazel.

Gamache, D., & Giobbe, E. (1990). *Prostitution: Oppression Disguised as Liberation.* Minneapolis: National Coalition Against Domestic Violence.

Greenman, M. (1990). At the agency. *Families in Society: The Journal of Contemporary Human Services* 71 (2): 110-13.

Hughes, D. M., Sporcic, L. J., Mendelsoh, N X., & Chirgwin, V (1999). *The Factbook on Global Sexual Exploitation. http://www.catwinternational.org/fb.* Accessed March 2002.

Lifton, R.J. (1978). Advocacy and corruption in the healing professions. In Figley, Charles R. (Ed.), *Stress Disorders Among Vietnam Veterans: Theory, Research and Treatment.* New York: Brunner/Mazel. pp. 209-230.

Lykes, M. B., Brabeck, M. M., Ferns, T., & Radan, A. (1993). Human rights and mental health among Latin American women in situations of state-sponsored violence. *Psychology of Women Quarterly* 17: 525-44.

Martin-Baro, I. (1988). War and mental health. In Martin-Baro, A. Aron & Corne, S. (Eds.) *Writings for a Liberation Psychology*. Cambridge: Harvard University. pp. 108-121.

Turner, F. (1996). *Echoes of combat: The Vietnam War in American Memory*. New York: Anchor/Doubleday.

Wetzel, J. W. (2000). Women and mental health: A global perspective. *International Social Work* 43(2): 205-215.

Living in Longing:
Prostitution, Trauma Recovery,
and Public Assistance

Margaret A. Baldwin

SUMMARY. Building on the extensive research documenting the traumatic impact of prostitution on survivors, this paper addresses the opportunities and challenges facing prostituted women who seek public assistance from state family welfare programs and from the federal Social Security disability system. Prostituted women often face complex risks to their safety, must struggle to recover trust in a world that has of-

---

Margaret A. Baldwin is Associate Professor of Law, Florida State University College of Law.

The author thanks Dr. Melissa Farley for her commitment to the well-being of prostituted women, and for the invitation to contribute to this volume. She is indebted to Margaret Gast, Barbara Lackner, Murdina Campbell, April Cherry, Paul Hoppe, Gregory Thompson, Elissa Peterson, Jennifer Greenberg, Lois Shepherd, and her family.

A research grant from Florida State University College of Law supported the author's work on this article, for which she is grateful.

My title is from Dante's Inferno, describing the eternal punishment suffered by unbaptized souls consigned to Limbo, the First Circle of Hell. These verses capture something about the spiritual dimension of the problems she addresses in this paper. The poet Virgil, himself a soul in Limbo, explains:

We are lost, afflicted only in this one way:
That having no hope, we live in longing.

DANTE ALIGHIERI, THE INFERNO OF DANTE 37 (Robert Pinsky, trans., 1994). My own hope is that the hopelessness afflicting prostituted women and girls can be lifted, during their lifetimes.

Printed with permission.

[Haworth co-indexing entry note]: "Living in Longing: Prostitution, Trauma Recovery, and Public Assistance." Baldwin, Margaret A. Co-published simultaneously in *Journal of Trauma Practice* (The Haworth Maltreatment & Trauma Press, an imprint of The Haworth Press, Inc.) Vol. 2, No. 3/4, 2003, pp. 267-314; and: *Prostitution, Trafficking, and Traumatic Stress* (ed: Melissa Farley) The Haworth Maltreatment & Trauma Press, an imprint of The Haworth Press, Inc., 2003, pp. 267-314. Single or multiple copies of this article are available for a fee from The Haworth Document Delivery Service [1-800-HAWORTH, 9:00 a.m. - 5:00 p.m. (EST). E-mail address: docdelivery@haworthpress.com].

http://www.haworthpress.com/store/product.asp?sku=J189
10.1300/J189v02n03_16

fered them no protection in the past, and at the same time find a way to survive materially. This paper details the public assistance eligibility issues that may affect prostituted women's ability to gain access to program benefits, how a woman's prostitution history might bear on her ability or willingness to comply with program requirements, and how the process of applying for benefits can serve as a vehicle for a survivor's recovery. The author further recommends reforms of existing assistance programs to better serve the needs and interests of prostitution survivors.

I. INTRODUCTION

Two decades of research document the gruesome rates of sexual violence, childhood physical and sexual abuse, impoverishment, compromised health, substance dependency, and spiritual despair endured by prostituted women and girls.[1] This research, and the clinical experience from which it emerges, enriches our understanding of the healing relationships and resources that prostitution survivors need, and should be entitled to receive, from their communities. A prostituted woman faces financial emergency, must struggle to recover trust in a world that sacrificed her body and soul with impunity, and needs time and support to imagine a different future. Public assistance benefits programs may be available to help her, but may also place obstacles in her path. In this paper, I explore how survivors' recovery needs can both be furthered, and impeded, by two important benefits programs: the Supplemental Security Income ("SSI") program, and the Temporary Assistance to Needy Families ("TANF") program. The SSI program is a federal program, adminis-

---

1.   Recent research by Farley and colleagues has documented prostitution's traumatic effects on women. *See* Melissa Farley, Isin Baral, Merab Kiremire, & Ufuk Sezgin, *Prostitution in Five Countries: Violence and Post-Traumatic Stress Disorder*, 8 FEMINISM & PSYCHOLOGY 415 (1998); Melissa Farley & Howard Barkan, *Prostitution, Violence, and Post-Traumatic Stress Disorder*, 27 WOMEN AND HEALTH 37 (no. 3, 1998). For summaries and citation to earlier data revealing the high incidence of sexual violence, forced imprisonment, beatings, and sexual humiliation among prostituted women, *see* Vednita Carter & Evelina Giobbe, *Duet: Prostitution, Racism and Feminist Discourse*, 10 HASTINGS WOM. L. J. 37 (1999) (reporting and summarizing data); Margaret A. Baldwin, *Split at the Root: Prostitution and Feminist Discourses of Law Reform*, 5 YALE J. OF LAW & FEMINISM 47 (1992) (compiling and summarizing data). For literature detailing the traumatic impacts of rape, political torture and captivity, combat, and domestic violence generally, *see e.g.* JUDITH L. HERMAN, TRAUMA AND RECOVERY (1992); TRAUMATIC STRESS: THE EFFECTS OF OVERWHELMING EXPERIENCE ON MIND, BODY, AND SOCIETY (Bessel A. van der Kolk, Alexander C. McFarlane, and Lars Weisaeth eds., 1996).

tered by the Social Security Administration, that provides cash assistance to needy people who are unable to work because of a disability.[2] The TANF program is the federal "welfare reform" family assistance program. TANF also provides cash assistance, but recipients must become employed, and meet other program mandates.[3]

My discussion develops three themes. First, I provide basic information about eligibility under these assistance programs, with special attention to information particularly useful to women and girls with histories in prostitution. This information should help clients find appropriate benefits programs about which they may be confused or unaware. I also explain the kinds of documentary support that will be of the greatest help in establishing a client's eligibility. Familiarity with eligibility and documentation requirements is especially crucial because, unfortunately, the agencies responsible for administering these programs may fail to communicate this information adequately to applicants. Women seeking help face a discouraging tangle of changing rules, stereotyping assumptions, and understaffed agencies. Many women in a recent welfare study characterized their interactions with TANF caseworkers as "If we don't ask, they won't tell."[4] Applicants for TANF assistance too often are kept in the

---

2.   The SSI program is a companion to the Social Security retirement and disability programs, but SSI benefits are available without regard to the applicant's previous contributions through employment.

3.   The TANF program replaced the Aid to Families with Dependent Children (AFDC) program in 1996, and represents a significant shift in federal family assistance policy. Under the old AFDC program, poor mothers were entitled to financial support for raising children, could care for their children at home, and were not required to seek outside employment.

4.   Equal Rights Associates, *The Broken Promise: Welfare Reform Two Years Later,* 15 BERKELEY WOMEN'S LAW J. 14, 22 (2000) (analyzing information collected from state-wide focus groups of women participating in the CalWORKS welfare-to-work program). The report offers the following explanation for these problems:

> One woman offered a possible explanation for this practice. Caseworkers "assume we know all this stuff. Assume that we've been manipulating the system all this time. When you ask them something they look at you like you are crazy." The participants reported that the caseworkers both look down on them as ignorant and lazy AND assume that they know an extraordinary amount about the system and have the know-how to manipulate it. Meanwhile, crucial information about available services is kept from recipients. Available resources remain largely unused.

Id.

dark about available programs, are unaware of eligibility pitfalls, and are left uninformed about resources and exemptions specially marked for survivors of violence.[5] SSI applicants confront similar barriers, especially applicants coming into the system from long-term unemployment or homelessness.[6]

My second theme organizes the analytic scheme of the paper. I begin with the assumption that you are establishing a therapeutic relationship with a survivor, at the same time that she is applying for public benefits. These aims–therapeutic and bureaucratic–interact in complicated ways. I explore that interplay here in detail. In each arena, the survivor's fundamental objectives are similar. She is trying to achieve a safe, healthy environment for herself and her family, trying to build new relationships supporting her interests rather than exploiting her, and trying to reconnect with her communities in empowering ways. Working towards these goals in the therapeutic context, though, can be both assisted and burdened by the bureaucratic demands placed on a survivor as she seeks government assistance. For brevity's sake, I focus on the initial therapeutic task facing a survivor–achieving safety–and explore how a survivor's involvement with the SSI and TANF programs can both promote, and complicate, the survivor's safety needs.

My third theme is more tacit. As this paper reveals, mental health diagnostic criteria have come to play an increasingly weighty role in determining a person's eligibility for public assistance. Our social safety net is being rewoven to catch the fall only of those who can prove that they have suffered severely debilitating, objectively measurable, medical or psychiatric conditions.[7] Diagnoses bearing on a person's ability to work, in particular, increasingly shape national social policy on poverty, maternal and children's wellness issues, and access to drug and alcohol treatment. This policy emphasis places tremendous

---

5.   *Id.* at 22-28. Women may also not be receiving adequate information regarding their child care rights under the new welfare law. *See* Roslyn Powell & Mia Cahill, *Nowhere to Turn: New York City's Failure to Inform Parents on Public Assistance About Their Child Care Rights*, 7 GEO. J. ON POVERTY LAW & POLICY 363 (2000).

6.   *See* Leonard Adler, *SOS for SSI: The Unfulfilled Promise to Homeless Americans*, 1 GEO. J. ON FIGHTING POVERTY 304 (1994).

7.   Addressing this development in the context of welfare reform, Sheldon Danziger and Harold Pollock observe: "Now, much attention has been focused on the extent to which recipients have clinically diagnosable conditions. Such conditions provide an acceptable explanation for welfare dependence and also require enhanced treatment services and possible exemption from time limits." Sheldon Danziger & Harold Pollock, *Welfare Reform, Substance Use, and Mental Health*, 25 J. OF HEALTH POL., POL'Y, & LAW 623, 629 (2000).

power in the hands of mental health and medical professionals, as the arbiters of whose needs, and which needs, will be deemed worthy of public aid.

With this power, comes the responsibility to appreciate the plights of women and children whose needs are the most urgent; among them, prostituted women and girls. I sincerely hope that this paper will deepen your solidarity with them. Moreover, as mental health professionals take on these responsibilities, we must all consider whether issues of social justice, citizenship, and equality should be resolved entirely by resorting to the diagnostic criteria of the DSM-IV-TR.[8] No therapist I know thinks that,[9] but our political culture seems increasingly entrenched in that position. I hope that the statutory and legislative material supplied in this paper will aid readers in making an informed judgment about the wisdom of these policy preferences.

In any event, every therapist I know is devoted to the loving task of healing the pain and distress of survivors. This paper is dedicated to that aim, in the hope that we can further those commitments within our social and political worlds. But we must begin with individual recovery, as do I here. The first stage of recovery for a trauma survivor is achieving safety.[10] A survivor faces multiple safety tasks, including naming the problem, and establishing a safe

---

8.   AMERICAN PSYCHIATRIC ASSOCIATION, DIAGNOSTIC AND STATISTICAL MANUAL OF MENTAL DISORDERS (4th ed., Text Revision 2000) (hereinafter DSM-IV-TR).

9.   Nor do the editors of the DSM-IV-TR, who explicitly caution that "[t]he clinical and scientific considerations involved in categorization of these conditions as mental disorders may not be wholly relevant to legal judgments, for example, that take into account such issues as individual responsibility, disability determination, and competency." *Id.* at xxxvii.

10.   The following summary is drawn from HERMAN, *supra* note 1, at 156-159, and from other sources as noted.

environment. How does the public benefits system implicate those safety tasks, together with the survivor's therapeutic work?[11]

II. NAMING AND BEING NAMED

Clinical assessment and diagnosis are threshold "naming" steps in the therapeutic relationship.[12] Trauma survivors must overcome daunting obstacles, both in naming their own experience, and in being named by others. Traumatic events sear the mind and the memory. Consequently, the diagnostic process may be complicated by "disguised presentations" of symptoms, by problems of recall, and by the effects of dissociative disorders. The survivor may not connect past traumatic events with present symptoms, may not remember those events, or may present symptoms that neither the therapist nor survivor can, or wishes to, address.[13] While a survivor may find comfort and validation from the information conveyed by the diagnosis,[14] she may also feel stigmatized by the diagnostic label, or feel otherwise diminished by it.[15] Moreover, survivors may experience a psychiatric diagnosis as a "moral victory to the

---

11. I do not separately address a third safety need identified by Herman, restoring the survivor's control over her body. Those needs include "basic health needs, regulation of bodily functions such as sleep, eating and exercise, management of post-traumatic symptoms, and control of self-destructive behaviors." HERMAN, *supra* note 1, at 160.

Access to medical services and care is crucial for survivors attempting to take care of their medical needs. Medicaid benefits may be available to survivors for medical support. The Medicaid eligibility process is beyond the scope of this paper, though; for a good general treatment of the health care access problems confronting prostitution survivors, *see* Tracy M. Clements, *Prostitution and the American Health Care System: Denying Access to a Group of Women in Need*, 1996 BERKELEY WOMEN'S L. J. 48.

Ultimately, restoring a prostitution survivor's control over her body is inseparable from empowering her to escape prostitution. In that sense, the recovery issues I address throughout this paper represent smaller steps toward that larger aim.

12. *See generally* HERMAN, *supra* note 1, at 156-159.

13. *See* Bessel Van Der Kolk, Alexander McFarlane & Onno Van Der Hart, *A General Approach to the Treatment of Post-Traumatic Stress Disorder, in* TRAUMATIC STRESS, *supra* note 1, at 417, 420-423 (special attention should be paid to the impact of intrusive re-experiencing, autonomic hyperarousal, numbing, intense emotional reactions, learning difficulties, memory disturbances, aggression, psychosomatic reactions on the assessment process).

14. *See* Marten W. de Vries, *Trauma in Cultural Perspective, in* TRAUMATIC STRESS, *supra* note 1, at 398, 405-407 (discussing the legitimizing and normalizing function of medical labelling on individual response to trauma); *see also* HERMAN, *supra* note 1, at 158.

15. *See* HERMAN, *supra* note 1, at 158.

perpetrator, in a way that acknowledging physical harm [is] not," and the act of seeking help as "compound[ing] the survivor's sense of defeat."[16]

Work between a prostitution survivor and a caregiver will arouse all of these complicated, tangled feelings–on both sides. Both caregiver and survivor may bring intense fear to the whole terrain of the survivor's prostitution history. Survivors deeply dread recalling the ugly events and unbearable emotions they carry with them from their days and nights in prostitution. Survivors are likely to suffer severe numbing and avoidance symptoms. These symptoms impede a survivor's ability to recall and describe events and feelings associated with prostitution.[17] Survivors expect to be shamed by outsiders, often feel their humanity has been irretrievably maimed, and fear that interviewers will eroticize their stories rather than empathize with their suffering. Prostituted women suffer a strongly stigmatized sense of self, believing that "people can 'tell' that they are prostitutes merely be looking at them."[18] Having endured terrible humiliations, survivors often feel dismissive of, and abandoned by, the "straight" women whose nice husbands may have bought them. You may be identified as such a wife or husband. This is the voice of one survivor:

> I was one such girl. I can tell you some of the things they did to me and other girls and women, but there is still much that I cannot speak of. . . . Survivors are split into pieces, fragmented, broken, filled with despair, pain, rage and sorrow. We have been hurt beyond belief. We are silent; we are numb. Our eyes see, our ears hear, but we do not tell. Our voices are non-existent, but even if they did exist, who would believe what we have to say? Who would listen? Who would care? We are dirty, ruined, despised, the whores of the earth. The men who use us throw us away. . . . The rest of you turn your backs, avert your eyes, pretend not to see, go on your way. You leave us to the predators.[19]

---

16. *Id.* at 158-59.
17. *See* Farley & Barkan, *supra* note 1, at 42 (reporting that prostituted women scored highest on C symptoms for PTSD, including numbing and avoidance; 79% of the sample suffered from three or more C symptoms).
18. Carter & Giobbe, *supra* note 1, at 48. One woman reported that she felt that "people look at me . . . like I'm dirty . . . just a funny look they give you when they know you have been on the streets." Evelina Giobbe, *Prostitution: Buying the Right to Rape,* *in* RAPE & SEXUAL ASSAULT III 144, 157 (Anne Wolbert Burgess ed., 1992).
19. Christine Grussendorf (Stark), *Surviving Sexual Slavery: Women in Search of Freedom, in* MAKING THE HARM VISIBLE: GLOBAL SEXUAL EXPLOITATION OF WOMEN AND GIRLS–SPEAKING OUT AND PROVIDING SERVICES 315, 315-316 (Donna M. Hughes & Claire Roche, eds., 1999).

Caregivers may initially respond to survivors' distress by feeling overwhelmed, defensive, and confused–reactions that compound, rather than soothe, the survivor's anxieties and fears. These powerful reactions can quickly generate patterns of interaction that I call "Hide the Prostitution." There are several versions. First, there is the "bury it" version: Either caregiver or survivor may simply feel unable to approach the survivor's prostitution history, or may do so only in the most superficial terms. While the survivor may have locked her prostitution experiences away or dread the emotional costs of recalling them, caregivers may feel that they lack the basic vocabulary, tact, and insight to explore the survivor's history respectfully. Second, there is the "me, too" version: This version hides the prostitution by treating the experience as no different from other abusive conditions that prostituted and non-prostituted women may confront, like rape, domestic violence, or sexual harassment–and not as its own painful world. Also forfeited in this version is the anguish and rage that prostituted women feel about the ways they see themselves as different from other women, and used by them. The loss of their children, crippling and exhausting struggles with drugs and alcohol, and memories of incarceration haunt survivors profoundly. A caregiver's well-meaning efforts toward intimacy and identification with the survivor can easily misunderstand and dishonor these wounds. Finally, there is the "let's pretend" version: This version hides the prostitution behind cultural myths, especially myths about money. Caregivers and survivors alike may express allegiance to the idea that prostitution is a real job that pays a great deal of money, even if the working conditions are poor. Confusing to a survivor is why she probably never felt like what she was doing was a job, why she never had any money–and why she always had to be drunk or loaded to turn a trick. For survivors, all of these versions of "Hide the Prostitution" freeze and and alienate the survivor's history, in manner sadly reminiscent of prostitution itself.

Similar naming issues confront survivors in the benefits eligibility process. SSI and TANF eligibility evaluators will want to know why the survivor is need of help, will explore her powers and potential for earning money, and raise special obstacles for applicants with alcohol and drug abuse histories. The SSI and TANF programs frame these issues in quite different ways, based on different eligibility criteria and procedures. At first glance, as I explain further below, each program seems to mimic at least one version of the "Hide the Prostitution" dynamic in deciding a survivor's eligibility. This might suggest that the survivor's isolation and anguish will only intensify as she moves through these bureaucratic systems. That prediction tells just part of the story, however. For both eligibility procedures create some important opportunities for the survivor and caregiver to transform the "Hide the Prostitution" dance into occasions for more authentic disclosure and relationship, greater safety, and stronger support from program services.

1. DESCRIBING NEED

The first questions a survivor will have to address when applying for SSI or TANF benefits have to do with the particular circumstances that have brought her to a condition of need.

a. SSI: the medicalized self

To qualify for benefits under the SSI disability program, the answer to the question "Why are you needy?" must be "Because I am currently disabled, unable to work very much, and my disability has or will last for a year or more." The legal definition of disability is as follows:

> [A]n individual shall be considered to be disabled . . . if he is unable to engage in any substantial gainful activity by reason of any medically determinable physical or mental impairment which can be expected to result in death or which has lasted or can be expected to last for a continuous period of not less than twelve months.[20]

Paradoxically, a survivor's prostitution history is both factually crucial, and legally irrelevant, to proving these requirements. On the one hand, most prostitution survivors are likely to suffer the kinds of impairments which qualify as disabilities under the law–as a result of her exploitation in prostitution. In that sense, a survivor's prostitution history is factually fundamental to her disability claim. On the other hand, the medical and psychiatric evidence necessary for documenting her claim need not directly refer to her prostitution history at all. In that sense, the evaluation treats her history as legally irrelevant to her disability status. Of the three versions of "Hide the Prostitution," the SSI system therefore seems to favor the "bury it" version: never inquiring about the biographical details lying below the surface of the survivor's symptoms, and never having to face the connection between the prostitution and the survivor's current pain and distress.

---

20. 42 U.S.C.A. 1382(c)(a)(1)(B)(3)(A). *See generally* Frank S. Ravitch, *Balancing Fundamental Disability Policies: The Relationship Between the Americans With Disabilities Act and Social Security Disability*, 1 GEO. J. ON FIGHTING POVERTY 240 (1994).

This pattern of denial emerges vividly in the agency's treatment of two of the three crucial issues used to determine if the survivor has a disabling impairment.[21] The first step is the "severity" determination; the second step, the determination whether the applicant suffers from a "listed impairment."[22] The "severity" inquiry asks whether the survivor's disabling condition restricts her ability to perform basic work-related activities.[23] In SSI jargon, those restrictions are called "functional limitations." When a survivor's impairment is mental or psychological, the survivor's "functional limitations" are evaluated in four main categories, including: activities of daily living; social functioning; concentration, persistence, or pace; and episodes of decomposition.[24] Survivors of prostitution are likely to experience significant distress in all of these areas, as a result of their involvement in prostitution. For example, the first factor, evaluating the survivor's "activities of daily living," takes into account how the survivor performs such tasks as cleaning, shopping, cooking, paying bills, taking public transportation, grooming and hygiene, and using the telephone. The agency will inquire whether she performs these tasks on a routine basis, the amount of supervision she may need to perform them, and whether she can perform them without undue distraction.[25] Many survivors of prostitution, like many battered women, struggle with these daily tasks as a conse-

---

21. The agency structures the determination whether an applicant suffers a sufficiently severe impairment to qualify as disabled through a 5-step inquiry. *See* 20 C.F.R. 920(a)-(e) (setting out the five-step inquiry used by the agency to decide if the applicant is disabled). The fourth and fifth steps are not addressed here, because the agency's determination of disability is likely to be made on the basis of the first three, at least for survivors whose PTSD symptoms are as persistent as those measured by Farley and colleagues in research among prostituted women. *See generally* Farley *et al., supra* note 1, *passim.* The third criterion assesses the applicant's income, which I discuss together with other matters relating to survivors' economic status *infra* notes 33-45, and accompanying text.

22. *See* 20 C.F.R. section 920(a), (b).

23. *See* 20 C.F.R. section 404.1520(c). It is important that the survivor also show that her medical impairment caused the restrictions on her capacity to work. *See* U.S. SOCIAL SECURITY ADMINISTRATION, DISABILITY EVALUATION UNDER SOCIAL SECURITY: MEDICAL CRITERIA FOR EVALUATING SOCIAL SECURITY DISABILITY CLAIMS 65 (2002) (Section 12.00B) (hereinafter THE BLUE BOOK) (available at *www.ssa.gov/disability/professionals/bluebook*) (functional limitations must be the result of mental impairment).

24. *See* 20 C.F.R. section 416.920a(c)(3)(evaluation of mental impairments; listing areas of functional limitation to be assessed; THE BLUE BOOK, *supra* note 23, at 66-68 (Section 12.00C, Paragraphs 1-4).

25. *See* THE BLUE BOOK, *supra* note 23, at 67 (Section 12.00C(1)) (discussing evaluation criteria for "activities of daily living").

quence of major depression. This is especially true for women recruited into prostitution as girls or young teenagers. For them, the developmental and social steps ordinarily taken during adolescence and young adulthood, preparing us to perform these tasks independently, were sacrificed to years of compulsory sex with strangers:

> A girl who enters prostitution at fourteen will have submitted to the sexual demands of four thousand men before she is old enough to drive a car, eight thousand men before she is old enough to vote and twelve thousand men before she is deemed mature enough to buy a single beer in many states.[26]

> Most Black women used in prostitution . . . lost their childhood to the streets. Many came of age in juvenile detention centers and matured in adult correctional facilities.[27]

Impaired social functioning, in turn, may be shown through a "history of altercations," evictions, firings, fear of strangers, avoidance of interpersonal relationships, and social isolation.[28] These kinds of difficulties are typical in the lives of women in prostitution and other trauma survivors.[29]

Despite the relevance of the survivor's prostitution history to producing these symptoms, they may be explored and presented in terms which shield that history from view. The "functional limitations" evaluate the survivor's current functioning, rather than the etiology of these symptoms. Indeed, the Social Security Administration has declared that an applicant's employment history is irrelevant to the evaluation of the severity of his or her impairment.[30]

The same denial pattern emerges in the agency's second evaluation step, whether the survivor suffers from a "listed impairment, which asks whether the survivor's condition is "presumptively disabling." A person who suffers from such a condition, when also functionally limited, is presumed to be un-

---

26. *Vednita Carter & Evelina Giobbe, Duet: Prostitution, Racism and Feminist Discourse,* 10 HASTINGS WOM. L. J. 37, 46 (1999).

27. *Id.* at 55.

28. *See* THE BLUE BOOK, *supra* note 23, at 67 (Section 12.00C(2))(assessment of social functioning).

29. Prostitution survivors are also likely to have difficulty in third and fourth areas, "concentration, persistence and pace," and "deterioration or decomposition in work or work-like settings."

30. *See* 20 C.F.R. section 404.1520(c) (agency will not consider age, education, or work experience in assessing functional limitations).

able to work.[31] The agency publishes an actual list of these conditions, and their diagnostic requisites; hence the term "listed impairment." The listed "mental impairments" include affective disorders, anxiety-related disorders, and personality disorders. The diagnostic criteria for each impairment is drawn extensively from the DSM-IV.[32] Prostituted women suffer these conditions at very high prevalence rates[33]; so, too, do women eligible for maternal assistance programs generally.[34] Here again, a survivor's prostitution history need not be addressed directly in making these assessments, since the relevant diagnostic criteria refer to current symptoms and quality of life. The "listed impairment" of major depression, for example, is based on observation of current depressed mood, diminished pleasure, weight loss, and insomnia, together with restricted life activities.[35] Even post-traumatic stress disorder, while diagnostically anchored in past exposure to traumatic events,[36] is identified principally in terms of the survivor's ongoing response to the trauma, and

---

31.   *See* 20 C.F.R. section 404.1520(d) (if severe impairment is among those listed in pertinent section of agency rules and meets duration requirement, agency will find applicant disabled); 20 C.F.R. section 416.920a(d)(2) (describing process of combining results of functional limitation criteria with medical findings related to impairment).

32.   *See* THE BLUE BOOK, *supra* note 23, at 75-77 (Affective Disorders)(Section 12.04); 77-78 (Anxiety-Related Disorders) (Section 12.06); 79-80 (Personality Disorders) (Section 12.08).

   For purposes of this discussion, I am stressing the trauma-related psychological disorders that prostitution survivors may experience. Caregivers should be aware, however, of the many physical health impacts that prostitution entails, including poorly healed broken bones and wounds, head injuries, severe damage to feet and legs, severe dental problems, hearing loss, and long-term malnutrition.

   These medical conditions may also constitute SSI impairments, and may be considered in combination with a survivor's psychological difficulties to determine the severity of the survivor's disability. The SSI evaluation is supposed to address the survivor as "the whole person, and not in the abstract as having several hypothetical and isolated illnesses." *Davis v. Shalala*, 985 F.2d 528, 534 (11th Cir. 1993).

33.   *See supra* notes 1-3, and accompanying text.

34.   One study indicates that 42% of welfare mothers report high levels of depressive symptoms; 53% of applicants to a welfare-to-work intervention program were documented to be at a high risk of depression. *See* Danziger & Pollock, *supra* note 10, at 630.

35.   *See* THE BLUE BOOK, *supra* note 23, at 75-77. For the parallel DSM-IV criteria, *see* DSM-IV-TR, *supra* note 8, at 356.

36.   *See* DSM-IV-TR, *supra* note 8, at 463-464 (summarizing diagnostic features of PTSD, giving examples of traumatic events that may precipitate the disorder); 467 (listing exposure to traumatic event as a diagnostic criterion).

her current symptoms.[37] Thus, a survivor may disclose all the information needed for an SSI assessment, without ever indicating that her condition might be linked to her prostitution history.

For several reasons, a survivor may find a measure of protection in shielding her prostitution history from the SSI system. A survivor may wish to avoid the distress of revisiting that history in the bureaucratic system, just as she may have wished to avoid that discussion in the therapeutic context. Any continuous, intrusive inquiry into her experience of prostitution, precedent childhood trauma and abuse, and ongoing struggles with the impact of those experiences will be difficult. Since the survivor's SSI eligibility may take up to two years to resolve,[38] a survivor may find the sustained vulnerability simply intolerable. In addition, since the benefits process is about receiving money, it may be especially important to a survivor that her eligibility not be linked to a demand that she disclose her prostitution experience. Otherwise, the whole process can start to mimic turning a trick: she presents herself as a prostitute, and then gets money for it. For all of these reasons, the buffer offered by the SSI process, between disclosing need, and disclosing the prostitution that made her needy, may feel like a soft landing for a survivor.

Nevertheless, these buffers can also exact a terrible price. Durston and Mills have described how walling-off the SSI diagnosis, from the cause and context of the survivor's distress, silences and oppresses survivors in the guise of protecting them. They give as an example an SSI hearing involving a woman suffering from chronic depression, the consequence of a history of severe childhood sexual and physical abuse:

In most disability hearings, it is the depression, not the history of abuse, that would be the subject of the hearing. In questioning the claimant, both the representative and the judge would focus on such factors as the severity of the depression, how often [the claimant] had attempted therapy, and how the depression has affected her ability to function at work. There would be little or no mention of the history of abuse, an omission

37. *See id.* at 463-464 (detailing responses to traumatic events, symptoms indicating PTSD); 468 (diagnostic criteria relating to response to trauma, current symptoms). The traumatic event criterion is defined loosely in the DSM-IV to include many forms of violence and threats of violence. The specific context in which the traumatic event occurred is not diagnostically crucial.
38. *See* Linda S. Durston & Linda G. Mills, *Toward a New Dynamic in Poverty Client Empowerment: The Rhetoric, Politics, and Therapeutics of Opening Statements in Social Security Hearings*, 8 YALE J. OF LAW & FEMINISM 119, 139 (1996).

of truth that would likely further the claimant's shame and exacerbate the pain of her public denial.[39]

Thus, just as the survivor may need ultimately to uncover her prostitution history with you in her therapy, it may empower her to do the same in the course of her SSI eligibility procedure.

Yet, to affirm that disclosure may be a good idea does not necessarily guide us in how to speak, or listen, to each other—much less to bureaucratic decision makers. Of course, survivors should be invited and supported to make disclosure choices that are the most empowering for them as the eligibility process unfolds. Caregivers and survivors need to learn a balance between deferring and engaging the survivor's prostitution history. Both must respect the time it takes to develop trust and tolerance, while accepting the significance of the prostitution experience in the survivor's painful world. In my experience, the strongest bridge across the gaps and fears and evasions, when a caregiver's impulse to "bury it" rears its head, is in the caregiver's willingness to attend to the survivor's present feelings and needs. It can be remarkably helpful to pay close attention to a survivor's requests for attention to her immediate medical concerns. Prostituted women's bodies are usually seen only as sexual and sexualized, even by their advocates. Talking with her about how her body feels in the here and now, and about how her body might be in pain, trust gradually develops. When the survivor can trust the caregiver to appreciate the physical harm that has been done to her, she may feel greater safety revealing how those injuries were inflicted in the first place.[40]

The SSI evaluation process has the potential to open up these channels for exploration and healing of the survivor's prostitution experience. The "listed impairment" assessment, focused as it is on current symptoms, encourages both caregiver and survivor to attend the survivor's immediate distress as the primary concern of both. For the survivor, the assessment process may be the

---

39. *Id.* at 139.
40. I learned this lesson working with a survivor who was "recruited" into prostitution by first being forced to perform in a strip club. At my initial meeting with her, she told me that a prison doctor had mistakenly amputated her toe while treating her painful bunions. Our discussions about her foot continued as I tried to get medical attention and proper shoes for her. Gradually, she was able to tell me that her foot was injured from years of stripping. This was the thread on which she began to tell me what happened to her in the strip clubs, and later in prostitution. For a period of time, she even had to perform on crutches while a broken leg healed. She needed very much for me first to appreciate that she had been hurt, in a clear physical way, and trust that I would take the injury seriously, before she was comfortable sharing with me how she had sustained the damage to her feet.

first time anyone has respectfully and seriously discussed symptoms she finds shameful, or has been encouraged to minimize, or has had little vocabulary to describe. Proceeding in this way, a deeper level of interpersonal trust, and a greater openness to the scope and impact of the prostitution, can develop over time. Evaluation of the survivor's "functional limitations" can yield similar fruit. By building understanding of the survivor's current circumstances and needs, both survivor and caregiver can bring into focus the chaos and disappointments that may have shaped the months and years she spent in prostitution, without necessarily immediately resolving the role played by prostitution in creating and exacerbating them. In turn, the caregiver can come to a fuller understanding of how the survivor experienced prostitution, challenging her own preconceptions and stereotypes along the way. In a culture that denies the reality of prostitution for women as vigorously as ours does, the opportunity offered by the assessment process to frame the experience from the standpoint of the survivor's world is an invaluable one. And the survivor's empowerment in the process will strengthen her resilience and resolve in pursuing her benefits claim, as well.

b. TANF: the domesticated self.

TANF evaluators will also want to know whether a survivor is needy, and why. Since the TANF program is a family financial assistance program, eligibility typically hinges on two factors: financial need, and family status. The two important family status issues are: whether the applicant is a mother or caretaker of children, and whether the applicant has been a victim of abuse.

Both questions are likely to raise difficult and unresolved issues for survivors, bearing on how survivors see themselves as different from normal, "straight" women. That survivors feel this alienation around motherhood and violence may seem surprising. We often assume that motherhood and victimization by violence–especially domestic violence–are conditions that many women share in common. Caregivers may make the same assumption, and attempt to create intimacy with a survivor on this presumed common ground. But for a prostitution survivor that shared terrain may not exist, or the geography of her life may look like Iceland to your Missouri. To assume common ground on these issues may instead begin the "me, too" version of the "Hide the Prostitution" dynamic: suppressing the ways prostitution has distinctively shaped a survivor's experience of maternity and of violence, while asserting connection based on shared experience. The TANF eligibility process, too, partakes of the "me, too" version, demanding that women present specific conforming family relationships, and anticipating that certain forms of violence and exploitation will have accompanied those relationships. The TANF eligibility process also has a kind of compulsory intimacy about it, involving face-to-face encounters with local caseworkers, and continuous "hands-on" monitoring of the recipient as a condition of assistance.

Survivors often adapt to these expectations in polarized ways. A survivor may try to conform to a caregiver's expectations, or instead focus solely on the differences dividing them. Both of these reactions can be motivated by strong feelings of shame, hopelessness and anger. In this section, I explore how the survivor's history of motherhood and violence can be mirrored with more genuine understanding: how prostitution creates "non-conforming" family circumstances, and how these distinctive circumstances can yet support a stronger connection among survivors, caregivers, and services staff.

i. Maternity

What kinds of families are "conforming" for purposes of TANF eligibility? The TANF statute defines a family as a household that includes a minor child who lives with the family, or a pregnant woman.[41] This definition is consistent with the primary purpose of the statute, to make it possible for children to be cared for in their own homes or in the homes of relatives.[42] For many survivors, though, achieving the status of poor mother has already become an unreachable goal, or has faded like a broken promise. Many prostituted women are childless. Among prostituted women who have children, most become pregnant and give birth before becoming enmeshed in prostitution.[43]

---

41. *See* 42 U.S.C.A. section 608(a)(1).

Other TANF family status rules may have special implications for prostitution survivors. The TANF program now permits two parent families to receive assistance, unlike the earlier AFDC progam, to encourage poor women to marry. *See* 42 U.S.C.A. section 601(a)(2),(3). This policy is of dubious merit as applied to women enmeshed in relationships with men who are pimping them.

Young mothers may also be required to live in 'adult-supervised settings." *See* 42 U.S.C.A. section 608(a)(2) (barring assistance to teenage parents not living in adult-supervised settings). The statute contemplates that teenage mothers live with adult relatives, including parents, legal guardian, or other relative. *See* 42 U.S.C.A. section 608(a)(5). Many of these relatives may be unsafe for prostitution survivors and their children. They may have abused the survivor, pimped her, or pushed her out of the family by neglect.

42. *See* 42 U.S.C. A. section 601(a)(1).

43. *See* ELEANOR M. MILLER. STREET WOMAN 138 (1985) (noting that women with children usually had children early in their involvement in prostitution). There is very little empirical work on pregnancy and fertility among prostituted women, perhaps reflecting an unconscious replication of the mother/whore dichotomy in our research agendas.

There are several reasons why. Untreated sexually transmitted disease may be a primary factor reducing prostituted women's fertility, as Eleanor Miller's research suggests.[44] But disease is not the only factor. For those who profit from women's prostitution, pregnancy and motherhood reduce a woman's economic worth.[45] Coerced abortions are sometimes the only form of medical care to which a woman in prostitution has had access.[46] Brutal beatings impair fertility and cause miscarriage.[47] Children may be exposed to the same violence and distress as their mothers, sometimes lethally. One survivor reported to me that her daughter had been killed by a trick, the child's body found stuffed in a garbage can.

Prostituted women who do have children seldom are able to keep them. Some women lose custody of their children outright, by divorce, by adoption, or by dependency or neglect proceedings brought by the state. Other women lose their children by degrees. Prostituted women often arrange for other family members to take care of the kids, with whom they have inconsistent and often painful contact. Family caretakers may ultimately seek formal custody of

---

44. *Id.* One survivor describes the damage to her reproductive system caused by several years of being pimped by her mother as a girl:

> Because of the damage done in my pre-pubescent years, I never had a period, but I never thought about it and my mom never said anything about it. It turned out that my uterus and ovaries had so much scar tissue that they pretty much atrophied. I found out I had tumors throughout my urinary and reproductive systems. Most were benign, but a few were in the cancerous stage, so I had to go through chemotherapy at twenty-one.

Minerva Kalenandi, *You Need Some Place to Escape To, in* MAKING THE HARM VISIBLE, *supra* note 19, at 222, 223.

45. The economics of pregnancy in prostitution may be changing. Many johns apparently believe that HIV-positive women cannot become pregnant. Pregnancy is seen consequently as a sign of health in women, and of reduced risk for the john. "Pregnant pussy is good pussy" is the street slogan.

46. This is extremely difficult for many women to discuss. The number of abortions is sometimes very high (6-8), and may have involved humiliating procedures.

47. Eleanor Miller notes that, among the 64 women she interviewed, "[m]any of these women also had had several pregnancies that had resulted in miscarriages or abortions." MILLER, *supra* note 43, at 33. Survivors who participated in Ruth Parriot's study of the health impacts of prostitution reported miscarriages resulting from beatings inflicted by partners/pimps. RUTH PARRIOT, HEALTH EXPERIENCES OF TWIN CITIES WOMEN USED IN PROSTITUTION: SURVEY FINDINGS AND RECOMMENDATIONS 19 (1998).

the children, especially if the mother has been incarcerated.[48] For women in these circumstances, who have never had children or who have lost them, TANF benefits are not legitimately available. As Miller points out, survivors deprived of assistance "become completely vulnerable to the 'men' who control the streets and/or to their drug habits."[49]

Over time, these circumstances may change. Survivors are most likely to restore contact with their children in their thirties and forties, sometimes as caretakers of grandchildren.[50] Survivors may become eligible for TANF benefits at this time, even if they had not been eligible before. These new relationships and options raise new uncertainties. Often deprived of their own childhoods, survivors may need ongoing support and attention to the impact of the years of separation and compromised care that a survivor may have had to offer her children in the past.[51] In terms of the survivor's TANF eligibility, the survivor's history and current relationship with her child may arise in connection with proving that the child presently lives with her, and does not continue to live in another household. Legally, the residency standard looks to the continuity of contact between caretaker and child.[52] For the survivor, achieving that continuity may be an important goal in the process of healing. By assisting survivors to become the mothers they wish to be, caregivers and TANF staff can create "me, too" alliances of genuine value to survivors.

---

48.   MILLER, *supra* note 43, at 138. Miller explains this as a consequence of the bonds between the prostituted woman and their children's caretakers weakening over time. *Id.*

49.   MILLER, *supra* note 43, at 125. Remember that SSI benefits are available whether or not a woman is a mother. If the survivor is not eligible for TANF, she may still be eligible for SSI.

50.   *Id.* at 138-139.

51.   *See generally* JOYCELYN M. POLLOCK, COUNSELING WOMEN IN PRISON 95-119 (1998); Kathy Boudin, *Lessons from a Mother's Program in Prison: A Psychosocial Approach Supports Women and Their Children, in* BREAKING THE RULES: WOMEN IN PRISON AND FEMINIST THERAPY 103 (Judy Harden & Marcia Hill, eds. 1998).

52.   Under the federal standard, a child does not live with a caretaker when the child has been absent for 45 consecutive days, or for any period between 30 and 180 days, as the state may choose. *See* 42 U.S.C.A. section 608(a)(10) (setting out the standard for family residence).

ii. Violence

The second eligibility question confronting a survivor applying for TANF benefits is whether she has been subjected to "battery or extreme cruelty."[53] The stakes are these. The federal TANF law contains a provision called the Family Violence Option (the "FVO")[54], that addresses the special recovery needs facing violence survivors, and the special obstacles those victims may face in meeting TANF program requirements.[55] The FVO authorizes the states to take three steps to assist victims.[56] The first is a "naming" step. States may "screen and identify individuals receiving assistance with a history of domestic

---

53. I put the phrase in quotation marks, because the term has a specific legal meaning under federal and state law. For the federal definition, *see infra* note 59 and accompanying text.

54. *See* 42 U.S.C.A. section 602(a) (7).

55. For an excellent bibliography of the published research tracing the links between violence against women and poverty, *see* Maria L. Imperial, *Self-Sufficiency and Safety: Welfare Reform for Victims of Domestic Violence*, 5 GEO. J. ON FIGHTING POVERTY 3, 10-12 (1997).

For analysis of the implications of welfare reform on battered women generally, *see* Sheryl L. Howard, *How Will Battered Women Fare Under the New Welfare Reform?*, 12 BERKELEY WOM. L. J. 140 (1997); Elspeth K. Deily, *Working With Welfare: Can Single Mothers Manage?*, 12 BERKELEY WOM. L. J. 132 (1997).

56. *See* 42 U.S.C.A. section 602(a)(7)(A)(i)–(iii). The states have responded nearly universally, if unevenly, to Congress' invitation to enact FVO legislation. According to a 1997 survey conducted by the NOW Legal Defense and Education Fund, thirty states have adopted the FVO in their new welfare plans, and 18 more have some form of domestic violence coverage. Six states, however, have declined to adopt any domestic violence exemptions at all. *See* Imperial, *supra* note 55, at 26 (summarizing NOW LDEF information). Maria Imperial's own survey produced somewhat different results. *Id.* at 27-34 (state-by-state analysis, including breakdown of which of the federal FVO components each state had adopted). For more information on FVO state implementation, *see* JODY RAPHAEL & SHEILA HAENNICKE, KEEPING BATTERED WOMEN SAFE THROUGH THE WELFARE-TO-WORK JOURNEY: HOW ARE WE DOING? A REPORT ON THE IMPLEMENTATION OF POLICIES FOR BATTERED WOMEN IN STATE TEMPORARY ASSISTANCE FOR NEEDY FAMILIES (TANF) PROGRAMS, FINAL REPORT <http://www.ssw.umich.edu/trapped/pubs_fvo1999.pdf>.

violence." Second, states may "refer such individuals to counseling and supportive services." Finally, states are authorized to waive program requirements, where enforcing them would compromise a survivor's safety or
penalize her for having been a victim of violence.[57] Unless a survivor has the
misfortune to live in a state with no FVO, she will be asked whether she has or
is experiencing violence, or should volunteer that information, to be eligible
for these significant services.[58]

There are two threshold issues survivors should anticipate in the course of
the initial screening. This first is whether the survivor's history satisfies the
criteria set out in her state's FVO statute defining "battery or extreme cruelty."
In states that follow the federal model, "battery or extreme cruelty" is defined
as follows:

I. physical acts that resulted in, or threatened to result in, physical injury
    to the individual;
II. sexual abuse;
III. sexual activity involving a dependent child;
IV. being forced as the caretaker relative of a dependent child to engage in
    nonconsensual sexual acts or activities;
V. threats, or attempts at, physical or sexual abuse;

---

57. The statute does not limit the kinds of program requirements that may be waived
under this section, but recites as examples "time limits (for so long as necessary) for
individuals receiving assistance, residency requirements, child support cooperation
requirements, and family cap provisions." *See* 42 U.S.C.A. section 602 (a)(7)(A)(iii).
58. I cannot overstate the importance of preparing a survivor for the possibility that
she may have to raise these issues herself in meetings with her caseworker. Procedures
for screening and referral may be inconsistent or nonexistent in some areas, even in
states which have enacted comprehensive FVO provisions. A RAND Corporation
survey of implementation procedures in California indicated, for example, that only
43% of large counties in California had operational domestic violence screening
procedures in place as of 1998. RAND CORP., WELFARE REFORM IN CALIFORNIA:
RESULTS OF THE 1998 ALL-COUNTY IMPLEMENTATION SURVEY 13-14 (Patricia A.
Ebener & Jacob Alex Klerman eds., 1999). In a study of CalWORKS recipients
conducted in 1999, "most participants did not know about the availability of other
supportive services, such as domestic violence, substance abuse treatment, or mental
health counseling." Equal Rights Advocates, *supra* note 6, at 21. One study participant
reported that, "I didn't find. . . out [about domestic violence services] until after they
almost dumped me out of the GAIN program." *Id.* at 20. Only 15% of participants had
received information about domestic violence services; 13% about mental health
counseling, and only 10% about substance abuse treatment. *Id.* at 21.

VI. mental abuse; or

VII. neglect or deprivation of medical care.[59]

Sadly, most women with histories in prostitution will have little difficulty identifying incidents like these in her own life. These criteria for brutal violence describe routine events for prostituted women.[60]

More difficult to grasp is how much worse it has been for them: the sadistic torture, the thousands of prostitution encounters an individual woman may have experienced, the aggression and contempt she has had to absorb day after day after day. The "me, too" hazard, in this context, is that the survivor has suffered so much violence–so much more than women who haven't been prostituted–that its impact is denied and the survivor's continued risk of injury underestimated. "Ordinary" abuse, like that contemplated by the FVO, can feel trivial by comparison, for survivor and caregiver both. More than once, I have found myself nodding as a survivor told me a pimp had "only" raped and beaten her, colluding with her minimization of the violence she has suffered. The challenge is not in identifying incidents in the survivor's history that fall within the scope of the FVO, but to hold the survivor's memories and feelings with respect and compassion.

The TANF staff may be less accepting of the survivor's account, either because the survivor is not believed, or because the bureaucracy requires more documentation to justify FVO assistance. In either case, the survivor must convince the agency of the facts on which she wishes to rest the determination of extreme cruelty. Again, the states have adopted a variety of forms of proof sufficient for this purpose, from simple sworn statements by the survivor, to mandates that women support their allegations with medical, psychological, or mental health reports, court orders, or police reports.[61]

---

59. 42 U.S.C.A. section 608(a)(7)(C)(iii). California has adopted a slightly more inclusive definition, adding stalking to the list, and deleting the phrase "as the caretaker relative of a dependent child" from (IV). CAL. WEL. & INST. SECTION 11495.12. The latter change would include pregnant women who are not yet mothers, and dependent children themselves, among those who might be covered by the clause. For an overview of the California legislation, *see* Rebecca S. Engrav, *CalWORKS: California's Response to Welfare Reform*, 13 BERK. WOM. L. J. 268 (1998).

60. *See generally supra* note 1, and accompanying text.

61. *Compare* CAL. WEL. & INST. section 11495.25 (victim sworn statement sufficient) *with* NEW MEXICO STAT. 27-2B-6 (documentation required to substantiate victim statement).

The more rigorous proof requirements can present a myriad of difficulties for survivors. Medical documentation may be lacking, since prostituted women are routinely deprived of access to medical care, or have been afraid to seek it for fear of retaliation. No police reports may exist, since prostitution survivors rarely report violent incidents to law enforcement. Survivors benefit infrequently from supportive services available to other women through battered women's shelters, and often feel that shelters are not available to them.[62] Survivors may feel trapped in a dilemma: their credibility impugned if they disclose a prostitution history, but impugned again if they withhold the very information that makes sense out of their experience and choices.

This may be a crucial point at which the survivor and her therapist need to address the therapist's role in advocating for the survivor. Both need to decide if the therapist should disclose information and session records to substantiate the survivor's account. From a practical standpoint, a letter from her therapist may be crucial to establishing the survivor's entitlement to FVO programs and waivers.

Finally, a survivor may face tremendous obstacles in identifying publicly as a victim of violence, especially prostitution violence, and especially in a social services setting.[63] "It took me three years just to be able–in a support group with other women–to be able to talk about what happened."[64] Years of minimizing the assaults, coercions, and losses she endured in prostitution, or feeling that her difficulties are minor or self-inflicted, may impede her willingness to access services and support. Too, the survivor may fear that these disclosures will be used against her, that she will lose her children (again) if staff knows she has a history in prostitution. She may also fear that she will be forced immediately to sever all connections with perpetrators, before this seems to be a workable or desirable goal to her:

---

62. Prostitution survivors have difficulty accessing battered women's shelters. Even a telephone call can be difficult to negotiate safely. Transportation is unreliable, and keeping scheduled appointments practically impossible. Prostituted women often feel stigmatized and out of place in shelter environments, and shelters may be unresponsive to survivors' chemical dependence and legal vulnerabilities.
63. *See* Howard, *supra* note 61, at 146 (discussing reluctance of battered women to so identify within the CalWORKS application process); Patricia Cole & Sarah M. Buell, *Safety and Financial Security for Battered Women: Necessary Steps for Transitioning from Welfare to Work*, 7 GEO. J. ON POVERTY LAW & POLICY 307, 323-326 (2000) (addressing barriers to communication between advocates and survivors in addressing issues of violence in social service settings).
64. Martha Davis, Prema Mathai-Davis, Diane Dugon, Dorothy Roberts & Sarah Buell, *Four Cornerstones to Ending Women's Poverty*, 7 GEO. J. ON POVERTY LAW & POLICY 199, 218 (2000) (remarks of Sarah Buell).

We assume that for battered women their number one goal must be leaving the batterer, getting a protective order, filing for divorce. I wasn't ready to make those kind of decisions. He's saying: "I'm going to kill you if you go to court." Are you going to move in with an AK-47 and ten state troopers? Then don't talk to me about how I need to go to court and get a protective order.[65]

On all of these fronts, caregivers need to strategize with survivors regarding how, and if, these disclosures can serve as a source of power, and not as occasions of vulnerability and revictimization.

2. ECONOMIC ASSETS AND CAPACITIES

A survivor's economic status is the second major "naming" issue that both the SSI and TANF programs compel her to address. Both SSI and TANF programs require applicants to declare their incomes, and will deny benefits to applicants whose incomes exceed a certain amount. The two programs define those income limits in different ways, though, creating different kinds of eligibility concerns for prostitution survivors. These concerns have to do with how the money she has received , or could receive, in prostitution will be treated under each benefit system. Under the TANF program, income is treated as a measure of how needy the recipient family is. Under the SSI program, income is treated instead as a measure of how disabled the recipient individual is. For prostitution survivors, income has a perverse relationship both to neediness, and to disability. The more enmeshed she is with prostitution, the more money may be coming into her hands; yet, at the same time and for the same reason, the more truly needy and disabled she may have become. Fair evaluation of her benefits eligibility will depend on clear explanation of these circumstances.

In this section, I explore how caregivers can assist survivors in presenting their financial situation to agency staffs. The process is complicated, because everyone involved–caregiver, survivor, and the agencies–may begin with strong commitments to the "let's pretend" version of the Hide the Prostitution dance, when it comes to the theme of prostitution and money. All may assume that prostitution has been a lucrative occupation for the survivor, beneficial to her financially if in no other way. This is rarely, if ever, the case.

---

65. *Id.* at 219.

a. TANF: income as presumptive independence.

The primary goal of the TANF program is to provide assistance to needy families.[66] Once a survivor qualifies as a family, as we examined in the previous section, she must then show that her family is financially needy.[67] TANF evaluators will look to family income and the valuation of property to determine need.[68] By measuring need by the yardstick of income, Congress assumes–sensibly in most cases perhaps–that the higher a person's income, the less needy the person is. For women in prostitution, though, this correlation, between income and neediness, holds only weakly. The higher a survivor's apparent income, the more needy–even materially–she may be. A survivor may perceive this disconnect, but have genuine difficulty disentangling why she is so achingly poor, when so much money passes through her hands. Caregivers may share this confusion. Further exploration of how money really works in the survivor's life can help the caregiver grasp her vulnerable economic position, and also help the survivor to more clearly describe her situation to TANF caseworkers.

An important question to raise with the survivor is what she thinks would happen if she stopped making the money. For many prostituted women, the answer is that she will be beaten or otherwise "disciplined" for failing to bring enough money home. For a woman in this position, her so-called "income" functions as a key element in a forced labor system. Clearly, there is no connection between the survivor's level of income, and her need. For others, prostitution and substance dependency have become enmeshed, such that the drug and alcohol use that got her through the prostitution, has become one reason that she continues to prostitute.[69] Further, increasing shame and feelings of defeat can accompany a woman's progressive economic involvement in prostitution. The prostitution money mires survivors ever more deeply in a downward spiral of despair, illness, and isolation. Survivors may also overstate the amounts of money they ever actually possess, even setting aside the sums

---

66. 42 U.S.C.A. section 601(a)(1).

67. State law, not federal law, fixes the standard for need eligibility. Federal law requires only that the state fix objective criteria for eligibility, and provide some procedure for review of benefit denials. *See* 42 U.S.C.A. section 602.

68. Income limits vary widely among the states. Ceilings range from $1,641 in Hawaii, to $205 in Alabama, for families of three. If a family has an income above these ceilings, the family is presumptively ineligible for benefits. *See* THE URBAN INSTITUTE, INITIAL TANF INCOME ELIGIBILITY THRESHOLDS (2002) (available at http:\\www.urban.org).

69. *See infra* notes 91-94 and accompanying text for more detailed discussion of alcohol and drug use among prostituted women.

given over to pimps and boyfriends. Prostituted women are constantly robbed, having their clothes stolen or damaged, and losing their homes. Among the "hurts" of prostitution, as one woman painfully explained, are "being raped, getting beaten up and stuff," and also "[g]etting stranded, having your clothes stolen, having your money stolen, robbed at gunpoint, whatever, all of that. Just hurt."[70] Daily living expenses are enormously high. Clothing costs, strip club stage fees, the outlays for palliative drugs and alcohol, and the more "hidden" costs of shelter (often temporary motel rooms), fast food, and the recurring replacement costs of abandoned or stolen possessions add up quickly. In all events, the money is not available for meeting a survivor's basic survival needs; and compromises her ability to escape sexually and physically violent conditions in her life.[71] Her income, in other words, measures not escalating freedom and independence, but charts instead intensifying need, threat of violence, and loss of control.

But how to express these economic realities to a survivor's TANF caseworker in a meaningful way? Can the survivor's caseworker bend the TANF income limits, in light of the survivor's real poverty? I think she can. As we have seen, the Family Violence Option voices Congress' concern that the TANF program not be implemented in such a way so as to force women to choose between benefits eligibility, and continued risks to her safety. Survivors should explain to their TANF caseworkers that treating the survivor's earnings from prostitution as income places her in an even worse position: she loses both eligibility, and any hope of future safety. Her caseworker should be able to waive the income limits for TANF eligibility under the FVO, just like any other program requirement that puts a survivor at risk of abuse can be waived. Since income measures of need are not mandated by federal law, exceptions to the income limit are within the discretion of the states to grant.

70. Lisa E. Sanchez, *Boundaries of Legitimacy: Sex, Violence, Citizenship and Community in a Local Sexual Economy*, 22 L. & SOC. INQUIRY 543, 561 (1998).
71. In this discussion, I have focused on how the amount of a survivor's real income compares to her level of need, for purposes of evaluating her TANF eligibility. The approach I suggest here might also be helpful to a survivor who is grappling with the question whether she can afford to leave prostitution. Careful discussion about where the money actually goes may assist a survivor in coming to more centered understanding of the economic toll that prostitution actually takes on her. If she decides she can move out of prostitution by becoming eligible for assistance, the panic and loss of control she may feel about foregoing the cash associated with prostitution may become more manageable for her if she has come to terms with the real economic implications of her decision.

b. SSI: income as presumptively productive activity.

A different kind of "let's pretend" complication awaits survivors who apply for SSI benefits. As we have seen, the basic eligibility issue for SSI applicants is whether they suffer from a disability. In the SSI system, an applicant may be treated as non-disabled for the sole reason that her income is too high. Here is how it works. The first question the agency asks in deciding if an applicant is disabled is whether the applicant is engaged in "substantial gainful activity" ("SGA"), producing income of at least $740 per month.[72] If the applicant is earning $740 or more monthly, she will be presumed not to be disabled.[73] The only limit on this principle lies in the definition of what economic activities are "substantial" and "gainful." Generally, work that "involves doing significant physical or mental activities" is considered "substantial"; "gainful" work is "the kind of work usually done for pay or profit."[74] It does not matter, in and of itself, whether the work is legal or illegal.[75]

If the survivor is currently prostituting, the amount of money she takes in may well exceed the SGA limit. Here again, though, the correlation between disability and earning power, presumed by the law, is inverted for prostitution survivors. The law presumes that the more a person can earn, the less he or she is disabled. For prostituted women, the presumption runs the other way: the *more* exposure to prostitution a woman experiences, the *more* her traumatic stress, depression, and the greater her resulting disability, since post-traumatic stress symptoms, dissociative anxiety and depressive disorders are the emotional consequences of prostitution. Disabling dissociative symptoms are paradoxically more "functional" in prostitution: the more dissociated a woman is,

---

72. 42 U.S.C.A. section 423(e)(1) ("No benefit shall be payable . . . to an individual for any month . . . in which he engages in substantial gainful activity"); 20 C.F.R. 416.974(a)(b)(2) (indexing SGA ceiling to national average wage; fixed at $740 for 2001).
73. 20 C.F.R. section 416.920(a) ("If you are doing substantial gainful activity, we will determine that you are not disabled."); *see also* 416.920(b)("If you are working and the work you are doing is substantial gainful activity, we will find that you are not disabled regardless of your medical condition or your age, education, and work experience.").
74. *See* 20 C.F.R. section 416.972(a) (defining "substantial work activity"); 20 C.F.R. section 416.973(a) (substantial work activity is that which requires "expertise, skills, supervision, and responsibilities"); 20 C.F.R. section 416.972(b) (defining "gainful work activity").
75. *See* 1994 U.S.C.C.A.N. (108 Stat.) 1464, 1499(amending 42 U.S.C.A. section 423(d)(4)). *See* Margaret A. Baldwin, *"A Million Dollars and an Apology": Prostitution and Public Benefits Claims*, 10 HASTINGS WOMEN'S L. J. 189 (1999) (explaining the legality/ illegality distinction in SGA doctrine).

the "better" she can perform as a fantasy object for johns.[76] The same holds for drug and alcohol abuse:

> The most inebriated prostitutes on the street appear to be the most successful in attracting clients. Women who appear entirely powerless and incapable of setting the boundaries of sexual activity to take place will attract men who may wish to legitimate an act of sexual abuse by the payment of cash.[77]

The SSI rules confront a survivor with a bewildering, cruel, and demeaning view of herself. According to the federal government, a survivor must feel better, not worse, the more she prostitutes. In this way, the SSI program itself endorses and reinforces denial of the impact of prostitution on survivors.

The legal terrain here is discouraging. Three federal cases have addressed the question whether money received in prostitution counts toward the presumptive SGA income limit.[78] All three held that the claimant's income from prostitution barred her eligibility for benefits. All three survivors based their disability claims on drug and alcohol dependence. All three had prostituted for many years. Melinda Bell was 32 years old at the time of her SSI appeal, had eight or nine years of school, had never had a job other than prostitution, and had used drugs since she was fourteen. She prostituted 5 nights a week, and earned between $800 and $1,000 a month.[79] Cynthia Love was 44 when she applied for SSI, had a 10th grade education, and performed "four acts of prosti-

---

76. Vednita Carter and Evelina Giobbe describe how prostitution requires women to dissociate themselves from their bodies:

> The repeated act of submitting to the sexual demands of strangers, with whom she wouldn't otherwise choose to engage in even the most superficial of social interactions, necessitates that a woman alienate her mind from her body. To be a prostitute is to be an object in the marketplace: a three-dimensional blank screen upon which men project and act out their sexual dominance.

Carter & Giobbe, *supra* note 1, at 46.
77. RETHINKING PROSTITUTION: PURCHASING SEX IN THE 1990'S 175 (Graham Scambler & Annette Scambler eds., 1997), *quoting* C. L. Morrison, S. Ruben, & D. Wakefield, *Alcohol and Drug Misuse in Prostitutes*, 90 ADDICTION 292 (1995) (letter).
78. *See Speaks v. Sec'y of Health and Human Services*, 855 F. Supp. 1108 (C.D. Cal. 1994); *Love v. Sullivan*, 1992 WL 86193 (N.D. Ill. April 22, 1992); *Bell v. Commissioner of Social Security*, 105 F.3d 244 (6th Cir. 1996).
79. *See Bell*, 105 F.3d at 246-247.

tution a day," generating $45 to $80.[80] Veda Speaks had been in prostitution for over 20 years, and made over $600 a month.[81] All three cases rejected the survivors' claims, based on the statutory SGA income presumption. In Melinda Bell's case, the court expressly declined to consider "whether [Bell's] prostitution was symptomatic of serious mental disorder and driven by her drug addiction."[82] Nor did the court treat as relevant the question whether Bell was capable of earning money in any other way, while acknowledging that "the Secretary's denial of [Bell's] claim for SSI–without deciding that the plaintiff is capable of any other activity–is tantamount to telling her that it is expected that in the future she will earn her living through prostitution."[83]

There are paths through these legal thickets, based on three different legal arguments that question the link between a survivor's income, and her presumed well-being. One argument asks the court to take a genuine look at the relationship between the survivor's drug use, and the money she takes in prostitution. An argument can be made that the amount of a survivor's income that she uses to buy drugs should be treated like an occupational expense–a cost that she must incur to make the prostitution minimally tolerable.[84] For many prostitution survivors, this exactly describes how drugs function in her prostitution. Survivors take drugs to tolerate prostitution, and drugs cost money.[85] Explaining her income in these terms should assist SSI evaluators to look behind the cultural myths that treat prostitution as if it were a big party, or as if prostituted women's drug use is nothing but a lifestyle preference.

A second argument confronts the myth that prostitution is "work," thus challenging whether money derived from prostitution should be treated as income. The survivor's task here is to explain that the activities comprising prostitution are not "substantial" mental or physical exertions, as the SGA rule requires. A precedential case involving the earnings of a drug courier helps ex-

---

80. *See Love*, 1992 WL 86193 at *3.

81. *See Speaks*, 855 F. Supp. at 1112.

82. *Bell*, 105 F.3d at 246-47.

83. *Id.* at 1111.

84. This analysis is based on a suggestion offered by one court, that the amount of money a claimant spends on drugs might be deductible from SGA income, if drug costs are an occupational expense for the claimant. *See Dotson v. Sullivan*, 813 F.Supp. 651 (C.D.Ill. 1995). The court implied that the claimant, who made his income from stealing, might have been able to deduct the amount of money he used for drugs from his SGA income, but found that the claimant "did not use drugs *in order to steal.*" Prostituted women, in contrast , *do* use drugs in order to prostitute.

85. *See infra* notes 91-94 and accompanying text.

plain what is meant by "substantial" exertion.[86] The court held that the earnings made by the drug courier claimant did not come from "substantial" exertion, and therefore did not count toward the claimant's SGA. The claimant was described as functioning only as an "instrumentality" in drug deals, whose role it was to sit in a car for less than an hour a day. The claimant's activities "did not require any significant mental or physical exertion," he "did no planning," he "did not use his own money for the transactions," and received his payment in drugs.[87]

The non-occupational characteristics the court recites here are more typical of prostitution than is ordinarily acknowledged. Prostitution has become so shrouded in occupational jargon, often as a strategy for normalizing it as a job like any other, that the way prostitution is lived out in practice is usually entirely lost. Survivors often refer to the complete irrelevance of any skill or personal competency to what they are doing in prostitution, this being another demeaning aspect of the experience. Describing what it was like for her to strip, one woman said to me that she couldn't dance at all, not at all, but the men waved the money and shouted at her all the same. Being an "instrumentality" defines what prostitution is: control of the transaction in the hands of johns, the "work day" consisting of more or less provisional tactics to evade the prostitution as long as possible and to get through it as necessary. By explaining what the "work" of prostitution is in these real terms, the survivor can do a great service in eroding the myth that prostitution is a "job," and in providing a more authentic understanding of the nature of the "work."

Just because prostitution isn't a job, though, doesn't mean that prostitution is nothing at all. It's just more like a war, than a job.[88] And the strongest legal basis for challenging the SGA limit takes up that theme. The legal argument goes under the name of the"heroic effort" exception to the SGA rule. The "heroic effort" principle allows the agency to disregard the claimant's earning level, in cases where, "were it not for effort . . . far beyond the call of duty [s]he would not be employed at all."[89] The exception recognizes that:

---

86. *See Carrao v. Shalala,* 20 F.3d 943 (9th Cir.1994).

87. *Id.* at 949.

88. This is more than a metaphor from a mental health standpoint. In the Farley and Barkan study, prostitution survivors experienced PTSD symptoms more intense (54.9) than treatment-seeking Vietnam veterans (50.6), and Persian Gulf war veterans(34.8). Farley & Barkan, *supra* note 1.

89. *Storyk v. Sec'y of Health, Education and Welfare,* 462 F. Supp.152, 158 (S.D. N.Y. 1978) (holding that the statute does not require "a finding that a person merely able to tolerate life, mostly in a prone position, is capable of SGA").

Even a terribly disabled person might be able to scrape [the SGA income limit] together by occasional work done at great personal cost, and yet by any realistic criterion he would be permanently disabled and should not be punished for his extraordinary exertions.[90]

Many survivors do understand their own strengths in facing and enduring the conditions that brought them into prostitution, and their courage in managing their lives under extremely difficult and damaging odds. Survivors speak in terms of exceptional endurance, that they did what they had to do: to keep themselves alive, to salvage their families. Survivors who were recruited or coerced into prostitution as adolescents were usually the victims of sexual and physical abuse at home–and were the kids who saw themselves as tough and smart enough to take care of themselves on the street. These women's lives have demanded "extraordinary exertion" beyond what many people could manage or can imagine. Tragically, these efforts are rewarded little if at all, and ultimately expose survivors to unconscionable risks of emotional damage, drug and alcohol abuse, disease, and death.

Telling this story requires the survivor to integrate both the costs exacted from her in prostitution, and the feelings of courage and endurance that may have accompanied those terrible losses. Like other combat veterans.

3. STIGMA

Public assistance is stigmatized in our society. Accounts offered by SSI recipients suggest that fear of stigma deters and troubles eligible applicants, in deeply painful ways:

I have thought a lot about whether I want the tag "disabled." . . . Despite the reward of direct credit to my bank account, and the later Medicare coverage, I was humbled; I felt shamed.

I told him [case manager] that I felt bad about going on disability because I felt like it was giving up. . . . I still don't like the idea of having to be on disability, but at this point, I have no other way to go.[91]

---

90.   *Jones v. Shalala*, 21 F.3d 191 (7th Cir. 1994).
91.   Sue E. Estroff, Catherine Zimmer, William S. Lachicotte, Julia Benoit, and Donald L. Patrick, *"No Other Way to Go": Pathways to Disability Income Application Among Persons with Severe, Persistent Mental Illness*, in MENTAL DISORDER, WORK DISABILITY, AND THE LAW 55 (Richard J. Bonnie & John Monahan eds. 1997) (quoting SSI recipients).

Prostitution survivors must confront these feelings, in common with all SSI and TANF recipients. In addition, survivors must come to terms with special exclusionary rules in each program, that may have an especially harsh impact on prostituted women as a group: exclusions based on drug or alcohol dependency, and drug-related incarceration. These rules place survivors under a double stigma: already stigmatized for needing assistance, they are stigmatized again as undeserving and weak.

a. SSI: Prohibited diagnoses.

Women and girls rarely endure being used in prostitution without resort to the numbing effects of drugs and alcohol. Drug and alcohol dependency are to prostitution as black lung is to coal mining. In one study of the health impacts of prostitution, nearly all of the women described themselves as chemically addicted, most frequently to alcohol and crack cocaine.[92] Half the women reported that they were high "all the time" while soliciting and turning tricks; 34% said they were high at least half the time. Seventy-eight percent stated that they began using crack while involved in prostitution.[93] Women brutally beaten by abusers may resort to drugs and alcohol as a palliative for the pain of injuries and broken bones:

> I would be in serious pain and I couldn't stop screaming. At first I denied and tried to hide the abuse, but he would beat me up to keep me quiet! But sometimes I'd have broken bones, so I couldn't just be quiet. He would go out and come home with "medicine," which I think was initially legit, and I fell for his acting like he was taking care of me. He'd shoot me up with it. He started buying morphine on the street. It really helped the physical pain and the emotional pain. And soon I needed more and more to numb the pain of broken bones that weren't set, including a broken arm. Now I try to get it on my own even when he isn't beating me because I am addicted.[94]

---

92. *See* PARRIOTT, *supra* note 47, at 15.

93. *Id.*

94. BETH E. RICHIE, COMPELLED TO CRIME: THE GENDER ENTRAPMENT OF BATTERED BLACK WOMEN 125 (1996). *See also* JAMES A. INCIARDI, DOROTHY LOCKWOOD & ANNE E. POTTIEGER, WOMEN AND CRACK-COCAINE 24-26 (1993) (summarizing data on women's use of drugs for self-medication stemming from trauma related to sexual abuse, pre-existing depression).

Substance abuse recovery programs are crucial for women moving out of prostitution. In separate studies, 67% of U.S. respondents and 82% of Canadian respondents reported that they wanted and would participate in substance abuse recovery support, if programs were available to them.[95]

Current SSI policy, though, treats addiction in a strictly punitive way, no matter the cause or context. In 1996, Congress ordered that benefits be revoked entirely from persons for whom drug or alcohol addiction is "material to the determination of disability."[96] This does not mean, however, that a survivor will automatically be turned down for SSI benefits because she has experienced substance abuse problems in the past, or is currently dependent on drugs or alcohol. The agency will ask "whether [the agency] would still find [the claimant] disabled if [she] stopped using drugs or alcohol."[97] Thus, the survivor need not have actually stopped using drugs or alcohol under this test to qualify for assistance.[98] Further, whether the claimant's drug or alcohol addiction caused other physical or psychological impairments, which are currently disabling, is irrelevant.[99] "The issue is not whether those conditions

---

95. *See* Melissa Farley and Jackie Lynne, *Prostitution in Vancouver: Violence and the Colonization of First Nation's Women* (2002) (submitted for publication) (Canadian study); Farley & Barkan, *supra* note 1 (United States study).

96. Section 105, P.L. 104-121, enacted March 29, 1996; codified at 42 U.S.C.A. section 1382(c)(a)(3)(J). It has not always been so. Before 1994, drug and alcohol dependency disabilities were treated on a par with any other disabling condition. In 1994, Congress began to retreat from that position, limiting the length of time that persons disabled by drug and alcohol could receive benefits, and mandating treatment *See* P.L. 103-296; *see also* HOUSE REPORT 103-60 (describing provisions, intended effect of new transitional policy).

97. 20 C.F.R. section 416.935(b)(1). The test is applied as follows:

> In making this determination, we will evaluate which of your current physical and mental limitations, upon which we based your current disability determination, would remain if you stopped using drugs or alcohol and then determine whether any or all of your remaining limitations would be disabling.

20 C.F.R. section 416.935(b)(2).

98. *See Jackson v. Apfel*, 162 F.3d 533, 537(8th Cir. 1998). Courts have noted, though, that it is more difficult to apply the materiality test when the claimant is still using. *Id.*

99. *See Lee v. Callahan*, 133 F.3d 927 (9th Cir. 1998).

are alcohol related, but whether in his present condition [the survivor] would be disabled because of them if [s]he stopped drinking."[100] These are not hollow exceptions. The Social Security Administration's statistics indicate that 60% of people who had received benefits based on substance abuse related disability prior to 1996 have continued to receive benefits based on another psychiatric condition.[101]

Survivors face at least three hidden risks in presenting substance abuse issues to SSI evaluators. First, it will be hard to predict how the agency will evaluate her substance abuse history, since each decision will "strongly depend on the facts of each case."[102] Second, the survivor may already have applied for SSI under the prior law, claiming drug or alcohol addiction as the basis of her impairment. At that time, she may have chosen not to disclose her experience in prostitution as the context in which her substance abuse emerged. Now, she is put to the task both of coming forward with information about the prostitution, and explaining her prior reticence to do so.[103] Third, agency decision makers and judges do not like to apply formulas, they like to make judgments. And the judgment closest to hand–the moral censure of drug and alcohol dependence underlying the exclusion of addiction from SSI coverage–may

---

100. *Id.*; *see also Ball v. Masanqri*, 2001 WL 668941 (9th Cir. 2001); *Sousa v. Callahan*, 143 F.3d 1240, 1242 (9th Cir. 1998).
101. *See* Paul Davies, Howard Iams, & Kalman Rupp, *The Effect of Welfare Reform on SSA's Disability Programs: Design of Policy Evaluation and Early Evidence*, 63 Soc. Sec. Bulletin 3 (No. 1, 2000). Congressional staff statistics are less encouraging. The House Ways and Means Committee report on SSI for the year 2000 asserts that only 39.9% of people who previously received benefits for DA&A disabilities continued to remain eligible. *See* U.S. HOUSE OF REPRESENTATIVES, COMMITTEE ON WAYS AND MEANS, 2000 GREEN BOOK: BACKGROUND MATERIAL AND DATA ON PROGRAMS WITHIN THE JURISDICTION OF THE COMMITTEE ON WAYS AND MEANS 254 (hereinafter 2000 GREEN BOOK).
102. *See e.g. Brown v. Apfel*, 192 F.3d 492, 499 (5th Cir. 1999) (noting that SSI eligibility where claimant has drug or alcohol history will "strongly depend upon the facts in each case").
103. This seems to have occurred in one case, where a court found less than credible a claim brought by a woman who initially alleged alcoholism as the disabling condition affecting her, but later altered her claim to one based on PTSD. *See Molloy v. Apfel*, 77 F.Supp.2d 1009 (S.D. Iowa 1999).

spill over into agency fact-finding regarding her eligibility.[104] For example, decisionmakers may be inclined to substitute a morally-charged inquiry into causation (did the drug addiction cause the impairment?) for the legally proper question of reversibility (will the impairment persist if the claimant stops using?).[105]

Ruthless moralistic judgments, of course, always threaten to engulf justice claims made by prostitution survivors. The stereotype of prostituted women as dope-besotted parasites is especially dangerous and misleading in this context. This stereotype can be challenged by presenting an account of a survivor's substance abuse in an historically encompassing account of her experience in prostitution. Typically, survivors' alcohol and drug use escalate as a coping strategy for dealing with intensifying levels of abuse from johns, strip club clientele, and other consumers and users. Research indicates that onset of substance abuse among domestic violence victims occurs almost entirely *after* the first reported episode of violence.[106] The same reactive strategies are prevalent among prostituted women. Substance abuse should be framed as a consequence, not cause, of the survivor's impairment–explaining the substance abuse itself in a realistic and empathetic way.

104. The entire exclusion has been challenged twice as an unconstitutional violation of equal protection. *See Ball v. Masanari*, 2001 WL 668941 (9th Cir. 2001); *Blackison v. Chater*, 1996 WL 101567 (E.D. 1996). Both challenges were rejected, on the ground that Congress could constitutionally conserve government resources by disfavoring addicted people in benefits programs. *Id.*
105. In at least one case, a reviewing court seems to have made this error already. The court denied benefits, relying on testimony from a physician that the claimant's substance abuse "preceded the emergence of any other mental impairment." *Gould v. Apfel*, 2000 WL 1499802 (D. Mo. 2000) (evaluating materiality of claimant's alcoholism to her dysthymia, depression, and personality disorder). The court's logic suggests that any disabilities caused by drug or alcohol dependence should be treated with the same disfavor as the underlying addiction. *Id.*
106. *See* EVAN STARK ET AL., WIFE ABUSE IN THE MEDICAL SETTING: AN INTRODUCTION FOR HEALTH PERSONNEL 18-19, NATIONAL CLEARINGHOUSE ON DOMESTIC VIOLENCE MONOGRAPH SERIES NO.7 (1981).

b. TANF: prohibited histories.

Women are not precluded from receiving TANF benefits based on drug or alcohol use,[107] but states may *permanently* disqualify anyone who has been convicted of a drug felony from TANF eligibility, [108] and most states do.[109] The federal lifetime ban is breathtakingly harsh,[110] and affects prostituted

---

107. Recipients may be required to participate in drug or alcohol treatment programs prior to job placement. *See e.g.* 42 U.S.C.A. section 608(b)(2)(A)(v) ("Individual Responsibility Plan," fixing commitments required of TANF recipients, may include a mandate that the recipient "undergo appropriate substance abuse treatment"). Recovery programs are important resources for women. In a California study, 34 out of 58 counties reported that substance abuse was of "particular concern" as a barrier to women returning to work. (Thirty-two counties registered similar concern regarding mental illness.) RAND CORP., WELFARE REFORM IN CALIFORNIA: RESULTS OF THE 1998 ALL-COUNTY IMPLEMENTATION SURVEY (Patricia A. Ebener & Jacob Alex Klerman, 1999). *See also* U.S. DEPT. OF HEALTH AND HUMAN SERVICES, OFFICE OF THE INSPECTOR GENERAL, FUNCTIONAL IMPAIRMENTS OF AFDC CLIENTS (1992) (reporting that alcohol and substance abuse are "among the most frequently cited functional impairments preventing recipients from leaving welfare and completing job training programs").

108. See 21 U.S.C.A. section 862a. The drug felony exclusion has been upheld against constitutional challenge, on the ground that the exclusion may deter drug use, and reduce fraud in the food stamp program. *See Turner v. Glickman*, 207 F.3d 419 (7th Cir. 2000).

The sponsor of the provision, Senator Phil Gramm of Texas, explained that the measure was intended to "ask[ ] a higher standard of behavior of people on welfare." *See* Cynthia Godsoe, *The Ban on Welfare for Felony Drug Offenders: Giving New Meaning to "Life Sentence,"* 13 BERK. WOM. L. J. 257, 259 (1998).

109. *See* NATIONAL GOVERNOR'S ASSOCIATION CENTER FOR BEST PRACTICES, SELECTED ELEMENTS IN STATE PLANS FOR TEMPORARY ASSISTANCE FOR NEEDY FAMILIES 19 (Nov. 20, 1997). Only thirteen states have chosen to opt out of the ban. *Id.* Of those states that have opted out, many have adopted less draconian, time-limited bans which may be waived if the person receives appropriate drug treatment. For example, Minnesota bans receipt of benefits for five years after a person has served a sentence for a drug felony, unless the applicant is in drug treatment, has completed a drug treatment program, or has been assessed not to need treatment. *See* MINN. STAT. section 256D.124.

110. Indeed, Cynthia Goodsoe quotes one California opponent of the ban, State Senator John Burton, describing the ban as "a very stupid, mean-spirited approach" that is the work of people who "are basically political cowards." *See* Goodsoe, *supra* note 108, at 262.

women with special severity. Prostituted women are at significant risk of substance abuse as their only palliative recourse.[111] I have been told by many prostitution survivors that drug dealing was their only way out prostitution, and that the risks associated with drug dealing were far less terrifying than the rapes and beating that they faced every day in prostitution. In addition, prostituted women suffer multiple special risk factors targeting them for over-prosecution for drug offenses: as women, as victims of exploitation, and as women with no other place of protection from violence other than prison. The impact of the "war on drugs" has fallen much more harshly on women than on men generally,[112] and most harshly of all on African American women.[113] Like other battered women, prostituted women are often enmeshed in drug dealing by exploitative intimates. Batterers and pimps use the same tactics of control and domination to inveigle a woman's participation in drug dealing, that are used to keep her in prostitution. One woman describes being beaten and threatened for over three years, to force her to act as a drug courier: "Twice I ran away from them and both times I got almost killed by them, so I quit, I just did whatever they wanted me to do."[114] Selling drugs can provide a source of supply for addicted abusers, and a means of moderating abusive attacks. "When we didn't have money for the drugs, I was in real trouble because his abuse got really out of control."[115] Drug dealing may be the only source of funds available to women trying to escape battering and prostitution, as was the case for this woman who had been battered by her husband for nine years:

> There is one and only one reason I am here . . . I sold drugs to try to get an apartment. [. . .] I tried working, but my husband found out, beat me up,

---

111. *See supra* notes 91-93 and accompanying text; *see also* Norweeta Milburn & Ann D'Ercole, *Homeless Women: Moving Toward a Comprehensive Model*, 46 AMERICAN PSYCHOLOGIST 1161, 1167 (1991).

112. *See* STEPHANIE GREENHOUSE, FACTS ABOUT WOMEN AND CRIME (NATIONAL VICTIMS RESOURCE CENTER/NCJRS 1991) (reporting FBI statistics on relative incarceration rates for drug offenses, comparing men and women). In 1995, over 40% of women incarcerated in the California prison system had been convicted of drug offenses; only 25% of men had drug offense convictions. *See* CALIFORNIA DEPARTMENT OF CORRECTIONS, OFFENDER INFORMATION SERVICES BRANCH (1996).

113. The greatest increase in jail, prison, and supervised populations between 1989-1994 was among African American women. There was a 828% increase in the number of African American women incarcerated for drug offenses in state prisons during that period. *See* MARC MAUER & TRACY HULING, YOUNG BLACK AMERICANS AND THE CRIMINAL JUSTICE SYSTEM FIVE YEARS LATER (1995).

114. LORI B. GIRSHICK, NO SAFE HAVEN: STORIES OF WOMEN IN PRISON 71 (1999).

115. RICHIE, *supra* note 86, at 124.

and took my money. There were lots of drugs in my neighborhood, and so it wasn't hard to find customers and suppliers. I never had an identity as a dealer, but I was starting to save enough money to move out. No one, so far, has believed me that I only did it as a way to get away from him. Oh well, at least being here I'm away.[116]

For women who come from environments of severe abuse, the only available battered women's shelter is prison, and crime a necessary pathway to physical safety and basic survival resources:

> I would have never thought it was true, but it's much better for me here than on the outside. In addition to "three hots and a cot," I have protection from him. He tried to get to me, but since he can't call, and I can refuse visits, and they search visitors, I am as safe from him here as I have ever been. I'm not saying it's a good place to be, but for women like me, it's better than living without guards.[117]

It strains credulity that Congress meant for these women to be punished even more, by refusing them TANF benefits. In principle, a state TANF agency should have the discretion to authorize a FVO waiver for the drug conviction exclusion, just as any other program regulation may be waived. Caregiver and survivor should work together carefully to develop that strategy. In particular, a survivor should explore whether her involvement with drugs was a result of a relationship that was coercive, consider how her boyfriend or pimp treated any resistance on her part to participation in his dealing, and what aims of her own, if any, she hoped to meet with her drug-related behavior.

This inquiry should have important healing significance for the survivor. In addition, this therapeutic work can lay the foundation for a broader challenge to the drug conviction exclusion, based on the state's FVO provisions. Even if

---

116. *Id.* at 125-126.
117. *Id.* at 130. Explicitly framing her criminal behavior as a way to escape *into* prison, a woman explains:

> With my kids' father I was beat for everything. He gave me a curfew that I had to abide by. I had to be in at eight o-clock in the summertime and I had to be in at six o'clock in the wintertime. And I just got beat if I'd come outside or someone spoke to me. I went through that for so long I felt prison was the place for me. But I was wrong. I felt that is was the only way that I could get away. That was why my crime was committed.

GIRSHICK, *supra* note 117, at 67.

the initial caseworker turns down the survivor's request, the state is required to provide some right of appeal. If the survivor has the fortitude, and safety, to pursue such an appeal, the effort could have important consequences for women across the nation facing these exclusions. The survivor may gain a successful claim for benefits, gain the strength that comes from telling the real story about painful events, and gain greater public visibility of the plight of women in prison. It is regrettable, though, that prostituted, poor and battered women have to bear this burden.

B. Establishing a Safe Environment.

Our focus so far has been the survivor's past history, and how she can safely tell it. In this section, our focus is on the future: how survivors can build new lives apart from prostitution. Building safe refuge is a crucial recovery aim for a survivor.[118] For prostitution survivors, who may have had little past experience of safe relationships or environments, the challenges facing her in doing so are great.[119] For survivors presently involved in abusive relationships, safety must be firmly grounded in "the self-protective capability of the victim. Until the victim has developed a detailed and realistic contingency plan and has demonstrated her ability to carry it out, she remains in danger of repeated abuse."[120] For many survivors, prison has served as the closest semblance to an accessible safe environment. Incested and abused within their families of origin, often homeless, enmeshed in complex, exploitative social networks, a woman's safety planning must encompass virtually every dimension of daily living. What for some trauma survivors is crisis intervention, for prostitution survivors may mean a wholesale re-creation of her entire life. She must find shelter, protect herself from both intimates and strangers, manage legal vulnerability, face loneliness, and obtain adequate financial resources.

In this section, I discuss how three features of a survivor's participation in SSI and TANF benefits programs implicate these ongoing safety concerns: the amount and timing of benefits, the role of family and other social networks, and the impact of employment mandates. For the survivor, all three parts of her

---

118. See HERMAN, *supra* note 1, at 162-172; Stuart W. Turner, Alexander C. McFarlane & Bessel A. Van der Kolk, *The Therapeutic Environment and New Explorations in the Treatment of Post-traumatic Stress Disorder, in* TRAUMATIC STRESS, *supra* NOTE 1, AT 537, 546-547; JILL DAVIES & ELEANOR LYON, SAFETY PLANNING WITH BATTERED WOMEN: COMPLEX LIVES/ DIFFICULT CHOICES (Claire M. Renzetti & Jeffrey L. Edleson eds., 1998).

119. HERMAN, *supra* note 1, at 165.

120. *Id.* at 169.

life–money, family, and work–were probably strongly enmeshed with the life of prostitution from which she is now trying to separate. Thus, the support–or lack of it–that she receives in these areas will be crucial to her success. Sadly, we have as yet few shared stories of recovery and healing among prostituted women. Isolated in their own struggles, survivors and their advocates can feel there is no life after prostitution, and that "living in longing" is all that the future can hold. In the following discussion, I advocate for several law reform measures that I believe would contribute to survivors' chances of future success.

a. Financial safety: personal autonomy as a condition for security.

Having enough money is a core safety issue for women. Economic survival is "central to the way . . . battered women think about their options."[121] Lack of money was the weightiest factor cited by battered immigrant Latina women impeding them from leaving a current relationship.[122] And having money to feed kids may be the most important concern facing poor women and structuring their choices:

> The most terrifying moments in my life were actually not having a gun held to my head. It was the third night of feeding my kids macaroni and ketchup, realizing we are out of macaroni and we're out of food stamps. And we're not getting any more for about a month.[123]

The best reason for applying for government benefits is to keep that wolf from the door. Neither the TANF nor SSI systems do well in reaching these goals, severely compromising prostituted women's safety needs.

i. Benefit amounts available to survivors.

In the last decade's debates over welfare reform, little was said about the real dollar amounts that poor mothers and disabled people receive from our beleaguered public assistance system. Politicians and pundits preferred to muse about whose fault it is that people are poor, rather than consider whether any of our programs in reality provide a secure and stable way of life for any recipi-

121. DAVIES & LYON, *supra* note 120, at 54.
122. Mary Ann Dutton, Leslye E. Orloff & Giselle Aguilar Hass, *Characteristics of Help-Seeking Behavior, Resource and Service Needs of Battered Immigrant Latinas: Legal and Policy Implications*, 7 GEO. J. ON POVERTY L. & POLICY 245, 269-70 (2000).
123. Davis *et al.*, *supra* note 76, at 219 (remarks of Sarah Buell).

ent. Neither SSI nor TANF does so. In 2000, the maximum SSI benefit for eligible individuals was $512 per month.[124] In the same year, the median TANF benefit was $421.[125] New babies born into TANF families fare even worse. Many states have adopted so-called "family cap" provisions, which eliminate or limit any increase in benefits with the addition of a new child born after a woman begins receiving assistance.[126] The Center for Law and Social Policy reports that more than 83,000 children have been born into families subject to family cap provisions, meaning that family members must get by on an even lower per-capita income.[127]

These are pitiful sums, given grudgingly. Benefit levels are inadequate to build financial security for any poor woman, and pose special safety risks for prostitution survivors. A prostitution survivor knows that these benefit levels signify contempt for her and her family. The family cap provisions, intended to deter survivors from having new babies and punishing them if they are born, impede survivors efforts to build new families and new futures. A survivor's ability to begin a relationship with a new baby may be the most hopeful and satisfying moment of her life, and aid her in stabilizing her exit from prostitution. Starved for family connections, and for financial security, women's safety needs go unmet and complicate her efforts to achieve a secure environment and manage dangerous relationships.

---

124. *See,* 2000 GREEN BOOK, *supra* note 101, at 213 (detailing basic benefit). A supplementary benefit is provided in all but seven states. *Id.* at 233. SSI has always been a better financial option than maternal assistance programs, though, and the gap grows increasingly great.

125. *Id.* at 389. In nineteen states, benefits for a parent and two children ranged from $350 to $450 per month. The most generous state is Alaska, with a monthly benefit of $923. The lowest benefit state is Alabama, where a mother with two children receives $164 per month. Texas comes in very low, at $201 per month for a family of three. The large urban states do little better than the national range, if at all. The Illinois benefit is only $377 monthly. New York City sets monthly benefits at $577; California, the largest system in the country, pays a monthly benefit of $626. *Id.* at 389-90.

126. Twenty-three states have adopted family cap provisions, eliminating or limiting any increase in benefits when a new child is born into a family already receiving assistance. Seventeen of these states prohibit any additional assistance for new children. *See* U.S. DEPARTMENT OF HEALTH AND HUMAN SERVICES, ADMINISTRATION FOR CHILDREN AND FAMILIES, TANF REPORT TO CONGRESS, Table 9.1, part B <http://www.acr.dhhs.gov/news/welfare/congress/tanft9.1b.htm>.

127. SHELLEY STARK & JODIE LEVIN-EPSTEIN, CENTER FOR LAW AND SOCIAL POLICY, EXCLUDED CHILDREN: FAMILT CAP IN A NEW ERA (1999), http://www.clasp.org/pubs/teens/excluded children.htm>; *see also* Diana Romero & Paul H. Wise, *Sex, Reproduction and Welfare Reform,* 7 GEO. J. ON POVERTY L. & POLICY 379, 381-83 (2000).

ii. Waiting for SSI; running out of TANF

The process of securing and retaining benefits is a difficult and risky journey. For SSI applicants, the eligibility process is fraught with delay and discouragement. The agency routinely denies benefits to nearly 70% of all applicants on their initial application,[128] in "denial letters so cursory in content and tone that many claimants are so devastated that they become suicidal."[129] An applicant must return to seek an agency "reconsideration," bolstered with extensive medical evidence documenting her condition, and endure several months of delay. Few denials are reversed at this stage; approximately 85% of reconsideration requests are again denied.

If a survivor can hold out for another level of appeal–scheduled sometimes years after her initial application–her patience may ultimately be rewarded. The reversal rate at the third stage is as high as 68%, and the formal hearing process convened at that stage can be a forum for a dignified and responsive consideration of her circumstances:

> [T]he persistent effort to secure benefits to alleviate poverty and obtain desperately needed medical care constitutes the first concerted effort many disabled individuals have ever made as agents on their own behalf. . . . For such claimants the experience of hearing their representative stating their claim in a positive light before a judge can be tremendously empowering. It can substantially restore to such historically disempowered claimants the voice and, with that, the spirit needed

---

128. U.S. GENERAL ACCOUNTING OFFICE, SOCIAL SECURITY DISABILITY: SSA MUST HOLD ITSELF ACCOUNTABLE FOR CONTINUED IMPROVEMENTS IN DECISION-MAKING (1997); *see also* 2000 GREEN BOOK, *supra* note 101, at 30 (reporting similar statistics for 1999). For a detailed examination of the process of SSI decision making, *see generally* LINDA G. MILLS, A PENCHANT FOR PREJUDICE: UNRAVELING BIAS IN JUDICIAL DECISION-MAKING 27-37 (1999) (detailing adjudicative process and statistical decision patterns).

129. Durston & Mills, *supra* note 43, at 140. They report that:

> In the early 1980's when the Reagan Administration terminated benefits of over 500,000 disability recipients, at least six suicides were directly attributable to what amounted to mostly illegal terminations.

Id. at 144 n.101 (citing MARTHA DERTHICK, AGENCY UNDER STRESS: THE SOCIAL SECURITY ADMINISTRATION IN AMERICAN GOVERNMENT (1990)).

to tell their stories fully and openly at the hearing and to view themselves as effective public personae.[130]

Survivors need to be prepared–emotionally and financially–for the "long haul" commitments and short term rejections characteristic of the SSI adjudication system. Serving up this confusing stew of sticks and carrots, mixed signals and stubborn refusals, no wonder the disability determination system is "probably the largest adjudicative system in the world."[131] No one knows when they have really lost, or when they might really win, so continuing to try is always the best policy.

TANF recipients may find the benefits system responsive in the beginning, but face discouragement if they continue to need help over an extended period, as prostitution survivors likely will. All federal benefits will be withdrawn after a specified period, under a provision of the TANF law called the "durational limit." The durational limit places a 60-month lifetime cap on the length of time a TANF family can receive federal funds.[132] The 60-month limit is a ceiling, and does not restrict states from imposing even more restrictive time limits. Twenty-one states have done so.[133] Many women and children across the country have now reached the end of their assistance eligibility. Those families must find immediate alternative assistance, or explore whether the state durational limit can be extended.[134]

---

130. Durston & Mills, *supra* note 38, at 140-141. *See also* Lucie E. White, *Subordination, Rhetorical Survival Skills, and Sunday Shoes: Notes on the Hearing of Mrs. G.*, 38 BUFF. L. REV. 1 (1990); Anthony V. Alfieri, *Reconstructive Poverty Law Practice : Learning Lessons of Client Narrative*, 100 YALE L. J. 2107 (1991).

131. *Heckler v. Campbell*, 461 U.S. 458, 461 n. 2 (1983) (quoting JERRY L. MASHAW ET AL., SOCIAL SECURITY HEARINGS AND APPEALS: A STUDY OF THE SOCIAL SECURITY ADMINISTRATION HEARING SYSTEM xi (1978).

132. *See* 42 U.S.C.A. section 608(a)(7)(A); *see also* 45 C.F.R. section 264.1 (reiterating 60 month durational limit; specifying families to whom the limit applies; clarifying which months "count" toward the 60 month total).

133. *See* 2000 GREEN BOOK, *supra* note 101, at Table 7-33, 452-59 (detailing state durational cap policies).

134. For women facing a permanent termination of benefits, the availability of alternative supports must be explored quickly and thoroughly. State-funded assistance programs, as well as SSI eligibility, may provide an additional safety net for women whose federally funded welfare eligibility is rapidly coming to an end. Caregivers may wish to explore with survivors whether they can and should seek legal services assistance to investigate options for maintaining assistance.

In some states, the durational cap may be waived, on either of two grounds. The limit may be exceeded "by reason of hardship or if the family includes an individual who has been battered or subjected to extreme cruelty." Federal law does not define the term "hardship," but state statutes might.[135] We have already encountered the phrase "battered or subjected to extreme cruelty," in the text of the Family Violence Option. The same definition applies in this context, as well. Prostitution survivors should have a strong claim for both of these exemptions.[136]

In order to qualify for these exceptions, though, the survivor must disclose the violence or hardship justifying a longer eligibility period. The burdens of identifying as a victim of violence, or as a person who suffers from a disabling condition, have already been addressed. The durational limits place especially brutal disclosure burdens on a survivor. As we have seen, a survivor may elect to defer services available to victims of violence, without jeopardizing her basic eligibility, in favor of strategizing disclosure at a later time. Likewise, the protracted SSI disability process has the virtue of giving the survivor time to integrate and explain her history over an extended period of time. Survivors reaching the limit of their TANF eligibility, though, enjoy no such leeway. Once the durational limit nears, she must disclose, or lose her assistance. Caregivers should be aware of the emergency conditions surrounding these disclosure issues for survivors, as well as the broader safety implications accompanying drastic change in the survivor's financial circumstances when her assistance eligibility expires.

---

135. For example, California law specifies the following 5 reasons for granting hardship exemptions:

   –the recipient is age 60 or older;

   –is caring for an ill or incapacitated family member, which responsibility makes it impossible for the recipient to work;

   –is receiving government disability benefits;

   –the county has determined that the individual is incapable of maintaining employment;

   –the recipient is a foster parent or custodian of a ward.

See CAL. WELFARE & INST. section 11454.

136. Survivors should be cautioned, though, that the states are not obliged to authorize hardship or "extreme cruelty" waivers unless they choose to do so. Indeed, many states that adopted the full 60-month limit have declined to authorize waivers beyond the limit for any reason. Most of the states that shortened or modified the 60-month limit, though, do allow either hardship or "extreme cruelty" waivers, or both. *See* THE URBAN INSTITUTE: ONE YEAR AFTER FEDERAL WELFARE REFORM: A DESCRIPTION OF STATE TEMPORARY ASSISTANCE FOR NEEDY FAMILIES (TANF) DECISIONS AS OF OCTOBER 1997, at IV-2, IV-5 tbl. IV.1 (1998) (http://www.urb.inst.org).

b. Domestic safety: protection from intimate abusers.

Forging safe, respectful family ties, while building strong boundaries against family exploitation, are important goals for survivors creating new futures. A study of the SSI application process indicates that family members are often forceful players within it. "Family members initiated almost as many SSI/SSDI applications as did mental health providers."[137] Prostitution survivors may be subjected to predatory behaviors by family members and intimates who intend to use the survivor's benefits for their own purposes. The survivor should be encouraged to explore with caregivers what options she has for achieving control over her benefit money, while maintaining safety.

The TANF program risks re-enmeshing a survivor with men who may have impregnated her, threatening her recovery and safety. Women receiving TANF benefits must cooperate with the state in establishing paternity[138] and in securing support orders,[139] and must assign support rights to the state with regard to any minor child in the family.[140] "Cooperation" may entail a significant commitment of time, information, and legal appearances.[141] Survivors should be aware of the need to raise objections to these procedures with TANF caseworkers, especially when cooperation would put a survivor's safety at risk, or reconnect her with dangerous people or retraumatizing experiences. Waivers for good cause may be granted, excusing a recipient from these requirements. Typically, waivers may be granted if the recipient is a victim of domestic violence, or if the child was conceived as a result of rape or incest.[142]

---

137. Estroff *et al.*, *supra* note 89, at 64.

138. *See* 42 U.S.C.A. section 608(a)(2) (reduction or elimination of assistance for noncooperation in establishing paternity or obtaining child support).

139. *Id.*

140. *See* 42 U.S.C.A. section 608(a)(3) (no assistance for families not assigning certain support rights to the state).

141. In California, for example, "cooperation" can mean requiring women to provide information about the man believed to be a child's father, giving the names of his relatives and associates, submitting to genetic tests, appearing at interviews, hearings and other legal proceedings. *See* CAL. WELFARE & INST. section 11477.04.

142. *See* 42 U.S.C.A. section 654(29)(A) (cooperation obligations subject to "good cause" and other exceptions which may take into account the best interests of the child); CAL. WELFARE & INST. section 11477.04 (specifying domestic violence, and rape or incest as grounds for non-cooperation).

Emotional and physical risks to the survivor are especially acute when the paternity determination involves a child born while she is, or was, practicing prostitution. In such a case, chances are great that the child's father is either a pimp/partner or a john. In either event, the survivor deserves to be treated as protectively as a woman whose child was conceived as a result of rape or incest, but it is unlikely that she will be. If the father is the survivor's pimp, the survivor may fear retaliation from him if she discloses his name, loss of her child to state child protective agencies if she discloses the nature of his relationship to her, or loss of her benefits if she declines to cooperate at all. If she suspects that the father is a john, she may have no idea who he is or where to find him. And she may fear losing her child if she discloses why she has so little information to offer. In a leading case applying the TANF paternity cooperation rules, the "non-cooperating" mother, Antoinette Walton, apparently confronted such a dilemma, and lost her benefits.[143] Caregivers and survivors need to explore and consider all of these problems, and the risks they pose to a survivor's safety, if the state makes a cooperation request.

c. Institutional safety: protection from risk environments.

The best-known innovation of the new welfare law is the "welfare-to-work" requirement, mandating employment as a condition of receiving assistance. The employment mandate is intended to advance Congress' policy preference for "job preparation, work, and marriage" over "dependence of needy parents on government benefits."[144] For many prostitution survivors, these are dubious aims. For her, a sustained period of dependence on someone other than a

---

143. *See Walton v. Hammons*, 192 F.3d 590, 591-92 (6th Cir. 1999). Ms. Walton identified her daughter's father as a "Mr. Jackson." She said she had little information about him, other than that she had seen him in a store, and that he lived on her block during her pregnancy. The state TANF agency deemed her statements uncooperative, and ended her assistance. The agency apparently assumed that Ms. Walton knew more about Mr. Jackson than she was disclosing, or that "Mr. Jackson" was a total fiction. There are many possible explanations for Ms. Walton's actions: that she was telling the truth, or that she had been raped by a Mr. Jackson whom she feared to identify, or that she feared disclosing someone else's name

Ms. Walton did not contest the agency determination that she had failed to cooperate in establishing her daughter's paternity, and did not challenge the termination of her benefits. The issue in the case was whether her children's benefits could be terminated on account of their mother's non-cooperation; the court held that the children's benefits could not be terminated for that reason and ordered the children's TANF and food stamp assistance reinstated. *Id.*

144. *See* 42 U.S.C.A. section 601(a)(2).

male intimate, in circumstances where she does not have to earn money for anyone, could be deeply healing. The survivor's history of "work and marriage," on the other hand, in relationships with intimate partners and with income-earning, may be steeped in violence and exploitation. The world of employment, as survivors have experienced it, is a bloody field of assault, sexual torture, gross humiliation, captivity, and risk of murder. What are the work requirements imposed on survivors receiving TANF assistance? What are the implications of this traumatic history on survivors' attempts to comply with them?

The work requirements come into play quickly, with only a few exceptions for urgent child care needs. States may exempt parents of children under 12 months from these requirements, and may not impose work requirements on custodial parents of children under six unless child care is available.[145] For mothers who fall outside of these exemptions, though, federal law now requires that mothers "engage in work,"[146] which may include a range of activities from paid employment, to community service, to vocational training, to high school equivalency preparation.[147] Within two months of receiving assistance, a mother may be required to participate in a community service activity if she is not otherwise employed at a job or enrolled in an authorized educational program.[148] All recipients must begin to work "once the State determines the parent or caretaker is ready to engage in work, or once the parent or caretaker has received assistance under the program for 24 months (whether or not consecutive), whichever is earlier."[149] A mother must generally work full-time to meet this requirement, defined as at least 30 hours per week.[150] Single mothers of children under six will be considered employed if she works

---

145. *See* 45 C.F.R. section 261.15(a).

146. *See* 42 U.S.C.A. section 602(a)(1)(A)(i) (state plan must require parent or caretaker receiving assistance to engage in work); 42 U.S.C.A section 607(e)(1) (fixing number of hours per week that an individual must work to meet annual federal mandates).

147. *See* 42 U.S.C.A. section 607(d)(listing placements that will meet the federal requirements for "work activities").

148. *See* 42 U.S.C.A. section 602(a)(1)(B); 45 C.F.R. section 261.10(b) (mandating community service after two months, "unless the State has exempted the individual from work requirements or he or she is already engaged in work activities"). States may opt out of this requirement. *See* 42 U.S.C.A. section 602(a)(1)(B)(iv).

149. *See* 42 U.S.C.A. section 602(a)(1)(A)(ii) (mandating work requirement, time-lines as quoted in the text); 45 C.F.R. section 261.10(a)(1)(same).

150. *See* 42 U.S.C.A. section 607(c)(1)(A) (mandating that individual be engaged in work for at least 30 hours per week, effective fiscal year 2000 and thereafter); *see also* 45 C.F.R. section 261.31(a)(1)(same).

a minimum of 20 hours per week.[151] Women face severe penalties for non-compliance, from a reduction in benefits, to termination of all assistance.[152]

An issue of great concern for survivors of prostitution is what kinds of jobs she may be required to perform to comply with TANF employment rules. At least three kinds of jobs are problematic for survivors. Survivors can explain why these work sites are dangerous to them, and seek exemptions under the Family Violence Option allowing them to refuse the employment. The grounds for granting FVO exemptions–where compliance would make it more difficult to escape abuse, would unfairly penalize survivors who have been victimized by such violence, or place the woman at risk of future abuse–are clearly present in these instances.

First, prostitution. A woman should not be required to return to prostitution as a condition of receiving benefits. This should be obvious, but for the doubts raised by the SSI cases treating prostitution as "substantial gainful activity." If prostitution is treated as gainful work under the SSI program, it could be treated the same way by TANF staff. If a survivor receives a suggestion from an agency caseworker that she could fulfill her work requirement by turning tricks, the survivor should be unequivocally supported in challenging such a proposal.

Second, TANF agencies could choose to treat legal sex work–stripping, pornography, or "soft core" Hooters-style waitressing, for example–as "work." This is clearly terrible policy, but not foreclosed by law. It should be. Compelled enlistment of women into these work sites should be expressly, legally prohibited, especially since it has proven difficult to document the kinds of jobs women are performing under the new work mandates. Fifteen to 20 percent of women who leave welfare are disappearing from visible or legitimate employment.[153] Many of these women are presumably now trying to support themselves in prostitution, stripping, and other commercial sexual exploitation which operate "under the radar" of legitimate employment reporting. Women currently receiving TANF benefits should be encouraged to decline such employment, and deserve support from agency staff for doing so.

Third, many other work sites create a substantial risk of retraumatizing women with prostitution histories. I recently assisted a survivor to refuse em-

---

151. *See* 42 U.S.C.A. section 607(c)(2)(B); *see also* 45 C.F.R. section 261.35.
152. *See* 42 U.S.C.A. section 103(a)(1).
153. *See* INSTITUTE FOR RESEARCH ON POVERTY, POST-EXIT EARNINGS AND BENEFITS RECEIPT AMONG THOSE WHO LEFT AFDC IN WISCONSIN 63 (1999) (20% of women who left welfare had no reported earnings in the state unemployment insurance system); THE URBAN INSTITUTE, WORK STATUS OF WELFARE LEAVERS (2002) (one in seven former TANF recipients has no visible source of income).

ployment, required by a prison aftercare program, working as a maid in a large hotel in central Florida. She had prostituted for years in hotels just like the one to which her supervisors now wanted her to return. She could not face the prospect of returning to the same place, again by compulsion, to clean beds. In my view, women with prostitution histories should not be compelled to work in any service occupation, no matter how superficially innocuous, or in any occupational role that requires the display of female submission, or in any job in which the pay is based on tips. In any event, caregivers should explore carefully the associations, and accompanying risks of symptom intrusions, to which a survivor may be exposed by accepting a job as a condition of her assistance eligibility.

IV. CONCLUSION

How do we work to end prostitution, and the damage prostitution inflicts on women and girls? As we have seen in this tour through the SSI and TANF systems, prostitution survivors are barely tolerated as eligible applicants, and must confront retraumatizing disclosure and safety risks as conditions of participation. These conditions should be changed, through public advocacy, on the harms of prostitution and the needs of its survivors. Throughout this paper, too, I have assumed a relationship that exists all too rarely in reality: an established, trusting, and continuing relationship between a prostitution survivor and her therapist. This is a crucial relationship to create and nurture, and one to which all prostituted women and girls should be entitled.

Ten Reasons
for *Not* Legalizing Prostitution
and a Legal Response
to the Demand for Prostitution

Janice G. Raymond

SUMMARY. Since the mid-1980s, the debate about how to address prostitution legally has become a subject of legislative action. Some countries in Europe, most notably the Netherlands and Germany among others, have legalized and/or decriminalized systems of prostitution, which includes decriminalizing pimps, brothels and buyers, also known as "customers or johns." Other governments, such as Thailand, legally prohibit prostitution activities and enterprises but in reality tolerate brothels and the buying of women for commercial sexual exploitation, especially in its sex tourism industry. Sweden, has taken a different legal approach–penalizing the buyers while at the same time decriminalizing the women in prostitution.

Janice G. Raymond, PhD, is Professor Emerita of Women's Studies and Medical Ethics at the University of Massachusetts in Amherst. She is also Co-Executive Director of the Coalition Against Trafficking in Women (CATW), an international NGO having Category II Consultative Status with ECOSOC, and with branches in most world regions. Professor Raymond is the author of five books and multiple articles including *Women as Wombs: Reproductive Freedom and the Battle Over Women's Bodies* (1994). She can be contacted at (jraymond@wost.umass.edu).
Printed with permission.

[Haworth co-indexing entry note]: "Ten Reasons for *Not* Legalizing Prostitution and a Legal Response to the Demand for Prostitution." Raymond, Janice G. Co-published simultaneously in *Journal of Trauma Practice* (The Haworth Maltreatment & Trauma Press, an imprint of The Haworth Press, Inc.) Vol. 2, No. 3/4, 2003, pp. 315-332; and: *Prostitution, Trafficking, and Traumatic Stress* (ed: Melissa Farley) The Haworth Maltreatment & Trauma Press, an imprint of The Haworth Press, Inc., 2003, pp. 315-332. Single or multiple copies of this article are available for a fee from The Haworth Document Delivery Service [1-800-HAWORTH, 9:00 a.m. - 5:00 p.m. (EST). E-mail address: docdelivery@haworthpress.com].

http://www.haworthpress.com/store/product.asp?sku=J189
10.1300/J189v02n03_17

This article offers ten arguments for not legalizing prostitution. These arguments apply to all state-sponsored forms of prostitution, including but not limited to full-scale legalization of brothels and pimping, decriminalization of the sex industry, regulating prostitution by laws such as registering or mandating health checks for women in prostitution, or any system in which prostitution is recognized as "sex work" or advocated as an employment choice. This essay reviews the ways in which legitimating prostitution as work makes the harm of prostitution to women invisible, expands the sex industry, and does not empower the women in prostitution.

What happens when prostitution is treated as "sex work" rather than when it is treated as sexual exploitation and violence against women? What happens when a country such as Sweden rejects legalization and addresses the demand for prostitution?

1. LEGALIZATION/DECRIMINALIZATION OF PROSTITUTION IS A GIFT TO PIMPS, TRAFFICKERS AND THE SEX INDUSTRY

What does legalization of prostitution or decriminalization of the sex industry mean? In the Netherlands, legalization amounts to sanctioning all aspects of the sex industry: the women themselves, the buyers, and the pimps who, under the regime of legalization, are transformed into third party businessmen and legitimate sexual entrepreneurs. Legalization/decriminalization of the sex industry also converts brothels, sex clubs, massage parlors, and other sites of prostitution activities into legitimate venues where commercial sexual acts are allowed to flourish legally with few restraints.

Some people believe that, in calling for legalization or decriminalization of prostitution, they dignify and professionalize the women in prostitution. But dignifying prostitution as work doesn't dignify the women, it simply dignifies the sex industry. People often don't realize that decriminalization means decriminalization of the whole sex industry, not just the women in it. And they haven't thought through the consequences of legalizing pimps as legitimate sex entrepreneurs or third party businessmen, or the fact that men who buy women for sexual activity are now accepted as legitimate consumers of sex.

In countries where women are criminalized for prostitution activities, it is crucial to advocate for the *decriminalization of the women* in prostitution. No woman should be punished for her own exploitation. But States should never decriminalize pimps, buyers, procurers, brothels, or other sex establishments.

2. LEGALIZATION/DECRIMINALIZATION
OF PROSTITUTION
AND THE SEX INDUSTRY
PROMOTES SEX TRAFFICKING

Legalized or decriminalized prostitution industries are one of the root causes of sex trafficking. One argument for legalizing prostitution in the Netherlands was that legalization would help to end the exploitation of desperate immigrant women who had been trafficked there for prostitution. However, one report found that 80% of women in the brothels of the Netherlands were trafficked from other countries (Budapest Group, 1999)(1). In 1994, the International Organization of Migration (IOM) stated that in the Netherlands alone, "nearly 70 % of trafficked women were from CEEC [Central and Eastern European Countries]" (IOM, 1995, p. 4).

The government of the Netherlands presents itself as a champion of anti-trafficking policies and programs, yet it has removed every legal impediment to pimping, procuring and brothels. In the year 2000, the Dutch Ministry of Justice argued in favor of a legal quota of foreign "sex workers," because the Dutch prostitution market demanded a variety of "bodies" (Dutting, 2001, p. 16). Also in 2000, the Dutch government sought and received a judgment from the European Court recognizing prostitution as an economic activity, thereby enabling women from the European Union and former Soviet bloc countries to obtain working permits as "sex workers" in the Dutch sex industry if they could prove that they are self employed. Non-governmental organizations (NGOs) in Europe report that traffickers use the work permits to bring foreign women into the Dutch prostitution industry, masking the fact that women have been trafficked, by coaching them to describe themselves as independent "migrant sex workers" (Personal Communication, Representative of the International Human Rights Network, 1999).

In the year since lifting the ban on brothels in the Netherlands, eight Dutch victim support organizations reported an increase in the number of victims of trafficking, and twelve victim support organizations reported that the number of victims from other countries has not diminished (Bureau NRM, 2002, p. 75). Forty-three of the 348 municipalities (12%) in the Netherlands choose to follow a no-brothel policy, but the Minister of Justice has indicated that the complete banning of prostitution within any municipality could conflict with the federally guaranteed "right to free choice of work" (Bureau NRM, 2002, p. 19).

The first steps toward legalization of prostitution in Germany occurred in the 1980s. By 1993, it was widely recognized that 75% of the women in Germany's prostitution industry were foreigners from Uruguay, Argentina, Paraguay, and other countries in South America (Altink, 1993, p. 33). After the fall of the Berlin wall, 80% of the estimated 10,000 women trafficked into Germany were from Central and Eastern Europe and CIS countries (IOM, 1998a , p. 17). In 2002, prostitution in Germany was established as a legitimate job after years of being legalized in tolerance zones. Promotion of prostitution, pimping, and brothels are now legal in Germany.

The sheer volume of foreign women in the German prostitution industry suggests that these women were trafficked into Germany, a process euphemistically described as facilitated migration. It is almost impossible for poor women to facilitate their own migration, underwrite the costs of travel and travel documents, and set themselves up in "business" without intervention.

In 1984, a Labor government in the Australian State of Victoria introduced legislation to legalize prostitution in brothels. Subsequent Australian governments expanded legalization culminating in the Prostitution Control Act of 1994. Noting the link between legalization of prostitution and trafficking in Australia, the US Department of State observed: "Trafficking in East Asian women for the sex trade is a growing problem . . . lax laws–including legalized prostitution in parts of the country–make [anti-trafficking] enforcement difficult at the working level" (U.S. Department of State, 2000, p. 6F).

3. LEGALIZATION/DECRIMINALIZATION
OF PROSTITUTION DOES NOT CONTROL
THE SEX INDUSTRY:
IT EXPANDS IT

Contrary to claims that legalization and decriminalization would control the expansion of the sex industry, prostitution now accounts for 5% of the Netherlands economy (Daley, 2001, p. 4). Over the last decade, as pimping was legalized, and brothels decriminalized in the year 2000, the sex industry increased by 25% in the Netherlands (Daley, 2001, p.4). At any hour of the day, women of all ages and races, dressed in hardly anything, are put on display in the notorious windows of Dutch brothels and sex clubs and offered for sale. Most of them are women from other countries who were probably trafficked into the Netherlands (Daley, 2001, p. 4).

In addition to governmental endorsement of prostitution in the Netherlands, prostitution is also promoted by associations of sex businesses and organizations comprised of prostitution buyers who consult and collaborate with the government to further their interests. These include the "Association of Operators of Relaxation Businesses," the "Cooperating Consultation of Operators of Window Prostitution," and the "Man/Woman and Prostitution Foundation," a group of men who regularly use women in prostitution, and whose specific aims include "to make prostitution and the use of services of prostitutes more accepted and openly discussible," and "to protect the interests of clients" (Bureau NRM, 2002, pp.115-16).

Faced with a dwindling number of Dutch women who engage in prostitution activities and the expanding demand for more female bodies and more exotic women to service the prostitution market, the Dutch National Rapporteur on Trafficking has stated that in the future, a solution may be to "offer [to the market] prostitutes from non EU/EEA [European Union/European Economic Area] countries, who voluntarily choose to work in prostitution . . . " These women would be given "legal and controlled access to the Dutch market" (Bureau NRM, 2002, p. 140). As prostitution has been transformed into "sex work," and pimps into entrepreneurs, so too this recommendation transforms trafficking into "voluntary migration for sex work." Looking to the future, the Netherlands is targeting poor women for the international sex trade to remedy the inadequacies of the free market of "sexual services." Prostitution is thus normalized as an "option for the poor."

Legalization of prostitution in the State of Victoria, Australia, resulted in massive expansion of the sex industry. Along with legalization of prostitution, other forms of sexual exploitation, such as tabletop dancing, bondage and discipline centers, peep shows, phone sex, and pornography, have all developed in much more profitable ways than before legalization (Sullivan & Jeffreys, 2001). Prostitution has become an integral part of the tourism and casino boom in Victoria with government-sponsored casinos authorizing the redeeming of casino chips at local brothels (Sullivan & Jeffreys, 2001).

A range of state-sponsored prostitution systems exist in Austria, Denmark, Germany, the Netherlands, and Switzerland. It seems likely that European state-sponsored prostitution countries serve as magnets and, ultimately, as conduits through which significant numbers of women are trafficked to other European nations. Europe has a high density of women trafficked per square mile compared to North America, for example. Given the porousness of national borders facilitated by the Schengen agreement (2), it is not surprising that high numbers of trafficked women are also present in other European countries that do not have legalized or decriminalized systems of prostitution. Although accurate numbers of women trafficked are difficult to obtain, the International Organization of Migration (IOM) has estimated that 500,000 women and children are trafficked in Europe annually (IOM, 1998). In contrast, it has been estimated that 45,000-50,000 women and children are trafficked annually into the United States (Richard, 1999, p. 3).

4. LEGALIZATION/DECRIMINALIZATON
OF PROSTITUTION
INCREASES CLANDESTINE, ILLEGAL
AND STREET PROSTITUTION

One goal of legalized prostitution was to move prostituted women indoors into brothels and clubs where they would be allegedly less vulnerable than in street prostitution. However, many women are in street prostitution because they want to avoid being controlled and exploited by pimps (transformed in legalized systems into sex businessmen). Other women do not want to register or submit to health checks, as required by law in some countries where prostitution is legalized (Schelzig, 2002). Thus, legalization may actually *drive some women into* street prostitution. Arguing against an Italian proposal for legalized prostitution, Esohe Aghatise has suggested that brothels actually deprive women of what little protection they may have on the street, confining women to closed spaces where they have little chance of meeting outreach workers or others who might help them exit prostitution (Aghatise, in press).

In the Netherlands, women in prostitution point out that legalization or decriminalization of the sex industry does not erase the stigma of prostitution. Because they must register and lose their anonymity, women are more vulnerable to being stigmatized as "whores," and this identity follows them everyplace. Thus, the majority of women in prostitution still operate illegally and underground. Some members of Parliament who originally supported the legalization of brothels on the grounds that this would liberate women are now seeing that legalization actually reinforces the oppression of women (Daley, 2001, p. A1).

Chief Inspector Nancy Pollock, one of Scotland's highest-ranking female police officers, established Glasgow's street liaison team for women in prostitution in 1998. Pollock stated that legalization or decriminalization of prostitution is "... simply to abandon women to what has to be the most demeaning job in the world" (Martin, 2002, p. A5). Countering the argument that legalized prostitution provides safer venues for women, Pollock noted that women in sauna prostitution, for example, "have even less control over what services they will perform. On the street, very few women will do anal sex and few do sex without a condom. But in the saunas, the owners, who obviously don't want their punters going away disappointed, decide what the women will do, and very often that is anal sex and sex–oral and vaginal–without a condom" (Martin, 2002, p. A5).

The argument that legalization was supposed to take the criminal elements out of sex businesses by strict regulation of the industry has failed. The real growth in prostitution in Australia since legalization took effect has been in the illegal sector. Over a period of 12 months from 1998-1999, unlicensed brothels in Victoria tripled in number and still operate with impunity (Sullivan & Jeffreys, 2001). In New South Wales where brothels were decriminalized in 1995, the number of brothels in Sydney had tripled to 400-500 by 1999, with the vast majority having no license to advertise or operate. In response to widespread police corruption, control of illegal prostitution was removed from police jurisdiction and placed under the control of local councils and planning regulators. However, the local councils do not have the resources to investigate illegal brothel operators (Sullivan & Jeffreys, 2001).

5. LEGALIZATION OF PROSTITUTION AND DECRIMINALIZATION OF THE SEX INDUSTRY INCREASES CHILD PROSTITUTION

Another argument for legalizing prostitution in the Netherlands was that it would help end child prostitution. Yet child prostitution in the Netherlands has increased dramatically during the 1990s. The Amsterdam-based ChildRight organization estimates that the number of children in prostitution has increased by more than 300% between 1996-2001, going from 4,000 children in 1996 to 15,000 in 2001. ChildRight estimates that at least 5,000 of these children in Dutch prostitution are trafficked from other countries, with a large segment being Nigerian girls (Tiggeloven, 2001).

Child prostitution has increased dramatically in the state of Victoria compared to other Australian states where prostitution has not been legalized. Of all the states and territories in Australia, the highest number of reported incidences of child prostitution came from Victoria. In a 1998 study undertaken by ECPAT (End Child Prostitution and Trafficking), who conducted research for the Australian National Inquiry on Child Prostitution, there was increased evidence of organized commercial exploitation of children (ECPAT Australia, 1998).

6. LEGALIZATION/DECRIMINALIZATION OF PROSTITUTION DOES NOT PROTECT THE WOMEN IN PROSTITUTION

In two studies in which 186 victims of commercial sexual exploitation were interviewed, women consistently indicated that prostitution establishments did little to protect them, regardless of whether the establishments were legal or illegal. One woman said, "The only time they protect anyone is to protect the customers" (Raymond, Hughes, & Gomez, 2001; Raymond, d'Cunha, Ruhaini Dzuhayatin, Hynes, & Santos, 2002).

One of these studies interviewed 146 victims of trafficking in 5 countries. Eighty percent of the women interviewed had suffered physical violence from pimps and buyers and endured similar and multiple health effects from the violence and sexual exploitation, regardless of whether the women were trafficked internationally or were in local prostitution (Raymond et al., 2002, p. 62).

A second study of women trafficked for prostitution in the United States yielded the following statements. Women who reported that sex businesses gave them some protection qualified it by pointing out that no "protector" was ever in the room with them. One woman who was in out-call prostitution stated: "The driver functioned as a bodyguard. You're supposed to call when you get in, to ascertain that everything was OK. But they are not standing outside the door while you're in there, so anything could happen" (Raymond et al., 2001, p. 74).

In brothels that have surveillance cameras, the function of cameras was to protect the buyer and the brothel rather than the women, with one brothel putting in cameras after a buyer died (Raymond et al., 2001, p. 74). Protection of the women from abuse was of secondary or no importance.

7. LEGALIZATION/DECRIMINALIZATION OF PROSTITUTION INCREASES THE DEMAND FOR PROSTITUTION: IT ENCOURAGES MEN TO BUY WOMEN FOR SEX IN A WIDER AND MORE PERMISSIBLE RANGE OF SOCIALLY ACCEPTABLE SETTINGS

With the advent of legalization in countries that have decriminalized the sex industry, many men who previously would not have risked buying women for sex now see prostitution as acceptable. When legal barriers disappear, so too do the social and ethical barriers to treating women as sexual merchandise. Legalization of prostitution sends the message to new generations of men and boys that women are sexual commodities and that prostitution is harmless fun (Leidholdt, 2000).

As men have a plethora of "sexual services" offered to them in prostitution, women must compete by engaging in anal sex, sex without condoms, bondage and domination, and other acts demanded by buyers. Once prostitution is legalized, for example, women's reproductive capacities are sellable products. Some buyers find pregnancy a turn-on and demand breast milk in their sexual encounters with pregnant women (Sullivan & Jeffreys, 2001, p. 10).

In the State of Victoria in Australia, specialty brothels are provided for disabled men. State-employed caretakers (who are mostly women) must take these men to the brothels if they wish to go and literally facilitate their physical sexual acts (Sullivan & Jeffreys, 2001). Advertisements line the highways of Victoria offering women as objects for sexual use. Businessmen are encouraged to hold their corporate meetings in clubs where owners supply naked women on the table at tea breaks and lunchtime. A Melbourne brothel owner stated that the client base was "well educated professional men, who visit during the day and then go home to their families" (Sullivan & Jeffreys, 2001). Women in relationships with men find that often the men in their lives are visiting the brothels and sex clubs.

8. LEGALIZATION/DECRIMINALIZATION OF PROSTITUTION DOES NOT PROMOTE WOMEN'S HEALTH

A legalized system of prostitution often mandates health checks and certification, but only for women and not for male buyers. Health examinations or tests for women but not men make no public health sense because monitoring prostituted women does not protect *them* from HIV/AIDS or STDs. This is not to advocate that both women in prostitution and male buyers should be checked. It is simply to point out the duplicity of a policy that implies, "We'll have safer sex and HIV/AIDS control if we examine the women under a regulated or decriminalized system of prostitution." Male buyers can and do originally transmit disease to the women they purchase.

It has been argued that legalized brothels or other "controlled" prostitution establishments protect women through enforceable condom policies. In one study, 47% of women in U.S. prostitution stated that men expected sex without a condom; 73% reported that men offered to pay more for sex without a condom; and 45% of women said that men became abusive if they insisted that men use condoms (Raymond et al., 2001, p. 72). Although certain sex businesses had rules that required men to wear condoms, men nonetheless attempted to have sex without condoms. One woman stated: "It's 'regulation' to wear a condom at the sauna, but negotiable between parties on the side. Most guys expected blow jobs without a condom (Raymond et al., 2001, p. 72)."

In reality, the enforcement of condom policy was left to the individual women in prostitution, and the offer of extra money was an insistent pressure. One woman stated: "I'd be one of those liars if I said 'Oh I always used a condom.' If there was extra money coming in, then the condom would be out the window. I was looking for the extra money (Raymond et al., 2001, p. 73)." Many factors militate against condom use: the need of women to make money; older women's decline in attractiveness to men; competition from places that do not require condoms; pimp pressure on women to have sex with no condom for more money; money needed for a drug habit or to pay off the pimp; and the general lack of control that prostituted women have over their bodies in prostitution venues.

"Safety policies" in brothels did not protect women from harm. Where brothels allegedly monitored the buyers and employed "bouncers," women stated that they were injured by buyers and, at times, by brothel owners and their friends. Even when someone intervened to momentarily control buyers' abuse, women lived in a climate of fear. Although 60% of women reported that buyers had sometimes been prevented from abusing them, half of those same women answered that, nonetheless, they thought that they might be killed by one of their buyers (Raymond et al., 2002).

9. LEGALIZATION/DECRIMINALIZATION OF PROSTITUTION DOES NOT ENHANCE WOMEN'S CHOICE

Most women in prostitution did not make a rational choice to enter prostitution from among a range of other options. They did not sit down one day and decide that they wanted to be prostitutes. They did not have other real options such as medicine, law, nursing or politics. Instead, their "options" were more in the realm of how to feed themselves and their children. Such choices are better termed survival strategies.

Rather than consenting to prostitution, a prostituted woman more accurately complies with the extremely limited options available to her. Her compliance is required by the fact of having to adapt to conditions of inequality that are set by the customer who pays her to do what he wants her to do.

Most of the women interviewed in the studies authored by Raymond et al. reported that choice in entering the sex industry could only be discussed in the context of a lack of other options. Many described prostitution as their last choice, or as an involuntary way of making ends meet (Raymond et al., 2001; Raymond et al., 2002). In one study, 67% of a group of law enforcement officials expressed the opinion that women did not enter prostitution voluntarily. Similarly, 72% of social service providers did not think that women voluntarily choose to enter the sex industry (Raymond et al., 2001, p. 91).

The distinction between forced and voluntary prostitution is precisely what the sex industry is promoting because it will give the industry more legal security and market stability if this distinction can be utilized to legalize prostitution, pimping, and brothels. Women who consider bringing charges against pimps and perpetrators will bear the burden of proving that they were "forced." How will marginalized women ever be able to prove coercion? If prostituted women must prove that force was used in recruitment or in their "working conditions," very few women in prostitution will have legal recourse, and very few offenders will be prosecuted.

Women in prostitution must continually lie about their lives, their bodies, and their sexual responses. Lying is part of the job definition when the customer asks, "did you enjoy it?" The very edifice of prostitution is built on the lie that "women like it." Some prostitution survivors have stated that it took them years after leaving prostitution to acknowledge that prostitution wasn't a free choice because to deny their own capacity to choose was to deny themselves.

There is no doubt that a small number of women *say* they choose to be in prostitution, especially in public contexts orchestrated by the sex industry. In the same way, some people choose to take dangerous drugs such as amphetamine. However, even when some people consent to use dangerous drugs, we still recognize that is harmful to them, and most people do not seek to legalize amphetamine. In this situation, it is *harm* to the person, not the *consent* of the person that is the governing standard.

A 1998 International Labor Organization (United Nations ILO) report suggested that the sex industry be treated as a legitimate economic sector, but still found that

> ... prostitution is one of the most alienated forms of labour; the surveys [in 4 countries] show that women worked 'with a heavy heart,' 'felt forced,' or were 'conscience-stricken' and had negative self-identities. A significant proportion claimed they wanted to leave sex work [sic] if they could. (Lim, 1998, p. 213)

When a woman remains in an abusive relationship with a partner who batters her, or even when she defends his actions, concerned people now understand that she is not there voluntarily. They recognize the complexity of her compliance. Like battered women, women in prostitution may deny their abuse if they are not provided with meaningful alternatives.

10. WOMEN IN SYSTEMS OF PROSTITUTION DO NOT WANT THE SEX INDUSTRY LEGALIZED OR DECRIMINALIZED

In a 5-country study on sex trafficking, most of the trafficked and prostituted women interviewed in the Philippines, Venezuela, and the United States (3) strongly stated their opinion that prostitution should not be legalized and considered legitimate work, warning that legalization would create more risks and harm for women from already violent customer and pimps (Raymond et al.,

2002). One woman said, "No way. It's not a profession. It is humiliating, and violence from the men's side." Not one woman we interviewed wanted her children, family or friends to have to earn money by entering the sex industry. Another woman stated: "Prostitution stripped me of my life, my health, everything" (Raymond et al., 2002).

AN ALTERNATIVE LEGAL ROUTE: PENALIZING THE DEMAND

There is no evidence that legalization of prostitution makes things better for women in prostitution. It certainly makes things better for governments who legalize prostitution and of course, for the sex industry, both of which enjoy increased revenues. The popular fiction that all will be well in the world of prostitution once the sex industry is legalized or decriminalized, is repudiated by evidence that the degradation and exploitation of women, as well as the harm, abuse, and violence to women still remain in state-sponsored prostitution. State-sponsored prostitution sanitizes the reality of prostitution. Suddenly, dirty money becomes clean. Illegal acts become legal. Overnight, pimps are transformed into legitimate businessmen and ordinary entrepreneurs, and men who would not formerly consider buying a woman in prostitution think, "Well, if it's legal, if it's decriminalised, now it must be O.K."

Governments that legalize prostitution as "sex work" will have a huge economic stake in the sex industry. Consequently, this will foster their increased dependence on the sex sector. If women in prostitution are counted as workers, then governments can abdicate responsibility for making decent and sustainable employment available to women.

Instead of abandoning women in the sex industry to state-sponsored prostitution, laws should address the predation of men who buy women for the sex of prostitution. Men who use women in prostitution have long been invisible. Legislators often leap onto the legalization bandwagon because they think nothing else is successful. But there is a legal alternative. Rather than sanctioning prostitution, states could address the demand by penalizing the men who buy women for the sex of prostitution.

Sweden has drafted legislation recognizing that without male demand, there would be no female supply. Thinking outside the repressive box of legalization, Sweden has acknowledged that prostitution is a form of male violence against women and children, and the purchase of sexual services is criminalized. The inseparability of prostitution and trafficking is recognized by the Swedish law: "Prostitution and trafficking in women are seen as harmful practices that cannot, and should not be separated; in order to effectively eliminate trafficking in women, concrete measures against prostitution must be put in place" (Ekberg, 2003, p. 69).

Sweden's Violence Against Women Government Bill (1997/98:55 (4), prohibits and penalizes the purchase of "sexual services" (Swedish Government Offices, 1998). This approach targets the male demand for prostitution: "By prohibiting the purchase of sexual services, prostitution and its damaging effects can be counteracted more effectively than hitherto" (Swedish Government Offices, 1998, p. 2). The Swedish legislation criminalizing the buyers is based on the policy that "Prostitution is not a desirable social phenomenon" and is "an obstacle to the ongoing development towards equality between women and men (Swedish Government Offices, 1998, p. 2)." Furthermore, the law against purchasing sexual services is part of a wider Violence Against Women Bill that allocates resources to support the development of alternatives for women in prostitution.

Results of the Swedish legislation thus far have been promising. The prohibition against men buying prostituted women has received strong social support. Several polls, conducted in 2000 and 2001, show that approximately 80% of the Swedish population support the law. Of those who want to repeal the law, the majority are men, with only 7% of women in support of repeal (Jacobson, 2002, p. 24). Most importantly, women who are attempting to leave prostitution support the law (Ekberg, 2001). Swedish NGOs that work with women in prostitution also support the law and maintain that since passage of the law, increased numbers of women contact them for assistance. The very existence of the law, and the fact that people know it will be enforced, they say, serve as an aid to young women who are vulnerable to pimps and procurers (Ekberg, 2001).

Street prostitution has declined in the three years since the law was passed. The number of prostituted women has decreased by 50%, and 70-80% of the buyers have left public places. Furthermore, a police representative maintained that there is no indication that prostitution has gone underground, or that prostitution in sex clubs, escort agencies, and brothels has increased (Björling, 2001). Police have also stated that the Swedish law prohibiting the purchase of sexual services has had a chilling effect on trafficking (5). According to police, were it not for the law, Sweden, like Norway and Finland, would experience major trafficking of Russian women across the border. In the northern regions of both Norway and Finland, trafficked Russian women are made to service Scandinavian men in prostitution camps (Bystrom, 2001).

Women's and human rights groups should be advocating for study and replication of the Swedish law. Instead of giving carte blanche to profoundly abusive sex industries, governments should respond to the male violence and

328 PROSTITUTION, TRAFFICKING, AND TRAUMATIC STRESS

sexual exploitation of women in prostitution by legally addressing the demand for prostitution.

Sweden has also focused on *preventing* the demand for prostitution by initiating a national campaign against prostitution and trafficking. One of the innovative aspects of this effort has been to take the campaign to the racetrack. In May 2002, the Swedish campaign against prostitution and trafficking was launched at the *Solvalla* Racetrack in Stockholm. Racing fans often celebrate their winnings at a brothel or by paying for sex acts with women in street prostitution. At *Solvalla*, pimps commonly hustle buyers at the racetracks or give them a ride to sex clubs after the races end (Ekberg, 2003, p. 72).The *Solvalla* racetrack dedicated its first race of the evening to the campaign against prostitution and trafficking, advertising the campaign in its racing program. After the first race, Swedish Vice-Prime Minister and Minister for Gender Equality Margareta Winberg spoke to the 5000 persons in attendance about the campaign and about its focus on the buyers of women and children in prostitution (Ekberg, 2003, p. 71). Opening a national campaign against trafficking and prostitution at a racetrack must rank as one of the most inventive "best practices" to prevent sexual exploitation, targeting a large population of men who actually and potentially buy women for sex acts.

Sweden also launched a nationwide poster campaign focusing on the demand for prostitution. Colorful posters publicizing the *Law Prohibiting the Purchase of Sexual Services* were displayed in bus shelters, subway stations and on streetcars throughout Sweden. The posters were designed to increase public awareness about prostitution and trafficking in women by spotlighting the men who buy women for sex. For example, one poster was a representation of Swedish sex tourists who travel to Baltic countries. The poster featured a well-dressed man in a suit, wearing a wedding band, with the caption, "Time to flush the johns out of the Baltic." Another poster depicted a young man surfing for Internet pornography. The poster reads: "More and more Swedish men do their shopping over the Internet (Ekberg, 2003, pp. 75-76)." The poster campaign attracted much public attention both within and outside Sweden (Ekberg, 2003, p. 72).

We hear too little about the role of the sex industry in creating a global sex market for women and children. Instead, we hear that prostitution could be made into a better job for women through regulation and/or legalization, through unions of so-called "sex workers," and through campaigns that provide condoms to women but fail to provide them with alternatives to prostitution. We hear much about how to keep women *in* prostitution but very little about how to help women get *out*.

Sadly, in several countries, labor unions have been encouraged to accept prostitution as work (Young, 2002). Rather than affirming prostitution as work, labor unions could follow the example of Denmark's Confederation of Trade Unions (LO) which, in June, 2003, prohibited its 1.5 million members (in a country of 5.4 million) from engaging in prostitution when they represent the union on business and travel abroad (Agence France Presse, 2003).

It would be a great leap forward in the campaign against sexual exploitation for governments and UN agencies to prohibit their diplomats, military personnel, UN police, and peacekeepers from engaging in prostitution activities on or off duty. Some agencies, such as the UN Inter-Agency Standing Committee (IASC) that brings together over 15 UN and multilateral agencies, have devised codes of conduct for their personnel in humanitarian crisis situations (Inter-Agency Standing Committee, 2002). One of the core principles of the IASC code of conduct states: "Sexual exploitation and abuse by humanitarian workers constitute acts of gross misconduct and are therefore grounds for termination." Another core principle makes clear that "Exchange of money, employment, goods, or services for sex, including favours or other forms of humiliating, degrading or exploitative behavior is prohibited" (Inter-Agency Standing Committee, 2002).

The way in which countries address the legal status of prostitution will have an enormous impact on efforts to combat trafficking. Anti-trafficking advocates and legislators must address prostitution as a root cause of sex trafficking, and not be silenced by those who insist that we must speak only about trafficking–not prostitution–in governmental or non-governmental forums. Many governmental and nongovernmental representatives have capitulated to *censorship* at international forums where pressure is exerted, not to mention prostitution, but only to talk about trafficking–as if this were possible.

Finally, rather than cashing in on the economic profits of the sex industry by taxing it, governments could seize assets of sex businesses and then use these funds to provide real alternatives for women in prostitution. Measures to prevent trafficking and prostitution, or to prosecute traffickers, recruiters, pimps, and buyers, will be inadequate unless governments invest in the futures of prostituted women by providing economic resources that enable women to improve their lives.

NOTES

1. Nearly 40 governments and 10 organizations participate in the Budapest process, initiated in 1991. Approximately 50 intergovernmental meetings at various levels have been held, including the Prague Ministerial Conference.

2. Citizens of European Union countries are guaranteed the right of common travel, among other measures, under the Schengen agreement. This means that trafficked

women entering one of the Schengen countries legally or illegally can easily be trafficked to another country within the Shengen territory.

3. The 5 countries studied in this report were Indonesia, the Philippines, Thailand, the United States, and Venezuela. The question about legalization of prostitution was not asked in the Indonesian and Thailand interviews. In the Philippines country report, 96% of the women interviewed recommended that prostitution not be legalized. In the United States country report, 56% of the Russian/Newly Independent States (NIS) women interviewed said that prostitution should not be legalized, with the remaining 44% stating that they were unsure or had no opinion; 85% of the U.S. women in prostitution who were interviewed stated that prostitution not be legalized. In the Venezuelan country report, 50% stated that prostitution should not be legalized, 29% stated that legalization would protect women, and 21% did not respond to the question.

4. All references to the Swedish Law Prohibiting the Purchase of Sexual Services, 1998, quote the English summary of the law from the Swedish Government Offices Fact Sheet, 1998, available at www.kvinnofrid.gov.se. The actual text of the law states: "A person who obtains casual sexual relations in exchange for payment shall be sentenced–unless the act is punishable under the Swedish Penal Code–for the purchase of sexual services to a fine or imprisonment for at the most six months. Attempt to purchase sexual services is punishable under Chapter 23 of the Swedish Penal Code" (Sweden, Law Prohibiting the Purchase of Sexual Services 1998, p. 408).

5. According to a 2002 report of the National Criminal Investigation Department (NCID) of the National Swedish Police, the Swedish National Rapporteur on Trafficking has stated:

> In recent years there have been obvious indications that the Act relating to purchase of sexual services have (sic) had a positive result as regards trafficking in human beings. Several women have in interrogations told that pimps and traffickers in human beings that they have been in contact with do not consider Sweden a good market for these activities. The women must be escorted to the purchasers and then they do not have time with as many purchasers as they would have in a brothel or in street prostitution. So pimps and traffickers in human beings do not earn money quickly enough. Another aspect is that the purchasers in Sweden are very afraid of being discovered and they demand that the purchases of sexual services take place with much discretion. To carry on the activities indoors it is necessary to have several apartments or other premises available. The necessity of several premises is confirmed in almost all preliminary investigations that are carried on in 2002. Some women have also stated that countries like Denmark, Germany, Holland, and Spain have appeared as more attractive for traffickers in human beings and pimps.

> Telephone interception has also demonstrated that Sweden does not stand out as a good market for selling women . . . criminals complain about the purchasers being afraid and about the fact that the activities in Sweden must be more organized to be profitable. On several occasions also the police from the Baltic States have informed that criminals in the native countries do not consider Sweden a good market for trafficking in human beings. (National Criminal Police, 2002, pp. 33-34)

In the NCID report, the National Rapporteur does not include any information about total numbers of victims trafficked into Sweden. She states that there is no available information to indicate " . . . that trafficking in human beings to Sweden has increased. But there is nothing that is indicating that trafficking in human beings has decreased" (National Criminal Police, 2002, p. 2).

REFERENCES

Agence France Presse (2003). *No More Prostitutes, Danish Union Says.* June 30, 2003.

Aghatise, E. (In press). Trafficking for Prostitution in Italy: Possible Effects of Government Proposals for Legalization of Brothels in Italy. *Violence Against Women.*

Altink, S. (1995). *Stolen Lives: Trading Women into Sex and Slavery.* London: Scarlet Press.

Björling, S. (2001). Gatuprostitutionen minskar i Stockholm. *Dagens Nyheter.* February 16, 2001.

Budapest Group (1999). *The Relationship Between Organized Crime and Trafficking in Aliens.* Austria: International Centre for Migration Policy Development. June 1999.

Bureau NRM (2002). *Trafficking in Human Beings: First Report of the Dutch National Rapporteur.* The Hague. November 2002.

Byström, M. (2001). Prostitutionen breder ut sig i Norrland. *Dagens Nyheter* (Sweden). February 16, 2001.

Daley, S. (2001). New Rights for Dutch Prostitutes, but No Gain. *New York Times.* August 12, 2002: A1 and 4.

Dutting, G. (2000). Legalized Prostitution in the Netherlands–Recent Debates. *Women's Global Network for Reproductive Rights*, 3. November, 2002: 15-16.

ECPAT Australia. (1998). *Youth for Sale: ECPAT Australia's Inquiry into the Commercial Sexual Exploitation of Children in Australia.* Available from ECPAT, Australia.

Ekberg, G. (2001, March 15-16). *Prostitution and Trafficking: The Legal Situation in Sweden.* Paper presented at the day of reflection on La mondialisation de la prostitution et du trafic sexuel. Comité québécois Femme et Développement, Montréal, Québec.

Ekberg, G. (2003). Nordic Baltic Campaign Against Trafficking in Women 2002. Final Report. Nordic Council of Ministers. Stockholm, Sweden.

Jacobson, M. (2002). "Why do Men Buy Sex?" Interview with Sven-Axel Mansson. NIKK magasin, (Journal of the Nordic Institute for Women's Studies and Gender Research), 1: 22-25.

Inter-Agency Standing Committee (IASC). 2002. Task Force on Protection from Sexual Exploitation and Abuse in Humanitarian Crises. *Plan of Action.* New York. June 13, 2002.

International Organization for Migration (IOM). (1995). *Trafficking and Prostitution: The Growing Exploitation of Migrant Women from Central and Eastern Europe.* Budapest: IOM Migration Information Program. May, 1995.

International Organization of Migration (IOM). (1998a). *Analysis of Data and Statistical Resources Available in the EU Member States on Trafficking in Humans, Particularly in Women and Children for Purposes of Sexual Exploitation.* Report for the STOP Program, Geneva, IOM.

International Organization of Migration (IOM). (1998b). *Information Campaign Against Trafficking in Women from Ukraine.* Research Report. July, 1998.

Leidholdt, D. (2000). Quoted in *So Deep a Violence: Prostitution, Trafficking and the Global Sex Industry.* Coalition Against Trafficking in Women (CATW) Video. Available at http://www.catwinternational.org.

Lim, L.L. (1998). *The Sex Sector*. International Labour Office (ILO). Geneva, Switzerland.

Martin, L. (2002). The Compassionate Detective. *The Herald*: [Glasgow] April 10, 2002: A5

National Criminal Investigation Department (NCID). 2003. Situation Report 5 on Trafficking in Women 2002. Sweden.

Raymond, J., Hughes, D., and Gomez, C. (2001). *Sex Trafficking of Women in the United States: Links Between International and Domestic Sex Industries*. N. Amherst, MA: Coalition Against Trafficking in Women (CATW). Available at http://www.catwinternational.org.

Raymond, J., d'Cunha, J., Ruhaini Dzuhayatin, S., Hynes, H.P., Ramirez Rodriguez, Z., and Santos, A. (2002). *A Comparative Study of Women Trafficked in the Migration Process: Patterns, Profiles and Health Consequences of Sexual Exploitation in Five Countries (Indonesia, the Philippines, Thailand, Venezuela and the United States)*. N. Amherst, MA: Coalition Against Trafficking in Women (CATW). Available at http://www.catwinternational.org.

Richard, A.O. (1999). *International Trafficking in Women to the United States: A Contemporary Manifestation of Slavery and Organized Crime*. DCI Exceptional Intelligence Analyst Program. Washington, DC: Central Intelligence Agency.

Schelzig, E. (2002). German Prostitutes Ponder Salaried Work. *International Herald Tribune*. May 13, 2002.

Sullivan, M. and Jeffreys, S. (2001). *Legalising Prostitution is Not the Answer: the Example of Victoria, Australia*. Coalition Against Trafficking in Women, Australia and USA. Available at http://www.catwinternational.org.

Swedish Government Offices. (1998). Fact Sheet on Government Bill 1997/98:55 on *Violence Against Women*. Available at www.kvinnofrid.gov.se

Tiggeloven, C. (2001,). *Child Prostitution in the Netherlands*. Available at http://www.catwinternational.org.

U.S. Department of State. Bureau of Democracy, Human Rights and Labor. (2000). *1999 Country Report on Human Rights Practices*, "Australia." Section 6F. February 25, 2000.

Young, R. (2002) Oldest Profession Says Yes to Union. *The Times* (UK). March 5, 2002.

Author Index

Ackley, K., 226
Aghatise, E., 320
Alexander, P., 179,188,189
Altink, S., 317
Altmann, M., 127-128
Alvarez, D., 77
Amnesty International, 1
Ananova.com, 170
Anderson, G., 61,200
Anderson, M. J., 79,80
Arabul, G., 200
Aral, S. O., 58
Arizona Coalition Against Domestic
  Violence, 171
Assistant Deputy Ministers'
  Committee on Prostitution
  and Sexual Exploitation of
  Youth, 240
Azaola, E., 149

Badgley, R., 240
Bagley, C., 35
Baldwin, M. A., 268n1,292n75
Ball, J. C., 62
Bandyopadhyay, S., 56
Baral, I., 19,37,127,134,171,172, 200,
  203,257,268n1
Barkan, H., 35,268n1
Baron, R., 62
Barry, K., xxiii,176,188,189,205
Bates, K., 144
Becker, D., 256
Belcher, L., 58
Bell, L., 188,189
Belton, R., 35
Bennett, L., 26
Benoit, C., 59,240,248

Benoit, J., 296n91
Biernacki, P., 189,230
Bird, Y. M., 154
Bishop, R., xx
Blanchard, E. G., 41
Bonnie, R. J., 296n91
Bosch, F., 56
Bosley, A., 117
Boudin, K., 284n51
Bownes, I. T., 56
Boyd, C., 189,190
Boyer, D., 258
Breton, M., 256
Briere, J., 97
British Broadcasting Company (BBC),
  149
Brom, D., 232,233
Brown, L., 143
Brownmiller, S., 2
Buckley, T. C., 41
Buell, S. M., 288n63,288n64
Buitrago, M. M. A., 39
Bunch, C., 133
Bureau NRM, 317
Burger, J., 94
Burgess, A. W., 59
Burris, A. B., 154
Burt, M., 76
Butters, J., 60
Buzawa, C. G., 10
Buzawa, E. S., 10
Bystrom, M., 327

Cambodian Women's Crisis Center,
  171
Campaign Against Trafficking in
  Women, 180

Campbell, J., 59
Caralis, P., 25
Cardwell, D., 172
Carlson, E. B., 204
Carroll, J. J., 57,63
Carter, C., 240
Carter, V., 9,172,268n1,273n18,
     277n26,293n76
Cassese, J., 97,98
Casteneda, M., 155
Castillo, D. A., 149,154,157
Castillo, M. L., 256
Chapkis, W., 188,189
Chattopadhyay, M., 56
Cheery, C., 58
Chiquiar, D., 148
Chirgwin, V., 257
City Club of Portland Report, 18
Clark, J. P., 240
Clements, T. M., 272n11
Codigo Penal de Colombia, 39
Coid, J., 4
Cole, P., 288n63
Cole, S., 98
Commonwealth Fund Survey of
     Women's Health, 25
Cone, E. J., 62
Connell, R. W., 95
Cooper, B. S., 200,203
Cotton, A., 62,77,154
Council for Prostitution Alternatives,
     20,24
Craft, N., 122
Crowe, C., 62
Crowell, N. A., 59
Cubbins, L. A., 87

Dada, Y., 61
Daley, S., 318,320
Dalla, R. L., 34,62
Danzinger, S., 270n7
Darrow, W. W., 190
Darves-Bornoz, J. M., 203
David, H., 226

Davidson, J. O., 34,177
Davis, M., 288n64
Davis, N. J., 226,227
Davis, P., 299n101
D'Cunha, J., 59,171,172,177,178,321
Degiovanni, A., 203
Deily, E. K., 285n55
Delacoste, F., 179,188,189
Delgado, B., 149,154,157
Delgado, R., 98
D'Ercole, A., 302n11
Dersks, A., 145
Derthick, M., 307n129
De Sanjose, S., 5
Desmond, D. P., 63
De Vries, M.W., 272n14
Diatkite, F., 171
Dienemann, J., 59
Dilorio, C., 102
Dines, G., 96,98,99
DiPaolo, M., 56
Ditmore, M., 176
Doezma, J., 176
DuBois, W. E. B., 205
Dugon, D., 288n64
Duncan, M., 56
Durston, L. S., 279,279n38,307n129,
     308n130
Duttagupta, C., 56
Dutting, G., 317
Dutton, M. A., 305n122
Dworkin, A., xx,xxii,19,20,96,98,
     99,100,110n5,170,205
Dzuhayatin, S. R., 59,171

Earls, C., 226
Ebener, P. A., 286n57
Edelstein, J., 207
Edleson, J. L., 304n118
Edmonson, R., 96,104
Edmunds, C. N., 76,78
Egendorf, A., 256
Ekberg, G. S., xxi,327,328
El-Bassel, N., 189,190

Elsass, P., 209
Epstein, D., 10
Equality Now, 177
Erickson, P. G., 60
Espitia, V., 56
Estroff, S. E., 296n91

Factum of the Intervener Women's
    Legal Education and Action
    Fund, 96
Family Violence Prevention Fund, 25
Farley, M., 19,77,89,97,127,134,173,
    188,194,226,248,257,268n1,
    298n95
Figley, C. R., 256
Finstad, L., xix,xxi,60,190,203,226,
    233
Flitcraft, A., 26
Foa, E. B., 76
Ford, D., 25
Forneris, C. A., 41
Foy, D. W., 37,56
Frankel, R. M., 57
Freed, W., 134,135,161
Friedman, M. J., 37,59
Frosh, S., 95
Fuchs Ebaugh, H., 225
Funari, V., 207-208
Fundacion Renacer, 39
Fung, R., 108
Funk, R. E., 62,95

Gaillard, P., 203
Gamache, D., 22,36,259
Gamble, N. C., 78
Garrity, R., 19
Gershuny, B. S., 76
Gielen, A. C., 59
Gill, M., 97,98
Giobbe, E., 19,21,22,36,57,65,170,
    174,206,259,268n1,273n18,
    277n26,293n76

Girschick, L. B., 302n112
Godsoe, C., 301n108,301n110
Goldsmith, B., 180
Goldstein, J., 2
Gomez, C., 24,57,123,154,321
Gomez, E., 256
Gomez, M. G. R., 149,157
Gonzalez de la Vega, F., 155
Gonzalez-Lopez, G., 156
Goodman, L. A., 24
Gorst-Unsworth, C., 56
Gossop, M., 63
Graaf, I. de, 35
Graham, D. L. R., 161
Granskaya, J., 58
Green, B., 37
Greenfeld, L., 78
Greenhouse, S., 302n112
Greenman, M., 258
Griffiths, P., 63
Grussendorf, C., 273n19
Gutman, R. A., xv
Gysels, M., 57

Hadden, G., 155
Hall, M., 134
Hansen, N., 102
Hanson, G., 148
Harbury, J., 155
Harden, J., 284n51
Hardill, K., 62
Harrigan, M., 22,36
Hartgers, C., 98
Hartman, A., 208
Hartwell, T., 102
Hass, G. A., 305n122
Hatch, J. P., 63
Haugaard, L., 2
Haver, B., 26
Hayashi, J., 56
Heber, S., 61,200
Hedin, U. C., 9,224,226,227,230,231
Heiman, J. R., 97,102
Heinzl, T., 149

Herman, D. S., 37
Herman, J. L., 6,58,97,209,210,268n1,
    271n10,272n11,272n12,
    304n118
Hernandez, A., 150
Hernandez, T. K., xxiii,65,162
Heslet, L., 59
Hessle, S., 228,230,232
Higgins, D. J., 97,102
Hills, M., 284n51
Hirsch, B., 228,234
Hodgson, C., 36,161,171
Hoigard, C., xix,xxi,60,190,203,226,
    233
Holland, G., 125,128
Holsopple. K., 22,61
Homan, B., 97
Horton, A. J., 107
Hotaling, N., 9,19,154,171,257
Houskamp. B. M., 37,56
Howard, O., 20,87,172,288n63
Howard, S. L., 285n55
Hoyt, D. R., 155
Hoyt, L., 226
Hubbell, A., 189,190
Hughes, D. M., 24,57,117,119,121,
    134,178,257,273n19,321
Hughes, T. L., 98
Human Rights Vigilance of Cambodia,
    134
Human Rights Watch Asia, 143
Hunter, S. K., 35,57
Huska, J. A., 37,41
Hynes, H. P., 59,171,321

Iams, H., 299n101
ICBF (Instituto Colombiano de
    Biensestar
    Familiar)-UNESCO, 39
Idol, Ryan, 103
Iliina, S., 127
Imperial, M. L., 285n55
International Human Rights Law
    Group, 176

Isherwood, C., 94,96,103,105,110n6
Island, D., 18

James, J., 35,240
Jayasundara, D., 77,79
Jeffreys, S., xx,65,170,179-180,319,
    321,323
Jenckes, M., 25
Jensen, R., 94,96,99
Johnson, B. J., 154
Johnson, C., 2
Johnson, T., 98
Jones, A., 21
Jones, A. S., 59
Jones-Alexander, J., 41
Jordan, M., 155
Jordan, P., 104
Joyce, R. A., 155

Kalenandi, M., 283n44
Kalichman, S. C., 58
Kalugin, I., 127
Kandel, M., 89
Karlsen, C., 226,233
Kashiwagi, S., 56
Katz, B., 76
Keane, T. M., 37,41
Kellog, B., 116
Kelly, V., xxvn2,55,200,226,
Kemp, A., 37,56
Kendall, C. N., 62,94,95,99,100,101,
    110n4
Kennedy, M. A., 200
Kilpatrick, D. G., 76,78
Kimerling, R., 98
Kingsley, C., 240,248
Kinsie, P., 66n3
Kiremire, M., 127,172,203,257,268n1
Kleber, R. J., 232,233
Klerman, J. A., 286n57
Kluft, R. P., 206
Koss, M., 2,59

Kovaleski, S. F., 154
Kovalskys, J., 256
Koverola, C., 203
Kramer, L., 34,63
Kristiansen, A., 230
Kub, J., 59

Lachicotte, W. S., 296n91
Lang, A. R., 87
Lange, W. R., 62
Langeland, W., 98
Larsson, S., 226,228
Lawson, M., 26
Lederer, L., 98,99,149
Leech, G. M., 39
Leidholdt, D., xxiii,171,322
Leigh, C., xxv
Leighton, J., 21
Letellier, P., 18
Levin-Epstein, J., 306n127
Lewis, J., 61,240
LifeSiteNews.com, 170
Lifton, R. J., 256
Lim, L.L., xix,64,65
Linehan, C., 128
Lira, E., 256
Litz, B. T., 37,41
Lizotte, A. J., 79
Ljokjell, T. R., 228,232
Loring, M.T., 24,25
Lostaunau, F., 153
Louis, M., 170,177
Lovelace, L., 4,96
Lowman, J., 240
Lykes, M. B., 256
Lynch, T., 78,79
Lynne, J., 63,77,154,248

McCabe, M. P., 97,102
McCauley, Y., 25
McFarlane, A., 58,268n1
MacKinnon, C. A., xx,xxi,xxiii,xxvn1,
        1,20,65,95,96,98,99,
        100,110n5

McLaughlin, J. F., 128,129
Madigan, L., 78
Maeda, Y., 56
Maher, L., 26
Maki, F. T., 154
Maltz, W., 97
Mandel, F., 58
Mann, J. M., 58
Mansson, S. A., 9,62,170,224,226,
        227,231
Marcovich, M., 175
Mark, M., 240,248
Martin, L., 320
Martin-Baro, I., 256
Mathai-Davis, P., 288n64
Maticka-Tyndale, E., 240
Mattsson, M., 233
McGrady, M., 4
Mebari, L., 56
Medrano, M. A., 63
Melbye, K. A., 154
Mendelson, N. X., 257
Meston, C. M., 97,102
Meyerding, J., 35
Milburn, N., 302n111
Millar, A., 59,240,248
Miller, E., 26,190,283,284,284n48
Miller, J., 35,77,78,79,89,90
Millet, K., xix
Mills, L., 10,307n129,308n130
Mills, Linda G., 279n38
Minami, K., 56
Minnesota Advocates for Human
        Rights, 171
Minnesota Coalition Against
        Prostitution, 22
Mitchell, K., 26
Mitchell, S. P., 103
Monahan, J., 296n91
Monto, M. A., 89
Moos, R. H., 98
Morgan, M., 39
Morse, D. S., 57
Motta, C., 39
Muecke, M., 144

Munczek, D., xxi
Munn, A. J., 117
Munoz, N., 56
Musialowski, R., 25
Muth, S. Q., 190

Nachimson, D., 58
Nadon, S. M., 203
Nakashima, K., 56
National Coalition for the Homeless
    Fact Sheet, 24
NCMEC (National Center for Missing
    and Exploited Children), 39
Nelson, V., 19
Nelson-Pallmeyer, J., 2
Network of Sexwork Projects, 176
Nnulasiba, B, 57
Norris, J., 87
Norton, G. R., 61,200

O'Campo, P., 59
O'Donnell, M., 157
O'Gorman, E. C., 56
O'Hare, P., 241
Ojeda, N. L., 157
O'Leary, C., 20,87,172
Orloff, L. E., 305n122
Ouimette, P. C., 98
Overmeyer-Velazquez, R., 156
Owen, R., 177
Ozden, S. Y., 200

Palacio, V., 56
Park, G., 154
Parker, J., 25
Parriott, R., 24,35,56,172
Pateman, C., 171
Patrick, D. L., 296n91
Patterson, O., 1,58
Paymor, M., 22
Pease, B., 95

Pelcovitz, D., 58
Pelzer, A., 56
Pennebaker, J. W., 233
Pense, E., 22
Pfeiffer, M. B., 62
Phan, H., 135
Pheterson, G., 233
Phillips-Plummer, L., 190
Phoenix, J., 203,207
Pick, W. M., 61
Pines, A. M., 19,35,57,77,171,172,
    203,226
Piot, P., 58
Pollock, H., 270n7
Pollock, J., 284n51
Pool, R., 57
Potterat, J., 190
Powis, B., 63
Prince, D., 190
The Protection Project, 170
Putheavy, P., 135
Putnam, F. W., 5,204

Quayle, E., 125,128

Rabinovitch, J., 9,154,240,242-244,
    251
Radomsky, N. A., 59
Ramirez Rodriguez, Z., 321
Ramsay, R., 56
Raphael, J., 60,195
Ravitch, F.S., 275
Rawlings, E., 37
Raymond, J. G., 24,57,59,63,123,171,
    178,321,325,326
Rechsteiner, R. J., 240
Reilly, C., 58
Renzetti, C. M., 304n118
Reyes, M. E., 39,77,154
Reynolds, D., 102,103
Richard, A. O., 64,149,319
Riggs, D. S., 76

Riley, D., 241
Roberts, D., 288n64
Robinson, L., xx
Roche, C., 273n19
Rodriguez, L. F., 39
Rodriguez, N., 37
Rodriguez, O., 157
Rodriguez, Z. R., 59,171
Roman, G., 56
Romero-Daza, N., 58
Roos, D., 124
Rose, F., 118,119
Ross, C. A., 57,61,161,200,203,204, 210
Ross, M. H., 61
Roth, S., 58
Rothenberg, R. B., 190
Rubenstein, S., 66n3
Ruhaini Dzuhayatin, S., 321
Rupp, K., 299n101
Russell, D. E. H., 1,4,19,99
Russo, A., 96,98
Ryan, J., 22,36
Ryan, S. W., 37

Salgado, X., 64
Sanchez, L. E., 291n70
Sanders-Phillips, K., 58
Santos, A., 59,171,321
Saunders, D. G., 37
Sawyer, R. G., 62,63
Sayers, A., 56
Scambler, A., 293n77
Scambler, G., 293n77
Schelzig, E., 171,320
Schilling, R., 189,190
Schiraldi, G. R., 62,63
Schludermann, E. H., 203
Schmidt, M., 62
Schnurr, P. P., 37
Schollenberger, J., 59
Schwartz, H. L., 57,161,206,210
Schwartz, M. D., 77,78,89,90
Scully, E., 63

Seitles, M. D., 39
Seng, M., 190
Sevim, M., 200
Seymour, A. E., 76,78
Sezgin, U., 19,37,77,134,154,172, 200,257
Shaboltas, A., 58
Shapiro, D. L., 60,195
Shaw, J., 98
Silbert, M. H., 19,35,57,77,78,79,171, 172,203,226
Simons, R. L., 35,188,190
SIPAZ, 155
Skee, M., 105
Smith, B., 240
Smith, R. W., 24,25
Snyder, F. R., 62
Southwick, S., 59
Spiwak, F., 39,77
Spiwak, S., 154
Sporcic, L. J., 257
Stang, J., 63
Stark, C., 21,26,36,162,171
Stark, E., 26,174
Stark, S., 306n127
Stiglmayer, A., xxi
Stoltenberg, J., 94,95,100
Stormo, K. J., 87
Strangelove, M. E., 117
Straver, C. J., 35
Stritzke, W. G. K., 87
Stychin, C., 94,104,108
Suchman, A. L., 57
Sullivan, M., 170,180,319,321,322, 323
Svensson, B., 230

Tafur, L., 56
Taino, S., 149
Taylor, M., 125,128,129
Thoennes, N., 77
Thompson, D., xx
Tibaux, G., 56
Tiggeloven, C., 321

Tjaden, P., 77
Torres, F. G., 105
Trapnell, P. D., 97,102
Trull, L. A., 57,63
Trulsson, K., 229
Turner, F., 256
Turner, S., 56
Turner, S.W., 304n118
Tutty, L. M., 97,98
Tyler, K. A., 155

UNICEF, 134,135,155
UNICEF Colombia, 39
U. S. Report of Trafficking in Persons, 39
Urabe, K., 56

Valentiner, D. P., 76
Valera, R. J., 62
Van de Kemp, H., 37
Van Der Hart, O., 272n13
Van der Kolk, B. A., 4,58,268n1, 304n118
Vanwesenbeeck, I., 35,61,144,226, 232
Van Zessen, G., 35
Vasconcelos, A., 171
Vasquez, S., 56
Vaux, A., 227,228,234
Visser, J. H., 35
Vranic, S., xxi

Waldorf, D., 189
Walker, L. E., 18
Waller, N. G., 204
Walton, M., 240
Watters, J. K., 189
Weathers, F. W., 37,41,42,56
Weeks, M., 58
Weine, S., xxi
Weisaeth, L., 268n1
Weisberg, D. K., 35
Wetzel, J. W., 256
Whitbeck, L. B., 35,155,188,190,226
Wilcox, B. I., 228,234
Williams, E. A., 58
Williams, J. L., 208
Wilsnack, S. C., 98
Winick, C., 66n3
Worth, D., 58
Wynne, C., 59
Wynter, B., xx

Yargic, L. I., 200,203,204
Yehuda, R., 59
Young, A. M., 189,190
Young, L., 35
Young, R., 328
Young, S., 240
Yuille, J. C., 200

Zarate, L., 158
Zimmer, C., 296n91
Zubick, J., 240
Zule, W. A., 63
Zumbeck, S., 77,154

Subject Index

Aboriginal peoples: struggles of, 248; women, in sex trade, 63,239, 249; youth, in prostitution, 240,249. *See also* First Nations, indigenous women

abstinence standard for drug/alcohol abuse, lack of, 260

abuse: denial of, 325; psychological consequences of, 171; reporting, lack of, 159; ritual, 19,28. *See also* emotional abuse; physical abuse; sexual abuse

acting out, sexual, 97

acupuncture, 261

addiction, 4,9-10,209; prostitution as cause of, 34; treatment for, xix,26. *See also* drugs; substance abuse

adolescent girls: age of at entry into prostitution, 134; from Nepal, 143; from Nigeria, 321; recruitment and sale of, 134-35; violence against, in Africa, 58. *See also* genital mutilation

"adult-supervised settings" for teenage mothers, 282n41

advocacy, need for, 161,221,247,256

Africa, violence against girls in, 58

African-American communities, cultural and social barriers within, 217

African-American men, stereotyped as sexual predators, 106-107

African-American women, 203; HIV/STD infection rate among, 215,216,217; as law enforcement target, 215; poverty and dependence among, 214,216,217; in prostitution, 213; services for prostituted, 216-18; stereotypes of, 215; and war on drugs, 302

agency relationships, collaborative, 261

AIDS, 105,145; age of infection with, 58; safer-sex and, 105; and sexual violence, 58. *See also* HIV; HIV/AIDS

Aid to Families with Dependent Children (AFDC), 269n3. *See also* Temporary Assistance to Needy Families (TANF)

alcohol. *See* substance abuse

alcohol abuse, maternal (FAS/FAE), 218,242

alienation, social, 12

amnesia, 206

anger: feelings of, 262,282; management of, 261

anti-rape organizations, 28

anxiety disorders, 57,140,142,189

appellate court decisions, 75-76

arrest, fear of, 216

Arte Sana, Dripping Springs, Texas, 147,158-59

art exhibit, by sexual assault survivors, 158

Asian men, as inferior, 106,108

Asian women: abuse of online, 119; trafficked, 168,177

Asia Watch, 143

Australia, xx; brothels in, 177,322-23; growth of child prostitution in, 321; growth of illegal prostitution in, 320-21; harm

reduction approach in, 241.
See also Victoria, Australia
Australian National Inquiry on Child
    Prostitution, 321
Austria: brothels in, 177;
    state-sponsored prostitution
    in, 319
autonomy, as insubordination, 4-5
avoidance, symptoms of, 273,273n17
Axis I diagnoses, range of, 204
Axis II diagnoses, 58,204

Babes4U, 127
Bangkok. *See* Thailand
Bangladesh, 173
battered women, 9,17-18,23-24,25,26,
    35,158
battered women's movement and
    prostitution, 221
battered women's shelters, 151,157; as
    prison, 303; services of, 288,
    288n62
batterers: control by, 21-22,302;
    multiple, 23,27; physical
    injuries from, 24-25; and
    pimps, similarities between,
    21-23,174
battering: and homelessness, 23-24;
    and prostitution, similarities
    between, 18,29n5; spousal,
    24,173-75; and substance
    abuse, 26; trivialization of, 20
battery or extreme cruelty: defined,
    286-87; forms of proof of,
    287-88; prostitution as, 18
*Bell v. Commissioner of Social
    Security*, 293-94
benefits: amounts and timing of, 304,
    305-306;SSI,306,307; TANF,
    306,306n125
Bilateral Safety Corridor Coalition
    (BSCC), San Diego,
    California, 147,151,152,153,

154,159-60; task forces in,
    160
bipolar disorder, 220
bisexual men, 96-97,100
Blacks. *See* African Americans
bodily functions, control of, 4
body awareness training, 233
bondage and discipline centers, 150,
    319,322
border crossing, illegal, 157
border factories, working conditions
    in, 162
Bosnia-Herzegovina, women in, xxi
Brazil, 149
breakaway from prostitution: in
    Canada, 239; economic
    implications of, 291n71;
    factors affecting, 225; phases
    of, 225; planning in, 260;
    pregnancy in, 229-30;
    preliminary stages of, 225,
    231; theory, 224-25. *See also*
    prostitution, leaving
Breaking Free service agency, in
    Minnesota, 216,217-219
brides, mail order, 19,28,63,150
brothel owners: deceptive practices of,
    135; dependence on, 144
brothels, 168,203,224,240; in
    Australia, 177,180,320-23;
    bawdy houses, 240;
    Cambodian, 133-45;
    Canadian, 177;
    decriminalizing, 315; for
    disabled men, 322-23; false
    identities in, 137; field, 151;
    high class, xviii; impact of,
    143; Indian, 143; legal, 168;
    lineup in, xvii,xviii; living
    conditions in, 136,138; in
    Nevada, xxii,60,117,121;
    relationships between women
    in, 141; "safety policies" in,
    324; in San Diego County,
    150; sexual trauma in, 138; as

socially sanctioned activity, 135; sources for, 177; terms for, xviii; in Thailand, 143; as traffickers' destination, 178; in Turkey, 39,202; Web sites of, 119,120-21.

Budapest process, 329n1
bureaucrats, attitudes of, 244
Bureau of Justice statistics, 78
Burmese women, 143
"bury it" hazard, 274,275,280
Butler, Josephine, 176

Cambodia: brothels in, 133-45; captivity in, 141; cultural context of, 143-44,145; fear and anxiety in, 140,142; research in, 136; sex industry in, 134; trends in, 134-35; women's identity in, 135
Cambodian Women's Development Association (CWDA), 134, 143
Canada, 33,37-38,200; Aboriginal prostitution in, 63,239,240, 248-49; brothels in, 177; studies in, 37-38,62; depression rate in, 140,142; economic impact of prostitution in, xix; harm reduction approach in, 241; health problems of women in, 47,50,51,54,55,59; neurological symptoms, 59; prostitution in, 239-41. *See also* PEERS
cancer, breast and cervical, 218
captivity: coping strategies in, 142-43; health consequences of, 151; torture in, 141
caregivers, initial response of, 274
Carrao v. Shalala, 294-95,295n86
case examples: Chris, 258; Chris J., 101; Culver, Cal, 104;

Elizabeth, xx-xxi; Guadalupe, 152-54; Jaget, Claude, xvii; Jenny, 5; Jim Y., 102; Joline, 219-20; Katarina, 7-8; Kevin, 11; Maria, 158-59; Nicole, 8-9; of rehabilitation, 9-10; Sara, xviii; Sofia, 151-52; Stefano, Joey Iacona, 94, 103-104,105,110n6; Yvette, 9-11
caseworkers, monitoring by, 282
Catholic Charities, 152
Catholic Church, influence of on gender roles, 155-56
CEDAW. *See* Convention on the Elimination of All Forms of Discrimination Against Women
Centers for Disease Control, 215
Center for Law and Social Policy, 306
chastity, as issue in U.S. rape law, 76, 79,90
chat, live video, as pimps' marketplace, 116
chemical dependence. *See* addiction; substance abuse
child abuse. *See* sexual abuse, childhood
child prostitution, 34,40,36,57,133-34, 150,152; in Australia, 321; in Canada, 40,240; frequency of in Mexico, 155; increase in, 321; legalized prostitution and, 321
Child Protective Services, 151,153, 219
child sex offenders, use of Internet by, 128
childcare, xviii,261; needs, exceptions for, 312
childrearing and prostitution, double life of, 157,229
children: biracial female, 214; importance of in breakaway, 229-30; loss of custody of,

229,283-84; meeting with for
sexual exploitation, 128; of
prostituted women, xviii,8;
sale of to brothels, 214;
supporting, 229. *See also*
child prostitution; sexual
abuse, childhood
ChildRight, Amsterdam, 321
China, as trafficking source country,
64
choice: involuntary, 324; personal,
251-52; legal prostitution as
rational and, 324
Chronic Health Problems
Questionnaire, 42,55
churches, African-American, 221
client-centered approach, 261
climate, therapeutic, 6-7
clinical assessment and diagnosis, as
"naming" steps, 272
Coalition Against Trafficking in
Women, 39,167,168,176
cognitive dissonance, reduction of,
206
Colombia, 33,37,39; age of consent in,
39; health problems of
women in, 55; legal
prostitution in, 39; rape in,
163n4
colonialism: harms of, 248; legacy of,
63
colonization: of body, 4; of indigenous
women, 155
Combating Pedophile Information
Networks in Europe Project
(COPINE), 125,129
commodification, 188,208,209. *See
also* depersonalization;
identity; objectification
Commonwealth v. Houston, 84
Commonwealth v. Joyce, 83-84
communities: Black, cultural and
social barriers within, 217;
poor and urban, prostitution
in, 214

community: involvement of, 245-48;
partners, activities with,
245-46; peer counseling
program in, 256
Community Health Clinic, 152
comorbidity, 200
condom policies, enforceable, 323
condom use, 136,140,161,168,216,
323-24; sex acts without,
168,322; in street
prostitution, 320
Confederation of Trade Unions
(Denmark), 329
conflict, reduction of internal, 206
consciousness, altered states of, 4,200,
205
consent: and bias, role of prostitution
in proving, 80-88; issue of, as
admissable evidence, 75,138
contempt: fear of, 216; for men, 233
control: by batterers and pimps, 21-23,
174; over body, 272n4;
coercive, 2,4,6,17,172
Convention on the Elimination of All
Forms of Discrimination
Against Women (CEDAW),
xxvn1,175-76
Convention on the Rights of the Child,
39
Convention for the Suppression of the
Traffic in Persons and of the
Exploitation of Prostitution
of Others (United Nations).
See 1949 Convention
Council for Prostitution Alternatives,
xxiv,xxv
counseling, 196,247; for chemical
dependency, 218; peer,
effectiveness of, 255
countertransference, 12,209,273-274
COYOTE (Call Off Your Old Tired
Ethics), 179
coyotes (labor traffickers), 149-50. *See
also* trafficking
crack cocaine, 26,87,216

criminal justice system: bias against
     prostituted women in, 90,
     241,252n1; prostituted
     womens' fear of, 76. *See also*
     law enforcement officers
crisis intervention, 160,217
cultural imperialism, defined, 221n2
cultural practice, harmful traditional,
     xx
culture, "compulsory heterosexuality"
     of U.S., 94; male supremacy
     in Mexican, 154-57; Western
     popular, xxii
customers, 19; age differential of, 173;
     criminal sanctions against in
     Sweden, 180;
     decriminalizing, 315; demand
     for novelty by, 178;
     gratification of, 171; innate
     inequality of, 173; physical
     violence from, 322; terms for,
     65-66n1. *See also* johns,
     tricks
cutting, 220
Czech Republic, as trafficking source
     country, 64

danger, inability to recognize, 97,205,
     208
debt bondage, tactics of, xxiii,176
decriminalization, prostituted womens'
     resistance to, 325-326
Deep Throat (film), 4,99,109n5
degradation, eroticized, 100,101,124
demand for prostitution, penalizing the
     response to, 326-29
denial: of abuse, 325; in African
     American community, 215,
     221; of childhood sexual
     abuse, 57; of harms of
     legalization, 169,179,319,
     321,326; "Hide the
     Prostitution" dynamic, 2-3,
     12,274,280,281,284; "let's

pretend" hazard, 274,289,
     292; of prostitution history,
     in SSI assessment, 278-79;
     social, of harms of
     prostitution, 60,206,256. *See
     also* prostitution, invisibility
     of; prostitution, myths about;
     rape, reporting
Denmark, state-sponsored prostitution
     in, 319
depersonalization, xviii-xix,115,124,
     127,206,207,240-41. *See also*
     commodification; identity;
     objectification
depression, 57,173,189,207,217,240,
     244; in Cambodia, 140,142;
     rates of, 201,202,204,206
derealization, 206
development, disruption of normal,
     138-39
diabetes, 218
diagnoses prohibited in SSI, 297-300
dichos (sayings), Mexican, about
     gender, 156
dichotomy, mother/whore, 282n43
DID. *See* Dissociative Identity
     Disorder
DIF. *See* Mexican Social Services
"dildo cams," 122
disability, 9; categories of assessment
     of, 276; determination of,
     276; and earning power,
     inverted correlation between,
     292; legal definition of, 275;
     prostitution history as part of
     claim, 275; stigma of, 296
disclosure: obstacles to, 279-80,288;
     prostituted women's fears of,
     25; psychological impact of,
     249-51; by therapist, 288
dissociation, xviii,5,57,66n3,138,161,
     199-210,262; as avoidance
     strategy, 205; of ego states, 4;
     function of, 206; personal
     history as, 251; by rape

victims, 173; range of
response in, 203; as response
to childhood trauma, 204; as
social norm, 1; somatic,
207-208,209,233; studies of,
200-203,205-10; symptoms
of, 292-93; trauma model of,
200
Dissociative Disorder Interview
Schedule (DDIS), 201,202
Dissociative Disorder Not Otherwise
Specified (DDNOS), 206
dissociative disorders, 272; rates of,
202,204
Dissociative Experiences Scale (DES),
201,202,204
Dissociative Identity Disorder (DID),
5,206
dolls, inflatable, xx
domestic service, 66n5,214
domestic violence, 202,257; causes
and effects of, 221; control
through use of, 171; defined,
16,18-19,27; and HIV, 58;
invisibility of, 1; policies for,
25; pornography and
prostitution, nexus of with,
19-21; and prostitution, 17,
173-74; screening for, 286,
286n58; as system of power
and control, 174,175;
victimization by, 281. *See
also* violence, adult
dominance: systems of male, 1,4,19,
154,155,157,170-71,322;
ideology of male, 2; ritual
display of, 2. *See also* power
Dominican Republic, 117
drugs: breakaway from addiction to,
230; costs, 294n84;
dependence on as disabling
condition, 298n96;
detoxification from, 161;
prior prostitution for as
evidence, 86-88; sex for,

86-88. *See also* substance
abuse
DSM-IV-TR, 271,271n9,278,279n37
durational cap, waiver of, 308-309,
309n135
Dutch National Rapporteur on
Trafficking, 319
dysfunction, sexual, 204
dysregulation, affective and somatic, 4

Eastern Europe, women trafficked
from, 168,177
education: culturally relevant, 158;
intensive, 218; peer model in,
263-64; staff opportunities
for, 263
El Salvador, civil war in, 155
eligibility for benefits, factor of in
TANF, 281; and mental
health diagnostic criteria, 270
emotional abuse, rates of in Turkey,
202
emotional distress, symptoms of, 57
emotions: of women in prostitution,
while performing, 192-194;
range of negative, 187; about
sexuality, 192
empathy, loss of, 124
employment: mandates, impact of,
304; restricted access to
through racism, 214
End Child Prostitution and Trafficking
(ECPAT), 321
entry into prostitution, age of, 35,
39-41,49,134,191,217; in
Canada, 240
Equality Now, 177
escort prostitution, 20,28,29n4,34,148,
187,189,190,191,203,224,
240; in Australia, 180; and
rape, 60; Web sites of, 117,
120-21
Estonia, prostitution in, xxi
European Women's Lobby, 177

evidence: bias or motive to fabricate, 83-84,85; types of admissability of, 81
exit planning, as ongoing process, 260
exotic dancing, 61,200-202,204,240
extortion, prior, 85-86
Eye Movement Desensitization Processing (EMDR), 261

Fall of Communism as Seen Through Gay Porn, The (film),107
family: betrayal by, 64,137,138,139; crisis support from, 227; groups on relationships in, 218; financial assistance program for (TANF), 281; as initiators of SSI/SSDI applications, 310; limitations of support from, 227-28; obligation to in Cambodia, 141-42,143,144; of origin, 226-28; role of, 145,304; separation from, 139; status, issues around, 281; TANF definition of, 282; two-parent, 282n41; violence in, 202; welfare programs, state, 267. *See also* parents
"family cap" provisions, 306,306n126
family planning services, 151,218,261
Family Violence Option (FVO) waiver, 285-89,285nn53,55, 291,303,308,313
"fancy girls," 214
fantasies, masturbatory, of johns, xix, 20-21
Federal Bureau of Investigation (FBI), 152,153
felony conviction, for drug dealing, 301-303,301n108
feminist perspective, xix,1,176
fertility, reduced, 53,283,283n44
fetal alcohol syndrome, prevention of, 218,242

film actors, pornographic, 94,96-98, 100,200. *See also* pornography
film industry, 104-105
Finland, trafficking of Russian women to, 327
First Nations, 37-38,63,248. *See also* Aboriginal peoples; indigenous people
fisting, 102,110n5
flashbacks, 36,173,240
Foundation Against Trafficking in Women (Netherlands), 169, 170
France, 203
"freaking," for cocaine, 87
freedom of speech and expression, used to minimize harms of pornography, 100
Fucked-Up (film), 104
"functional limitations" determination, 276,277,281

gang rape, 35,173
gay men. *See* pornography, gay male
gay rights, 100-104
gender identity and sexual orientation, difference between, 153
gender roles, in Mexico, 153,155-56
gender stereotypes: eroticization of, 94-95; reinforcement of, 96
genital mutilation, female, xx,xxvn1
Germany, xx,33,37,38,168-69; brothels in, 177; legal prostitution in, xxi,38,63, 168,179,315,317-18,319; pimps in, 174; profit from prostitution in, 171
globalization: lost jobs from, 162; of sex industry, 134,168-69,175
goals, interplay of bureaucratic and therapeutic, 270
government response, 178-80
grandparenting, 229

groups: body awareness, 261; on
family relationships, 218;
intensive education, 218; for
male survivors, 11;
non-confrontational support,
262; for prostituted women,
xix,189,234n1; structured
peer support, 11,154,251;
Women's Program support,
220
Guatemala, 149; rape in, 163n4
guilt, feelings of, 189

harm reduction model, 255; nations
using, 241 nonjudgmental,
260; strategies used in, 260
harm: focus on physical, xviii,188,
280,280n40; invisible, xix;
social denial of, 257. *See also*
physical abuse; sexual abuse
Health Canada, 242
health care, 247; availability of
preventive, 216; barriers to,
25,257; facilities, 28,152;
HMOs and, 25; system,
failures of, 215-16; for
trafficking victims, 152;
transportation to, 218
health checks, 320
health insurance, 216
health problems: in Canada, 55; of
formerly prostituted women,
232; among Mexican women,
53; in prostitution, 4-5,
49-55,215-16; in Thailand,
53; in Turkey, 53;
transnational study of, 49;
types of, 53-55; violence as
source of, 53,59,151. *See also*
symptoms
health professionals, "john-like"
behavior of male, 231
hepatitis C, 161
history, Black, impact of, 213-14,221

HIV, 103,105,136,145,151,161,258;
and domestic violence, 58;
positive women, 283n45; sex
as cure for, 58. *See also*
AIDS; HIV/AIDS
HIV/AIDS, 150-51; education, 218;
fear of, 140. *See also* AIDS;
HIV
homelessness, 11,65,153,155,171,174,
217,220,259,304; and
battering, 23-24,62
homeless shelters, 28,159
homicidality, 262
homophobia, 95,99,153; in
contemporary Mexico, 163n2
"Hookers Ball," 179
"Hooters-style" waitressing, as legal
sex work, 313
housing: emergency, 151; need for,
xix,248; safe, 144,196,209,
219,220,261; secure, 60;
supervised, 9; supportive,
247
Human Resources Development
Canada, 242
human rights, violation of, xxv,170
Human Rights Mexico, 152
Human Rights Watch, 176
humiliation, 35; during prostitution,
192; eroticized, 100,101,124,
192; as sexual expression,
101
"hunt, the," for women offline, 123
Hustler (magazine), 20
hypermasculinity, 98
hyperarousal, 12,36,37,61,272n13

identity: of Cambodian women, 135;
dissociative, 206; false, as
control mechanism, 137; loss
of, 58; primary, sex trade
history as, 251; problems of,
6; sexualization of, 94-95,
101; tools for new, 244. *See*

also commodification; depersonalization; dissociation; objectification

ideology: of male domination, 2, 154-57; of criminal class, 6

immigrants: exploitation of, 317; illegal economy in, 148-50; poor, 177; undocumented, 159; women, 256-57

immigration status: feared loss of, 64; jeopardized, 160,162

Immigration and Naturalization Service (INS), 152,157,160

incest, xxii,36,57,171,173,202,208, 304; conception through, 310; invisibility of, 1

income: annual median, 240; declaration of as "naming" issue, 289; disconnect of with neediness, 290; limits, by state, 290n68; as presumptive of independence, 290-91; as presumptive of productive activity, 292-96

Indigenous Community Empowerment Vision workshop, 249

indigenous women: colonization of, 154-55; prostitution of, 63; trafficking of, 62-63. *See also* Aboriginal peoples; First Nations; Native Americans

Indonesia, economic impact of prostitution in, 64,65

"indoor" prostitution, and street prostitution, 203-204

inequality: culture of gender-based, 170; race, sex, and class, 63; sex, 58,148,154-57,161-62

Inter-Agency Standing Committee (IASC), United Nations, code of conduct of, 329

international forums, censorship at, 329

International Human Rights Law group, 176

International Labor Organization (ILO), 64,325

International Organization of Migration (IOM), 317,319

Internet: collecting child pornography from, 125-26,128; and effects of global community forums, 115,116,120-25, 127-28; history of, 117; lack of accountability in, 125; new technologies for prostitution on, 116-20,128; pimps and, 116; pornography on, 21, 107,116,190,328; prostitution tourism and, 117; and sex industry, relationship between, 64,115,117-18,129; unsafe sexual practices on, 107. *See also* World Wide Web

Internet Business Journal, The, 117

interventions: client centered, 258; community based, 256; paternalistic, 10; psychosocial, 144-45

interviews, life story, 225

intimate partner violence. *See* domestic violence

Istanbul. *See* Turkey

Italy, proposed legalization in, 320

jail, women in, 161,189

"job description," WHISPER, xxvi

job training. *See* training, vocational

Johannesburg, South Africa, brothel in, xviii

johns: assault by, 24-25; behavior of, xviii; impregnation by, 311; masturbatory fantasies of, xix,20-21; perspective of, xxii; power of, 34; violence committed by, 233. *See also* customers, tricks

Johnson v. State (MD), 87

Justice Canada, 242

Karma, belief in, 143
kidnapping, 155
Kings County District Attorney's
    Office, New York City, 178

labor, sweatshop, 66n5
labor system, forced, 290
labor unions, on prostitution as work,
    328-29
language: Khmer, 136,145; misogynist,
    124; Spanish, 157
lap dancing, 34,61,148,168,240
Larsen, Ronnie, 103
Latin America: male supremacy in,
    154,155-57; women
    trafficked from, 149,154,
    168,177. *See also* Colombia;
    Mexico
law, of rape, 76,79-80; "rape shield,"
    80; chastity in, 90
law enforcement officers: inability to
    trust, 76,90,160-61;
    prejudicial treatment by, 90,
    241,252n1; and rape victims,
    78-79; racism of, 215;
    referrals by, 242
Law Prohibiting the Purchase of
    Sexual Services (Sweden),
    328,330n4
Lee v. State, 80
legal assistance, 51,261
legalization, resistance to, 330n3
legalized prostitution. *See* prostitution,
    legalized
Lewis, Megan (survivor account),
    242-44,250-51
liaisons, community, need for, 239
libertarian activists, 179
*Little Sisters Book and Art Emporium
    v. Canada*, 109nn1,2

"Lovelace, Linda," 4
Love v. Sullivan, 293-94

McLaughlin, James, 128-29
male beauty, Eurocentric definitions
    of, 98
male bonding, 2
male dominance. *See* dominance
Mali, 173
Månsson, Sven Axel, 170
Marciano, Linda, 4,99,110n5. *See also*
    "Lovelace, Linda"
marginality: barriers in, 255,257,264;
    permanent, 230,232
Marie Claire (magazine), xxii
marriage, servile, 66n5
massage parlors, 19,20,28,34,148,190,
    191,203,207,240
masturbation, 20-21,125,126
maternity, experience of, 157,229-30,
    281,282-84. *See also*
    pregnancy
Medicaid, 272n11
medical problems. *See* health problems
men: bisexual, 96-97,100,104; and
    boys, prostitution of, 34,62;
    contempt for, 233; disabled,
    322-23; as health
    professionals, 231; sexuality
    of and pornography, xxii,
    125. *See also* dominance
mental health diagnostic criteria and
    public assistance eligibility,
    270-71,270n7,272
mental health support, long-term,
    231-33
mentoring, 247
Mexican Federal Police, 152
Mexican Human Rights Commission,
    153-54
Mexican Social Services (DIF), 152,
    153,154,159
Mexico, 33,37,38,154-55; frequency of
    child prostitution in, 155;

gender roles in, 153,155-56; health problems of women in, 53; homophobia in, 155; pimps in, 174; prostitution in, 64,157; prostitution law in, 155; as stopover, 149; trafficking from, 64,148-49; types of prostitution in, 61

migraines, 240

migrant communities, 148,150

migrant sex worker, xxiii-xxiv

migration, facilitated, 176,318

military personnel, 148,150,168

minimization, "me-too" hazard, 274, 281,284,287

Minneapolis, Minnesota: racism of law enforcement in, 215; rape of prostituted women in, 35

Minnesota, frequency of prostitution in, 216

Minnesota Department of Health, 215

models, male, 103,109-10n3

money: management of, 218; myths about, 274,289; and prostitution, 289. *See also* income

mothers, relationship with, 226,227,262

multiple personality. *See* dissociation, Dissociative Disorder, DDIS.

murder, 149,240

myths: cultural, 274; about money, 274,289; about prostitution, 20,60,62,89,247-48,251,325

naming, 272-75,285-86

National Violence Against Women Survey, Center for Disease Control and Prevention, 77

Native Americans, 202,203

need: describing, in application process, 275-87; eligibility standard for, 290n67; financial, 281; for professional help, 224; of

women leaving prostitution, 60,154,247,261

needs assessment, importance of, 160-61

Nepal, adolescent girls in, 143

Netherlands, xx; brothels in, 177; harm reduction approach in, 241; legalized sex industry in, 179, 318; legal prostitution in, xxi, 169-70,315,317; prostitution in economy of, 318; PTSD symptoms in, 61; sexual assault in, 35; state-sponsored prostitution in, 319; stigma of prostitution in, 320

networks, social, after breakaway, 230, 233-34

neurobiological problems, in prostitution, 4-5,59

neutrality, moral *v.* therapeutic, 7-8

Nevada, brothels in, xxii,60,117,121

new life, barriers to, 230

New Life for Young Women Project, International Catholic Migration Commission (ICMC), 136,142

New Zealand, xx

Nicaragua, civil war in, 155

Nigeria, girls from, 321

1949 Convention, 175-76

nongovernmental organizations (NGOs), 170,181,317

Norway, xx-xxi; trafficking of Russian women to, 327

numbing, emotional, 12,36,37,190, 195,206,262,272n13,273, 273n17,297

objectification, xx,xxii,57,188. *See also* commodification; depersonalization; identity

offenders, race of arrested, 221-22n3

online communication, modes of, 117. *See also* Internet, World Wide Web

online communities, for perpetrators, 123-25. *See also* Internet, World Wide Web
oral sex, 88,89,117
Oriental Guys (OG) (magazine), 106
outcall services, 34,322

panic attacks, 8,240
parents: role as, 230,232,234,235n5; problematic relationship with, 227; skills of, 218. *See also* family
partners: poor choices of, 228; as primary support providers, 228; relationships with during breakaway, 228-29
paternity: of prostituted womens' children, 310-11,310nn138, 141; TANF cooperation rules about, 310,311,311n143
patient, prostitution history of, 209
pedophiles, 34,125
peep shows, 19,28,207-208,319
peer education model, 263-64
PEERS, 239-52; community involvement in, 245-47; history of, 242; mission and philosophy of, 241-44; as model, 251-52; staff of, 241, 242,251; as training opportunity, 241
peer support model, 258-63
People v. Abbot, 79
People v. Varona, 88-89
personality disorders, 6,202. *See also* symptoms
Personal Touch Services, A, 117
Philippines: interviews in, 325-26; pimps in, 174
Phoenix, Arizona, study in, 187-96
phone sex, 34,190,191,319
physical abuse, childhood, 44,45,226, 227,232; rates of, 201,202, 204

physical assault, in prostitution, 21,44, 45,214,215,257,286,297,322
pimp: and batterer, similarities between, 21-23,174; as child's father, 311; control by, 9-10,22,36,62,63,302; and coyotes, 149-50; criminalization of, 28; deceptive practices of, 135; decriminalizing, 315; defined, 19,66n2; dependence on, 23; euphemisms for, xxiv; as "friend," 259; as legitimate sexual entrepreneur, 316,326; protection from, 160; "seasoning" by, xx; "stable" of, 174; surveillance by, 119-20; systematic violence of, 2,4,36,233,322; as third party businessman, 316; use of pornography by, 21
PIMPS 'R' US, 117
Planned Parenthood, 151
Playboy (magazine), 20
police corruption, 321
Pollock, Nancy, 320
pornography, xxii,150,319;
- child, 34,125-26; collecting, from Internet, 125-26,128
- gay male, 93-110; as act of rebellion, 94,109; AIDS and, 105; dehumanizing epithets in, 95; and equality, 108; as form of male power, 95; male beauty and masculinity in, 95,98; men used to produce, 95-96; profitability of, 99,108; racism in, 106-108; sex-based harms of, 99-100,104; as traumatic re-enactment, 97,98; unsafe sexual practices in, 105-106; as validation, 101
- heterosexual, 96,98-100; escalation of, 125; inequality and

exploitation in, 104-106; on
Internet, 21,34,107,125; as
legal sex work, 313;
misogyny in, 99; pimps' use
of, 21; and prostitution, xxii,
19-21,44,46,99,125;
prostitution and domestic
violence, nexus with, 19-21;
role of, 28; as violence, 28
Portland, Oregon, study of rape in, 35
poster campaign, in Sweden, 328
posttraumatic stress disorder (PTSD),
5,44,47-49,173,188,204,209,
217,227,232,278-79,295n88;
causes of, 36; Checklist
(PCL), 41-42,44,48; complex
(CPTSD), 4,36,58; gender
differences in, 49; symptoms
of, 34,36-37,41-42,276n21
poverty, 22,56,133,226,227,251; as
channel to prostitution, xxiii,
204,319; and disease, 161
power: and control, domestic violence
as system of, 174,175;
imbalance, exploitation of,
97,120-23,257; of johns, 34;
male, and gay male
pornography, 95; sense of
from mastery of Internet,
126. *See also* dominance
pregnancy, 322; in breakaway, 229-30;
economics of, 283n45; by
pimp, 311; prevention of, 161
Pretty Woman (film), xviii-xix
prior prostitution, admissability of as
evidence, 80,81-83,85-88,90
prison, as safe environment, 304
problems: physical, persistence of, 59;
relational, 6; social, of
women in prostitution, 9-12.
See also health problems
procurement, experiences in, 123-24
programs: court referral, 258;
educational, 247; internship,
218,247; life skills training,

247; pre-employment,
241-42; recovery, 301n107;
self-defense, 261; specifically
for women in prostitution,
28; support, xix; youth,
218-19,247
prostituted women: development of
alternatives for, 327,329;
emotional responses of, xix,
25,189-90,192-94; forms of
abuse of, 20,27,29n1,76,
77-79; needs of, 48-51,60,
144-45,154,209,247,261;
roles of, 157,174-75,221;
services (social, medical and
legal) for, 151-52;
stereotypes of, 300
Prostitutes' Empowerment, Education
and Resource Society. *See*
PEERS
prostitution:
- characteristics of: as
commodification, 188; as
form of rebellion, 195;
invisibility of, 12,27,65,240,
245; objectification, 188; as
slavery, 205,213-15,216,
324-25; structural social
factors contributing to,
116-20,145,161-62,230; as
toxic cultural product, xxii;
as victimless crime, 3; as
violation of human rights,
xx-xxi
- defined, 19,175-77; euphemisms for,
xxiii,xxiv,176; myths about,
20,60,62,89,247-48,251,325;
terms for, 29n4; stereotypes
of, 215,251
- domination in, 167,170-172; by
pimps, 9-10,22,23,29n3,36,
62,63,302
- as economic activity, xix,35,64,65,
116-20,171,188,317,319;

pimps' changed role in,
315-16
- entering, 136,137,170,171,226,
235n3,240,319; age at, 35,
39-41,49,134,191,217
- harms of, xix,xxv,6-7,18,24-25,99,
171,220; multiple trauma in,
34,60,127; shame and stigma
in, 3,188,233,240; and
substance abuse, 62-63,220;
and verbal abuse, 35,43,44,
55,161,257
- and health, xix,3,4-5,12,206-207,
209,215-16,240,278n32,
323-24
- leaving, xviii,xix,9-12,65,144-45,
208-209,217-19,223,241-42;
economic status in, 289-96;
needs while, 60,154,247,
261; phases of, 224-25
- legalization of, xx,xxv,38,39,49,52,
63,170,179,310,321-22,326;
decriminalization of, in
Sweden, xxi,xxv,180; pimps
and, 315-16; resistance to,
330n3; and "sex work," xxiii,
60,170,176,294-95,313,316
- men and boys in, 26,34,62,103
- pornography and, xxii,19-21,44,46,
99,125
- and public assistance programs, 80,
267-314
- trafficking and, xxiii,133-34,154-55,
167,176,177-78,329
- types of, 18,28,177,190,195,202-203,
320,322,323
- violence in, xxii,18,24-25,27,35,
42-44,45,55-57,102,105,148;
domestic violence and, 17,
19-21,167,173-74,202
See also brothels; child prostitution;
escort prostitution; exotic
dancing; lap dancing;
massage parlors; outcall
services; peep shows; phone

sex; saunas; sex clubs; sex
tourism; street prostitution;
strip clubs; stripping
Prostitution Control Act of 1994,
Australia, 318
Prostitution Questionnaire, 41,42
psychological distress, persistence of,
59
psychotherapy, 154; confidentiality in,
8-9; need for, 231-33;
neutrality in, 7-8; rules of, 6;
safety in, 9. *See also* therapy
PTSD. *See* posttraumatic stress
disorder
public assistance: women in
prostitution and, 267-314;
eligibility issues, 268,
269-70; mental health
diagnostic criteria and,
270-71,270n7,272; state
funded, 308n134;
stigmatizing of, 296
public education campaign, in Sweden,
180
public health agencies, attention of to
HIV and STD, 151
public speaking, about prostitution
experience, 249-51
PunterNet (United Kingdom), 118

race/ethnicity, xix
racism: and African American women,
215; barriers created by, 216;
eroticized in gay male
pornography, 106,108; in law
enforcement, 215; and
restricted access to
employment, 214; and
sexism, as dual oppression,
221; and systemic conditions
creating poor health, 162,
215; in trafficking, 64,162
rap groups, 256,257

rape, 57,149,257; of African slaves, 213; and battering, 24; "bought and sold," 173; in Cambodian brothels, 135; camp, online, 119; charge, fabrication of, 80,85-86; conception through, 310; as crime in Latin America, 155, 163n4; date, 173; definitions of, 66n4; experience of, xviii; extrinsic injury in, 78,82-83; French survivors of, 203; frequency of, 35,60; gang, 35,173; of gay men, 102; invisibility of, 1; lack of consent in, 138; law of, 76, 79-80,90; myths about, 62; in prostitution, 35,44,45,60, 77-79,173; reporting, 76, 78-79,80,89,90; "second," 78-79,89; stranger, 173; "yes/yes" inference, 85,88,89

recovery, stages of, 261

red-light districts, 155,221n1

rejection, emotional, in childhood, 227

relationships: building positive, 223, 232,241,262; coercive, 2,4,6, 17-23,63; desire for affirming, 228; exploitive, 11; family, 5,218,227-28; gay, 11; imbalance of power in, 97; impact of breakaway on, 230-31; importance of supportive, 223-35; internalized view of, 232; with other women, 141,262; with partners, 227-28; peer, 217,218,241-42,256-63,264; among people in prostitution, 6-7; problematic, 6,230-31; social agency, 244-45,261; strategies for changing, 231; therapeutic, 2-3,6-7,12; transitional, 228;

research on prostitution, future, 128, 204-205

residency standard, 284,284n52

residential schools, First Nations, 248

retraumatization, 153; cycle of, 220; in prostitution, xxv; in service occupations, 313-14

revictimization, 4,57

Rich, Adrienne, 94

risks: in revealing substance dependence, 299-300; in sexual practices, 11

Robinson v. State, 82-83

Rochester, Minnesota, program for African Americans in, 217

Russia: boys and men in prostitution from, 107; immigrant women from, 178; as trafficking source country, 64,327

R v. Butler (Canada), 99

sadomasochism, 101,172

safety: achieving, 271-72; domestic, 310-11; financial, 305-309; institutional, 311-14; physical, 209,303; planning for, 5,304-14

SAGE project, San Francisco, 255-56, 258-63; circle, the, 263; counselors in as role models, 260; diverse staff of, 259; networking and collaboration in, 261; staff opportunities in, 263; staff training, in, 263

St. Paul, Minnesota, program for African Americans in, 217

San Diego: brothels in, 150; commercial sexual exploitation in, 150; trafficking in, 148-51

San Francisco: prostituted women in, 35; raped women in, xxi; SAGE project in, 255-56,

258-63; Task Force on
    Prostitution in, xxiv-xxv
saunas, 18,28,320,323
Schengen agreement, 319,329-30n2
School of the Americas, 2
screening: for domestic violence, 286,
    286n58; questions, 28,29n5,
    209
secrecy, 3,12
self: domesticated, 281-89;
    medicalized, 275-81;
    personified parts of, 205-206,
    209; stigmatized sense of,
    273
self-blame, 64,76,139-40,145
self-care, basic, 208-209
self-destructiveness, 103,104
self-esteem, 192,194,196,218,232,259
self-loathing, 58
self-mutilation, 173
services: coordination of, 10; delivery
    of, non-traditional, 255;
    investment of, 10; need for
    culturally relevant, 247-49;
    providers of,
    African-American, 217; for
    women leaving prostitution,
    196,241,258-63
sex clubs, 224. *See also* strip clubs
sex education, 161
sex industry: associations in, as interest
    groups, 318-19; "choice"
    rhetoric of, 176; expansion
    of, 180,318-19; global scope
    of, 134,168-69, 175; and
    Internet, 64,115,117,129;
    profiteers in, 179;
    prostitution rings in 19; types
    of business in, 34
sexism, 95; in Catholic Church,
    155-56; and racism, as dual
    oppression, 221
sex shows: live, 19,28; online,
    116-118,125; women's
    experiences in, 126-28

Sex Stop (magazine), 107
sex tourism, 28,34,117,134,150,168,
    179,315,319
sex trafficking. *See* trafficking
sexual abuse:
- as assault, 2,24,35,213; in childhood,
    188,206,207
- childhood, xviii,8-9,24,35,44,57,
    96-98,102,153,171,172-73,
    217,220,226,227,232; adult
    vulnerabilities from, 97;
    contradictory feelings about,
    97; frequency of, 42-44,57,
    201,202,203-204,235n7; and
    PTSD, 37; in Turkey, 204
- as entertainment, 108
- male survivors of, 11,96-97
sexual accessibility, increasing, 120
sexual exploitation: in wartime, 155;
    Spanish terms for, 158
sexual harassment, 35,154-57
sexual history evidence, and
    fabrication of rape charge,
    80; and prior convictions for
    prostitution, 80
sexuality: based solely on physical
    performance, 98; feelings
    about, 192,196; homophobic
    silencing of gay male, 99;
    and intimacy, problems with,
    232; misinformation about
    women's, xxii
sexual orientation and gender identity,
    difference between, 153
sexual pleasure, 171,194-95
sexual services: criminalization of
    purchase of in Sweden, 326,
    327; types of demanded by
    customers, 322
sexual trauma, 138,142; symptoms of,
    240
sex work, xxiii,60,170,178-79,274,
    294-95; legal, 313,316; as
    legitimate option, 188;

"voluntary migration" for,
xxiii-xxiv,319
sex workers: legal quota of foreign,
317; migrant, xxiii-xxiv,317,
319; prostituted women as,
174-75; work permits for,
317
shame, 3,156-57,259,273; barrier of,
215; family, 155; feelings of,
137,138,139,142,145,230,
273,282
Sheriff's Department, San Diego, 151
Shooting Porn (film), 103
silencing, as oppression, 279-80
skills, lack of office, 243
slave owners, 213-14
slavery, 2; history of, 213-14; and
prostitution, connections
between, 214-15,216;
redefined as penance, 144; as
violation of human rights,
xxv
social functioning, impaired, 277,
277n29
social networks: after breakaway, 230;
building heterogeneous,
233-34; role of, 304; work
on, 223,224,232
Social Security. *See* Supplemental
Income Security program
social workers: importance of, 232; for
TANF, interaction with,
269-70,269n4
solidarity, staff and client, 262
South Africa, 33-34,37,38; frequency
of physical violence in, 60;
studies in, 38-39,61-62
Spanish language, 157,158
speakers' bureau, volunteer, 247
*Speaks v. Sec'y of Health and Human
Services*, 294
SSI. *See* Supplemental Security
Income program
stalking, 9-10,35,287n59,289

Standing Against Global Exploitation.
See SAGE project
State v. Johnson (IA), 80
State v. Johnson (NM), 85-86
State v. King, 78
State v. Slovinski, 82
STD/HIV: among African American
women, 215-17; public health
agencies' attention to, 151;
social factors in transmission
of, 58-59,161
stereotypes: of prostituted women and
prostitution, 251,257,300;
sexualization of racist, 106,
108,162,215
stigma, 3,12,188,233,259,296-304
Stockholm Syndrome, 23,161
*Storyk v. Sec'y of Health Education
and Welfare*, 295,295n89
street liaison team, Glasgow, Scotland,
320
street prostitution, xxiii,19-20,28,34,
148,187,190,191,195,
200-202,203,214,224; and
brothel prostitution,
differences between, 60-61;
decline of, in Sweden, 327;
illusion of control in, 60,208;
increase in, 168,320-21; and
"indoor" prostitution,
203-204; legalization and,
320-21; myth about, 19;
preference for, 60,320;
profile of in Minnesota, 216;
rape and, 60; reality of,
88-89; in San Francisco, 226;
sexual assault and rape in, 35
strip clubs, xxiii,20,34-35,61,148,
168,190,191,203,204,206,
207,214,295; fetishized
sexuality in, 154; as
traffickers' destinations, 178.
See also sex clubs
stripping, 29n4; as legal sex work, 313;
live online, 116,127-28;

physical contact in, 61;
verbal harassment in, 128
substance abuse, 4,227,235n4,293; as
barrier to escaping
prostitution, 26; batterers' use
of, 26; cocaine, 26,87,216; as
coping strategy, 26,187,189,
190,191,195,196,220; as core
issue, 261; dependency on,
297,298n96; among domestic
violence victims, 300; and
eligibility determinations in
SSI, 298-300,298n97; as
facilitator of dissociation,
206; frequency of, 201,202,
204,240; in prostitution,
62-63,216,217,300; recovery
support for, 247,297-98;
TANF program and,
301-304; transnational, 48,
50,57; by traumatized people,
98. *See also* addiction, drugs
"substantial gainful activity": defined,
292,294-95; prostitution as,
313
suicidality, 5,173,240,244,262
Supplemental Security Income
program (SSI), 267,268-69,
269n3; availability of,
284n49; barriers to for
applicants, 270;
determination delays,
307-308; and income,
292-96; "listed impairment"
determination, 276,277-78,
280-81; the medicalized self
and, 275-81; prohibited
diagnoses in, 297-300
support: groups, for women in
prostitution, xix,189,234n1;
instrumental, 228; long-term
mental health, 231-33;
mobilizing, 223;
nonconfrontational, 262;
partners as, 228; peer, 11,

154,251,258-263; primary
provider of, 227-28; for
recovery from substance
abuse, 247,298; social
workers as, 228,232. *See also*
groups
surveillance cameras, 322
survivors: 242; caregivers for, 272-75;
French rape, 203; male, of
sexual abuse, 11; multiple
layers of trauma in, 12,161;
ongoing concerns of, 304-14.
See also breakaway;
prostitution, leaving
Sweden: decriminalizing women in
prostitution in, xxi,xxv,180,
315; Goteborg, interviews in,
224-25,234n1; legislation in,
xxi,180,326-27; national
education campaign in, 328;
support for legislation in, 327
Swedish National Rapporteur on
Trafficking, 330n5
Switzerland, state-sponsored
prostitution in, 319
symptoms, "disguised presentation" of,
272; of dissociation, 207,
292-93; neurobiological, 4-5;
59; of PTSD, 34,36-37,
41-42,276n21. *See also*
health problems

tabletop dancing, 319
Tampa, Florida, 124
TANF. *See* Temporary Assistance to
Needy Families program
TASINTHA, Lukasa, Zambia, 39
Taylor, Max, 125
Temporary Assistance to Needy
Families program (TANF),
268,269; the domesticated
self and, 281-289; "durational
limit" in, 308-309; eligibility
factors in, 281,301-304;

evaluation of economic status for, 290-91; "functional limitations" determination, 276,277,281; lifetime cap on federal funds in, 308. *See also* Family Violence Option

terror, function of, xx

Thailand, xx,34,37,38,45; brothels in, 143; economic impact of prostitution in, xix,65; health problems of women in, 53; sex tourism in, 315; as trafficking source country, 64

therapy: body, 233; goals of, 209-10; neutrality in, 7-8,256; relationship in, 6-7,232; safety in, 8-9. *See also* psychotherapy

Tokyo, terms for prostitution in, xxiv

Tom of Finland (exhibit), 107

torture, 35; in captivity, 141; strategies of political, xx,1-2; techniques of, 21-22

tourist destinations, 148,150. *See also* sex tourism

trafficking:
- defining, 162-63n1,168,175-77; euphemisms for, 176,318; as gender-neutral, 176; as human rights violation, 170; as "voluntary migration for sex work," 319
- factors of: cultural and economic forces in, 148; economic enslavement in, 135; physical and emotional sequelae of, xix,64; resources needed to combat, 157-60,162; structural social factors contributing to, 161-62
- law of: in Sweden, 326-27; Trafficking Victims Protection Act, 177; in U.S., 148

- and prostitution, xxiii,167,168-70, 177-78,326-27; promotion of, 317-18
- trends in: from Eastern Europe, 177; increase in, 134,179; increase of in Germany, 168,318; increase of in Netherlands, 317; reduction of in Sweden, 180,327,330n5
- venues for, xxiii; domestic, 57,63-64, 167,322; in Finland, 327; international, 57,63-64, 151-52,160,169; in Latin America, 149,154,177; from Mexico, 64,148-49; source countries for, 64
- volume of, 148-49; in Europe, 319; international, 163n5; in U.S., 319

transgendered people, 39,49,62, 152-54,258

translators, lack of bilingual, 157; need for, 224

Transnational Convention Against Organized Crime, Trafficking Protocol to, 176

trauma: childhood, 202,207; "clean," 3; complex syndromes in, 3; contagion of, 12; multiple layers of survivors', 161; treatment, principles of, 12; vicarious, 209

traumatic event criterion, 278-79, 279n37

treatment: approaches for prostituted women, 154,209; culturally appropriate, 157; peer education in, 264; principles of trauma, 12

tricks, 19,28. *See also* customers, johns

tuberculosis, 161

Turkey, 34,37,38,200; brothels in, 39, 202; childhood sexual abuse in, 204; health problems of

women in, 53; Istanbul, study
    in, 200,202
"turning out," 172. *See also*
    objectification
turning point, dependence on primary
    support at, 225,227,228. *See
    also* prostitution, leaving
12 Step meetings, 26

Ukraine, as trafficking source country,
    64
UNICEF, 159
United States, 34,37,38, brothels in,
    177; interviews in, 325-26;
    pimps in, 174; source
    countries for trafficking to
    64,148-49; study of
    dissociation in, 203;
    trafficking laws and, 148
United States v. Harris, 81-82
Usenet, newsgroups on, 117

Vancouver, British Columbia, Canada:
    prostitution in, 38; study in,
    200,202
Venezuela, interviews in, 325-26
venues for sex, wider range of, 322-23
verbal abuse, 35,43,44,55,161,257
victim: blaming the, 27,87; credibility
    problems of, 77; prostituted
    woman as, 221; witness
    advocacy service, 10
victimization, 6,145; risk of further, 205;
    and sexual trauma, 138,142
Victims of Violence Program (Cambridge,
    Massachusetts), 3,4
Victoria, British Columbia, Canada, 239
Victoria, State of, Australia, 179-80;
    increased sex industry in,
    319; legalized prostitution in,
    318,319,320-21. *See also*
    Australia

video, trophy, 121
video cameras, live, 120
video chat, live, 118-19
videoconferencing, live, 118
"video content, streaming," 119
Video Fantasy, 126
videos, pornographic, 103,190,191
Vietnam: as trafficking source country,
    64,134; veterans, 256
Violence Against Women Government
    Bill (Sweden), 327
violence, adult, xix,19,45,172-75,188,
    203,232-33,257-58; eligibilty
    for TANF and, 285-89;
    eroticized, 100,101,124; in
    family context, 2,202;
    frequency of, 42-44,268;
    health consequences of, 53,
    151; intimate partner, 21,57,
    58; by johns, 233; in
    prostitution, 35,43; by pimp,
    9,10; physical problems and,
    53,59,151; state-sponsored,
    1-2; threat of, 324; types of,
    44,45. *See also* domestic
    violence
virginity: loss of, 135,138,156;
    attitudes about, 135;
    restoring, 156
Virtual Dreams, 118
vocational training. *See* training,
    vocational
VoyeurDorm.com, 121,124,127
voyeurism: commercial online, 116,
    120,121,124; therapist, 2,209

waiver, for "extreme cruelty," 309,
    309n136
Walton v. Hammons, 311n143
war on drugs, impact of, 302
Web sites. *See* World Wide Web
welfare reform, federal, 269,285n55,
    311,312-13

"welfare-to-work" requirement, 311, 312-13
WHISPER (Women Hurt in Systems of Prostitution Engaged in Revolt), xxiv,xxv,xxvin4
white households, domestic service in, 214
wife beating, pornography and, 20
Winberg, Margareta, xxi-xxii,328
Winfield v. Commonwealth, 86
Winnipeg, Canada, study in, 200-202
women: Burmese, 143; economic exploitation of, 22,23; enslaved, as breeders, 214; immigrant and refugee, 256-57; lack of educational opportunity for Mexican, 156; online surveillance of, 119-20; as property, 162; in prostitution, decriminalizing, 315,316; subordination of, 162. *See also* indigenous people; prostituted women

Women's Legal Education and Action Funds (LEAF), 99
Women's Legal Education and Defense Fund, 99
World Sex Guide, The, 117,118
World Wide Web: amateur pornography Websites on, 21; brothels, Websites of on, 119,120-21; cams, 119-20; history of, 117; pornography sites on, 116,117; sex industry subscription sites on, 118; use of, for prostitution, 116-20. *See also* Internet
Wuornos, Aileen Carol. *See* dedication page

youth, bisexual, 97

Zambia, 34,37,38
Zapatista uprising, 155